Controversies in Healthcare

Volume I

Controversies in Healthcare Volume I. 2022.
All rights reserved.
ISBN: 9798362448271

No part of this publication may be reproduced, stored in a retrieval system, or transmitted in any form or by any means that is electronic or mechanical, including photocopying, recording, or otherwise, without written permission of the publisher.

For information regarding permission, contact Jennifer G Schnellmann at
schnellj@email.arizona.edu

Published by Caduceus Press

Foreword

This first volume of Healthcare Controversies is an expansion of the first three volumes of *Controversies in Pharmacology*, a collaborative writing effort of students at the University of Arizona who were enrolled in a rigorous scientific writing course, a requirement of the Bachelor of Science in Pharmaceutical Sciences. These young essayists are identified in the writing course at nine weeks, and they are invited to join the League of Ten, a talented writing group that has proven prowess in scientific writing. Each student is offered an independent publishing project or the choice of contributing to a "Controversies" collaboration. These essays follow the principles of thought, inquiry, and debate as outlined by the University of Chicago Dean of Students, John Ellison, when he sent a letter to the University's students in August of 2016. In this letter, he reaffirmed the school's "commitment to freedom of inquiry and expression," and he wrote that those admitted to the University "are encouraged to speak, write, listen, challenge, and learn, without fear of censorship". In this spirit, we were not hemmed by the groupthink or dogma that pervades social commentary today. In short, these students were free to express their feelings in writing after learning the science behind medical topics that give rise to controversy.

In the truest essence of inclusiveness, no student voices were edited in thought or word. Even so, when this work was in the editing phase, often the idea of changing a word to make it "less offensive" emerged. The reflexive query was then always, "Offensive to whom?" These ideas were given due consideration each time and the collective editorial response was almost always: leave the student's written words as they were. To change the writings of the students would be to suggest that they were incorrect, invalid, or unreal. This would diminish the value of their expressed thought and perhaps by extension, suggest that the life experiences that led the students to those points of view were unimportant. Because perception is a reality for every human, we chose to allow all perceptions to be expressed, whether they were potentially "offensive" or not.

Thus, enjoy the essays for what they are: student opinions and interpretations of controversial topics. It is often useful to remember that the purpose of a university education is to teach students how to think. This will almost always disrupt their psychological equilibrium as they are exposed to ideas that contradict or entirely upend their current beliefs. A university education has another purpose: the pursuit of truth and the truth is that we all do not speak and think alike. Thus, we must welcome the thoughts and speech of everyone without exception if we are to learn from one another.

Contents

Introduction and Purpose 1

Topic: Lethal Injection 5

Essay: Constitutionality and Humaneness of the Lethal Injection 13
    Faithe Elsberry 13

Essay: The Irony of Investigating Humane Ways to Kill 16
    Lauren Thompson 16

Topic: Right (or Wrong) to Die? 18

Essay: The Antithesis to the Hippocratic Oath 22
    Jason Canizales 22

Topic: The Journey of Ru-486—The Much-Maligned Mifepristone 26

Essay: Ru-486: Undeniable Healthcare 31
    Brianna Hunt 31

Essay: RU-486: The Most Controversial Pharmaceutical Miracle 33
    Sarah Wolff 33

Essay: Ru-486: Take It Like A Woman 36
    Karlie Flader 36

Topic: Conscience Clauses in Medicine—The Right to Deny Patient Care 39

Essay: Personal Beliefs vs. Professional Obligations 43
    Gabbi Ciadella 43

Essay: Conscience Clauses: The Marriage of Medicine and Morality 46
    Lauren Thompson 46

Essay: Conscience Clauses–The Weight of Reasoning 49
    Aileen Muñoz 49

Essay: Conscience Clauses—Discrimination and Stubbornness 54

   Baden Cruickshank 54

Topic: Drug Scheduling—The Government Assigns Risk 57

Essay: Drug Scheduling: Revision Required 62

   Alena LaBree 62

Essay: Hindered Scheduled Substance Research—The Case of Marijuana 64

   Nanase Toda 64

Essay: Drug Scheduling and Discrimination 67

   Aileen Muñoz 67

Essay: Drug Scheduling and Marijuana 70

   Baden Cruickshank 70

Topic: Addiction: A Fiction? 73

Essay: The Changing Etiology of Addiction 78

   Jason Canizales 78

Essay: How Do We Cure Addiction? 85

   Nanase Toda 85

Topic: Compassionate Use and Expanded Drug Access—Should the Dying Have the Right-to-Try? 89

Essay: The Uncompassionate Truth About Compassionate Use 95

   Hannah Ducasse 95

Essay: How Compassionate is Compassionate Use? 98

   Alena LaBree 98

Essay: Compassionate Use of Drugs 101

   Ines Studer 101

Topic: Medicating Others for Our Needs—Acceptable or Abuse? 105

Essay: Use of Antipsychotics in Nursing Homes 110

   Brianna Hunt 110

Essay: The Dangers of Moving Towards Treatment 113

Aileen Muñoz *113*

Topic: There is A Drug for That! **117**

Essay: Medicalization of Everything **121**
    Ines Studer *121*

Essay: The Risks of Overprescribing and Self-Medication **124**
    Baden Cruickshank *124*

Topic: Opioids and The Opioid Epidemic—How Did We Get Here? **127**

Essay: The US Opioid Problem: Overprescription and Overdose **130**
    Baden Cruickshank *130*

Essay: The US Opioid Problem—Expect the Expected **133**
    Lauren Thompson *133*

Essay: The Opioid Epidemic—What We Aren't Doing **136**
    Erica Day *136*

Topic: Black and Gray Market Drug Purchasing **139**

Essay: Black and Gray Drug Purchasing **143**
    Ines Studer *143*

Topic: Placebo and Nocebo Effects **146**

Essay: The Placebo Effect and Placebo Responders in Clinical Trials **151**
    Alena LaBree *151*

Topic: Drug Advertising, Sales, and Prescribing **154**

Essay: Deceptive Drug Marketing **158**
    Jason Canizales *158*

Topic: Supplements and Homeopathy **163**

Essay: Traditional Chinese Herbal Medicine as Dietary Supplements in the US **170**
    Nanase Toda *170*

Essay: Personal Choices and Consequences in Medicine **178**

Teresa Noll 178

Essay: Misinformation about Vaccination and Ethical Conundrums of Treating Unvaccinated Patients 180

Jason Canizales 180

Topic: Physical and Mental Enhancements—When is It Just Therapy? **187**

Essay: The Ethics of Human Enhancement **192**

Jason Canizales 192

Essay: Physical Enhancement in Response to Climate Change **200**

Erica Day 200

Essay: Designer Babies—Gene Editing and Enhancement **204**

Baden Cruickshank 204

Essay: Genetic Editing of Humans **207**

Brianna Hunt 207

Topic: Transgender Controversies **209**

Essay: Gender Dysphoria in Children **213**

Faithe Elsberry 213

About the Student Authors 219

Appendix 224

Introduction and Purpose

This book is the first volume of essays from students selected in a highly rigorous scientific writing program at the University of Arizona, PCOL 305: Scientific Writing. Every semester, the best writers in this course are invited to participate in a writing project of their own or to participate in a collaborative effort. To accomplish the collaborative effort, the selected writers are concurrently enrolled, mid-semester, in another unique undergraduate course—PCOL 325: Controversies in Healthcare and Medicine. In this reading- and discussion-based course, we cover topics rooted in science and medicine. Specifically, we focus on topics that are deliberately provocative, encouraging critical thinking and deep civic engagement. Students frequently find themselves turning on the news, reading local and national newspapers, or researching the scientific and medical literature as their interests dictate and they seek to know more. This is education at its most wholesome: student-driven learning due to a desire to understand.

Then along with organized information about a host of medical and scientific topics, here we have a curation of _thoughtful persuasive essays written by undergraduate students_ in which they share their ideas about controversies in medicine that confound and complicate our human existence. The student writings reflect the importance of these topics to young persons as well as their frank shock value to students who are in the prime "season" of formulating lasting opinions about life's problems and potential solutions. While these essays are individually interesting and entertaining, we hope that other uses of our materials may emerge. For instance, perhaps instructors of college scientific or bioethical writing programs will be potential users of this material in college courses, challenging young thinkers about current topics often featured in our daily newspapers. Alternatively, this material may be exceptionally educationally provocative and appropriate for highly gifted high school writing students who can adroitly accept the challenge of understanding society's deepest conundrums that are founded in healthcare and basic science which affect all of us directly or tangentially via decisions made by health and medical policy leaders. For academic scholars who seek to replicate this type of course, the topic list we used is described below and the rubric applied to the writing assignments is provided in the Appendix. The topic choices for this course and this essay collection were as follows:

Lethal Injection
For this topic, the finality of this medically derived form of capital punishment was presented with the pharmacological choices available for executions. Students learned of the history of capital punishment and some mishaps that are frequently encountered with each. In the end, students were often horrified to find that lethal injection was not the most humane and cruelty-free form of dispatching our worst offenders.

Right to Die
Here, we contrasted the finality of capital punishment with the choice many US adults wish to make: the right to be relieved of a painful life situation on their terms. Because both of these topics are based on almost identical pharmacology, but they diverge at legal and medical points, this pairing was a tremendous eye-opener to get students energized about the work to follow for the rest of the semester. Students were perplexed to learn that the right to die may instead be a privilege to die.

The Journey of Ru-486
This drug was the first of its class approved for medically induced pregnancy termination. Since its approval, it has been identified to have additional uses for treating specific diseases. However, the public is riveted by its historical significance because it changed the landscape of medical care and added a novel element to female reproductive rights.

Conscience Clauses in Medicine
This topic is complex and fraught with ethical and religious underpinnings. That we can develop and approve medications, devices, and procedures to improve human health and then deliberately deny these advances to specific groups of patients or subjects has enormous human rights consequences.

Scheduling Drugs
The US government does not always use science-based methods to schedule or restrict the use of approved and unapproved drugs and compounds. So, frequently decision-making is political and devoid of evidence-based rationalization. Students learned about the DEA drug scheduling system, the history of pharmacological agents that have been re-classified, and how this system of scheduling changes disease treatment and patient access to medications.

Addiction: A Fiction?
The concept of human agency and choice was explored as we discussed whether addictions to drugs and other substances (food, alcohol, cigarettes) are diseases or willful selections that were transformed into habits that become difficult to break.

Compassionate/Expanded Drug Use
Drug approval is a lengthy and formal affair. However, when a person's life will end prematurely, and an as-yet-unapproved drug might save that life, rules may be bent under compassionate or expanded use guidelines. Indeed, Right-to-Try legislation is under review at this moment. Students learned about the FDA's program of expanded access which partners with pharmaceutical companies to offer special access to drugs still under investigation. We also explored human rights, scientific research limitations, and government involvement in patient care.

Medicating Others for Our Benefit
In this session, we discussed the consequences of treating children and nonconsenting elderly for the "benefit" of others. This form of "social medication" is not uncommon but it is not well studied, and everyone has an opinion about it. Students also learned about the intricacies of medicating the young and the old and how these approaches differ from administering drugs to adults.

There's a Drug for That!
Here, learned about disease-mongering versus therapeutic expansion of drugs and we discussed whether making a drug for every inconvenience is a good idea. Students learned about diagnosis codes and how often hilariously inclusive they can be (such as injured at the opera, ICD-10 code Y92.253).

The US Opioid Problem
Students learned about the series of poor and/or fraudulent events that led to the opioid crisis and they offered opinions about how to reverse the trend. Students explored ideas regarding who was responsible for our current opioid predicament and who should fund the efforts required to reverse this.

Black and Gray Market Drug Purchasing
Virtually everything you could desire is for sale online, including legal and illegal drugs...but should they be? Students learned about black and gray drug markets and the downfall of Silk Road. They shared their thoughts about online sales of prescription and illicit drugs, associated legal issues, and human perceptions and needs that drive online purchases.

Placebo and Nocebo Effects
Often during a clinical trial, subjects who receive the "dummy pill" or the placebo state that they have adverse or "nocebo" effects. In contrast, others who receive the same inert, non-drug control substance report a therapeutic benefit. Students learned about the genetic determinants that create the experience of a placebo or nocebo effect and they discussed the ethics of giving someone placebos in clinical trials. They also explored how reporting placebo and nocebo effects may prevent a new experimental drug from being approved.

Drug Advertising, Sales, and Prescribing
Studies show that authorized prescribers such as physicians and nurse practitioners are influenced by drug company propaganda and that they will change their prescribing habits in response to flattery, gifts, trips, invitations to speak at industry events, and monetary "grants". Students reacted to the business side of medicine concerning pharmaceutical company influence and discussed their concerns arising from these practices. Because most students in the course are interested in careers in healthcare, the influence of Pharma on their future patient decisions was especially interesting.

Supplements and Homeopathy
Supplements by definition are not drugs, so they cannot contain written or implied claims that they change the body, mitigate disease, or can be used to diagnose illness. Moreover, homeopathic preparations often have little to no active ingredient at all. Still, the supplement industry is a billion-dollar enterprise and homeopathic and naturopathic "physicians" are becoming more common and vying for space in Western medicine circles. Students wrote about ethical concerns surrounding selling compounds with unsubstantiated claims and truth in labeling.

Cognitive and Physical Enhancement
Many are entranced by the concept of bettering our brains with drugs. What may be surprising is that the FDA bans the manufacture of any compound to improve otherwise healthy brains. Our current research into staving off the cognitive loss caused by dementias has been one of a few

avenues of legitimate study for improving memory and focus, but these studies have never panned out. Next, physical enhancement has been around since the Greek games, but our approaches are more refined and surgically precise. Steroids, SARMs, and other performance enhancers are all the rage as a topic of interest on college campuses, so this was easy to offer to eager minds. To this end, students wrote about their understanding of cosmetic neurology and physical enhancement and demonstrated keen insight into the small return on investment in study drugs and compounds that change our physique for greater beauty and social accolades.

Personal Choices and Medical Conundrums
When US adults do not care for themselves properly, they create expensive healthcare problems for others. We covered ideas about personal responsibility and personal choices and how those can affect others when medical care is required to solve the consequences of those decisions. Students shared empathetic and compassionate responses to these expensive issues in medicine and broadened their knowledge of healthcare delivery. In this session, students learned the consequences and costs of having consumers rely on pharmacology to solve their (often self-induced) problems and the consequences of having insurance pick up the tab for many health issues arising from lifestyle choices.

Tainted Data
In what may have been the most disturbing lecture, students learned about the historical abuse of marginalized people in the US in the context of medical care as we contrasted the treatment of these individuals with war atrocities from World War I in Japan and World War II in Germany. We covered the medical injustice of Henrietta Lacks and the Tuskeegee experiments in the south. Lastly, students learned how medical students often train by performing invasive and intimate exams on unconscious surgical patients without their consent.

Transgender Health Issues
In the final session, students learned of emerging trends in transgender or gender-affirming medicine. We covered the legislation being enacted by US states as they seek to block this type of medical care and we heard from those who were in these legal binds by sharing their personal stories. We covered the pharmacology required to transition between genders and the expected outcomes.

Topic: Lethal Injection

Pharmacology has given us lifesaving drugs as well as the chemical means to end a life for penological purposes—in the form of lethal injection. The controversy surrounding the use of therapeutic agents to kill humans began in 1977 under the assumption that a particularly well-selected chemical concoction would be a more humane (read: palatable to witnesses and others involved in the execution) method for fulfilling a sentence of capital punishment.[1] Ideally, this novel and drug-based method of killing the condemned would be swift, painless, and certain, unlike past attempts to punish those who violently disrupted the moral fabric of society.

For instance, hanging a prisoner by the neck until death, a previously common implementation of criminal punishment, was a vivid spectacle. The neck is often overlooked as a zone of major blood vessels and delicate structures such as the hyoid bone located at the base of the lower jawbone, which facilitates speaking and swallowing. More obviously, the neck houses the airway, the esophagus, and the spinal cord.[2, 3] Thus, when a person is executed by hanging, he is strangled via vascular compression as a rope or similar device pulls tight around the neck due to a function of body mass and gravity.[4] The cause of death due to hanging was often thought to be the fracture of the second spinal cervical (C2) vertebrae. A break here would sever innervation and spinal communication with the rest of the body below that point. Thus, this type of spinal break became known as the "hangman's fracture".[5] However, studies now suggest that a C2 break occurs in slightly half of all hangings and that death arises due to head and neck trauma and lack of brain blood flow due to blockade of vertebral arteries.[4]

Next, firing squads—which are still used around the globe today—often failed, producing agonizing wounds to the prisoner when squad marksmen missed the target of the exercise, the condemned man's heart. Also, because firing squads were associated with Nazi German executions of masses of humanity, shooting prisoners was unappealing to many civilians who were well-versed in this history.[6] Such distaste of death by firing squad was augmented by complications arising from requests for and the ethics surrounding organs "donated" by executed prisoners to fill donor organ shortages.[7] Because organ donation was thought to reduce the degree of atonement from punishment, and because prisoners could not legally consent to organ donation, this grisly avenue for addressing legitimate organ shortfalls was quickly and permanently closed.[7-9] Another approach to capital punishment, the use of asphyxiant gas chambers with carbon dioxide or cyanide, caused visible suffering of the condemned as he fought to breathe.[10] The gassing of prisoners was also used in Nazi Germany for brutal suffocation experiments and it was implemented in North Korea at Camp 22 to kill prisoners who had been condemned for political crimes.[11] For the Korean experiments, a family of three to four individuals was suffocated in a closed room and onlookers watched the horror of parents attempting to revive their dead children.[12] This repugnant historical footnote may explain why most US states have never implemented gas chambers for capital punishment, and why several have converted their old and unused gas chambers into lethal injection rooms.

Next, death by electric chair was equally problematic. Even though this form of execution was the most prominent method of issuing capital punishment until the mid-1980s (when lethal injection was popularized), the chairs often malfunctioned and failed to efficiently kill the prisoner.[13] Even worse, the chairs often set fire to the condemned person who was burned alive, screaming and fighting against the chair's arm, leg, and head restraints.[14] Also, the smell of burning flesh and clothing was a potent reminder to onlookers about the barbarity of killing prisoners. The original instructions for the electrocution of prisoners called for applying 7 amperes and 1,750 volts for 20 seconds, followed by the application of no current for 20 seconds, and then a repeat of the first shock.[15] This was postulated to be sufficient for guaranteeing death. Interestingly, alternating current (AC) was used for execution instead of direct current (DC), because AC created a "wave" that was more efficacious for un-coordinating the heart rhythm.[16] Also, six to ten times more DC than AC is required to induce ventricular fibrillation. Even so, the amperage used for lethal punishment was seven times that needed to cause severe burns and stop respiration, an outcome that can be achieved with less than 1 ampere alone.[16]

Although our early experimental approaches to killing prisoners were depraved, these measures often appeared less brutish than the psychic pain caused by an interminable "life sentence"

"I think the use of lethal injection is the way of lying to ourselves, to make it look like executions are peaceful, are benign, are sort of like going to sleep, and they're not. They're brutal things."

Alex Kozinski, former Circuit Judge of US Court of Appeals (9th circuit)

behind bars until failing health and death or suicide claimed the prisoner's life. This distinction appeared to matter to Gary Gilmore of Utah, who was on death row for a double murder and who requested that his execution be meted out by a firing squad.[17] His request and the court's consideration of it created a public outcry under the belief that executions would increase if Gilmore's request was granted.

Also, some argued about the inherent unfairness of Gilmore being able to schedule a state-assisted suicide. This event re-introduced the concept of prisoner's rights and raised the question of whether Gilmore, who was declared sane and competent, had the right to request his death.[17] These considerations coalesced to prompt a less violent approach to ending a life that was no longer deserved. Specifically, an innovative lethal injection drug combination was requested. Jay Chapman, MD, an Oklahoma medical examiner, was asked to formulate such a potion for killing a prisoner sentenced to death. Interestingly, traditional physician training includes only one to two semesters of pharmacology and rarely toxicology. Even though physicians, at the end of their training, can prescribe any drug for almost any indication they deem appropriate (with few exceptions), Dr. Chapman did not consult a pharmacologist (an expert in how drugs/compounds affect the body) or a toxicologist (an expert in how poisons/toxicants affect the body) during the development of such an important lethal concoction. This lack of thoroughness may explain some of the problems that persist with these drugs for execution.[18, 19]

Chapman's fatal "cocktail" was not tested on a prisoner until 5 years after it was conceptualized when it was used to kill Charles Brooks, Jr. in Texas in 1982 to fulfill a sentence for murder.[20, 21] Since that first use of the lethal injection, a mixture of three unique drugs with different mechanisms of action has been used to carry out death sentences across the nation, formally medicalizing the most severe of human penalties. That we have had injection failures, lethal drug supply shortages, and a frequent reluctance of qualified medical personnel to facilitate the capital punishment process has created additional problems. Also, because some states use different drug doses, substitute drugs from similar pharmacological classes, and frequently have untrained personnel handling the execution, there is a multi-layered complexity in standardizing capital punishment sentencing and follow-through across US prison systems for the 31 states that allow lethal injection.[22, 23] Therefore, because in the US, 1,290 people have been sentenced to die with a pharmacological approach, there is a need to scrutinize the method and allow improvement or adjustments as warranted.

For instance, since the inception of the lethal injection, the chemical combination used has consisted of drugs in three classes, but this could change based on emerging pharmacological science and the creation of novel drugs with greater efficacies (meaning more painlessly lethal). This is worthy of investigation because some researchers suggest that Dr. Chapman developed the lethal injection with no science to support it at all and that his mixture was only serendipitously effective.[19] Even with the right drug mix and the correct dose, unqualified personnel can produce unintended and distressing disparities in prisoner sedation and unintentional infliction of pain and suffering.[21, 24, 25]

These perceptions of differential prisoner experiences at death have resulted in multiple court challenges to ascertain whether the lethal injection is unjustly painful or cruel and in violation of the 8th amendment to the Constitution. This amendment prohibits the government from imposing unduly harsh penalties on criminal defendants or cruel punishment for convicted criminals.[1] In response to these challenges, some states suspended their capital punishment programs so that they could study shortcomings in their protocols. Such an intersection of politics, the pharmaceutical industry, and the justice system may change our lethal injection. However, at this time, we still rely on these three deadly elements: a sedative/anesthetic to produce unconsciousness, a paralytic compound to render the prisoner motionless, and a drug to stop the prisoner's heart.[26]

First, the intravenous anesthetic sodium thiopental has a long history of being used to induce unconsciousness. This rapidly acting but short-duration drug is reliable for sedation, reducing some but not all pain, and at sufficiently high doses, inducing anesthesia. When given intravenously, the drug effectively takes the prisoner through common stages of "drunkenness" over minutes instead of hours.[27] Sodium thiopental has been tested using much lower doses as a "truth serum" on suspected criminals, psychiatric patients, and government spies. This use exploited the drug's ability to sedate an individual to the degree that anxiety was reduced and inhibitions were lowered. This allegedly stimulated a "barbiturate-induced confession" of some type of desired truth. That the drug produced an amnestic state after administration was especially helpful because the person treated with the "truth serum" would not likely remember the drug administration or the questioning. This was considered to be a more humane method for extracting information than torture. However, after some studies of the drug's effects, it was deduced that the compound simply removed inhibitions so profoundly that people said all manner of things, some true and some entirely imaginative.[28] Thus, the drug, which was not a serum at all, produced a chatterbox, not a truth-teller. With no ability to sort fact from fiction, the person hearing the information was left with something more interesting than useful.

Protocols for sodium thiopental called for 2–5 g of the drug to be given intravenously and this was based on the dose needed to induce surgical anesthesia (210–350 mg for a 150 lb man with half of that given continuously to maintain unconsciousness).[29] So, the dose given for execution is often 10 times the amount used for anesthetic induction for medical unconsciousness. However, prisoner tolerances to sedatives can vary, and ideally, doses should be titrated or adjusted to each condemned person to ensure efficacy but this cannot be done. This inter-individual variation in drug tolerance fueled studies of inmate post-mortem blood thiopental concentrations and data suggested that insufficient drug was given to assure a lack of awareness on behalf of the prisoner.[29] However, not all researchers agree with this conclusion and such assertions have been contradicted by other investigators who report that differences in the timing of blood measurements, differences in sites of blood collection, and inconsistencies in documenting the time between death and blood analysis may misdirect assumptions about sedation, anesthesia, and prisoner awareness.[30] Thus, inmates may well be receiving sufficient anesthesia that may last more than 10 minutes. Given that a lethal injection protocol requires 8–15 minutes, this may be appropriate.

> *"Capital punishment kills immediately, whereas lifetime imprisonment does so slowly. Which executioner is more humane? The one who kills you in a few minutes, or the one who wrests your life from you in the course of many years?"*
>
> Anton Chekhov, Russian playwright

Sodium thiopental ceased being the mainstay for initiating lethal injection in the early 2000s, when the manufacturer, Hospira, discontinued making it in the US.[31] When Hospira attempted to have the drug synthesized at one of its facilities in Italy, the country denied the drug company its very own product if it was to be used to kill humans.[32] Soon after this incident, Europe began to restrict drug importation into the US if the product was used for lethal injections. Then, with legal and industrial pressure, Hospira stopped making sodium thiopental altogether in 2011, and pentobarbital is presently used to induce anesthesia for lethal injection.

The second drug in the lethal mixture is a very large dose of pancuronium bromide (100 mg) which is given to paralyze the skeletal muscles, including those involved in respiration such as the lungs and diaphragm. During surgery, pancuronium is used therapeutically to relax the patient's body sufficiently to have a surgical procedure and to allow intubation for mechanical breathing support (ventilator use). For this purpose, only a fraction of the lethal injection dose is used, and although a few minutes are needed for the onset of action, pancuronium lasts up to two hours after administration has ceased. Pancuronium does not provide analgesia (pain relief) and it has no sedating effects. Thus, when pancuronium paralyzes the lungs, a conscious prisoner would feel a profound burning sensation as his diaphragm was unable to assist the lungs to expand and contract, thereby causing oxygen deprivation and subsequent asphyxiation.[33] Worse, the prisoner would be unable to communicate this pain due to the paralysis. This image is impressive to death penalty opponents who criticize the inhumanity of this potential outcome.[33]

Finally, potassium chloride is administered and this drug causes cardiac arrest by preventing the initiation of new heartbeats. Potassium in the body is chiefly stored within cells (98%) and a small amount (2%) remains outside of the cell. Because unbalanced potassium can be fatal, its intracellular and extracellular ratio is carefully re-equilibrated by the body as we eat, drink, and eliminate water and waste during the day. Potassium chloride makes the resting potential or electrical charge on heart cells more positive. If the cells are more positive, they are not at the ideal potential for sodium to enter heart cells to initiate a heartbeat. If a heartbeat cannot be generated by sodium, then the heart may initially behave erratically as it attempts to initiate contractions by other means. Eventually, though, the heart will stop beating, leading to cardiac arrest. People who have survived a heart attack and who recall events before that attack describe the sensation as being very frightening and painful. Also, intravenous injection of potassium chloride is very uncomfortable because it is a severe tissue irritant. Dosing potassium as mEq—instead of using milligrams or grams—is typical for electrolytes such as sodium and potassium. For lethal injection, 100 mEq of potassium chloride is given which is approximately 7.5 grams.

The potassium used for lethal injection is the same electrolyte that is given as an oral drug (tablet) to treat low potassium. However, the tablet for raising low potassium is often dosed at 20 mEq (approximately 1,500 milligrams). This oral dose is less bioavailable than an intravenous drug that is delivered directly and immediately into the circulation. For this reason, hospitals cannot give intravenous potassium chloride unless they are following a strict protocol that involves sustained administration over hours (10–20 mEq/hour) to allow cells to re-equilibrate their potassium stores. Potassium chloride is so efficacious at causing death, it is often a procedure of choice for inducing fetal terminations via cardiac injection of the compound.[34-36] Thus, at 100 mEq, potassium chloride delivered intravenously is absolutely lethal.

So, each drug in the lethal injection "cocktail" if given alone in sufficient quantities could produce death, but aside from thiopental, an anesthetic, the other two drugs would induce undue pain and significant human suffering.[33] Thus, this regimen, given in this order, is designed to reduce pain and suffering such that the person does not experience an unconstitutional punishment as prohibited by law. Even so, the outcome of the protocol is an intentional, medically induced death. Thus, it would seem logical that healthcare providers would be needed for lethal injection oversight or guidance. However, few physicians are willing to participate, even though due to the legality of executions in some states, participating physicians in those regions are not disciplined by their licensing boards. Also, states can protect the identity of participating healthcare professionals when they are requested or required to be present. Nevertheless, some physicians boldly self-report participation in capital punishment, underscoring their perceived obligation to make the process pain-free.

No clinical trials to test the outcomes of lethal injection have ever been performed—for obvious reasons—so much of what we hypothesize about lethal injection has been gathered from small, isolated studies of the behavior of each drug in humans, case reports of accidents or overdoses, and witness and executioner testimony regarding the end of the inmate's life. Thus, in essence, a lethal injection-mediated execution is an impromptu clinical trial with one subject every time it occurs.[37] Because humans cannot be experimented on legally, and because prisoners actually have more protections than the non-incarcerated in this regard, the lethal injection procedure may constitute a violation of the inmate's rights regarding consent to human research. These rights are recognized in the Declaration of Helsinki which was developed by the World Medical Association to guide human experimentation. This document is based on a set of ten principles of the Nuremberg Code which were drafted after the Nuremberg Trials that exposed inhumane human research studies conducted on concentration camp prisoners during the Second World War.[38] The resulting Code includes provision for consent, reduced risk, the free will to cease being a research subject and the mandate that all experiments should stop when danger is obvious. The Declaration of Helsinki uses these principles as a foundation and these have been strengthened over time with policy revisions and clarifications.

Then, the US Health and Human Services department developed a federal policy for protecting human subjects, the Common Rule.[39] Under this Rule, prisoners are defined as being truly incapable of informed consent to medical or scientific human research because they have a dependency on the prison system (they are not free). Thus, prisoners can agree to participate in research when the risk of harm is minimal. However, it is understood that incentives to participate in research can be ethically problematic if those incentives are items the prisoner wants but otherwise has no method for accessing (phone calls, personal items, or sentencing or incarceration modifications).[40, 41]

Therefore, lethal injection is a pharmacological controversy that is multifactorial and complex. The intentional use of therapeutic drugs to kill people is a moral hazard for some. This is even more complicated because we have no proper means of studying best practices for executing criminals with injectable compounds and we cannot ever know if pain and suffering were a consequence of the execution. Finally, due to social and ethical constraints on healthcare professionals to guide or assist with lethal injection, we may never have truly qualified medical personnel on whom we can rely to offer the most humane death to a prisoner.

Writing Prompts

- Should we create and sell drugs expressly for killing human beings?
- Should capital punishment be legal?
- Has capital punishment run its course, and now it should be abolished?
- Should lethal injection as a capital punishment technique be outlawed?
  - Can it be improved or what should we do instead?
- Is the current system of killing condemned prisoners effectively a form of unauthorized human subject research?
  - Would modifying the execution process also be a form of human experimentation?
- Is lethal injection a medical procedure?
  - Do healthcare providers have a duty to participate?
  - Do healthcare providers have a duty NOT to participate other than certifying the dead?
  - Should a protected class of experts be empaneled instead?
    - Toxicologist, pharmacologist, or nurse, for example?

- Should states shield their professionals from the public to encourage their participation?
- Should board certification be revoked for medical professionals who participate in capital punishment?
- How is the lethal injection treated in contrast to euthanasia or self-directed suicide at the end of life?
- Is lethal injection humane and if so, for whom: the prisoner or the witnesses/legal justice and penal system?
- Have we really attempted to make this more just or have efforts been incomplete due to politics?
- Is capital punishment an effective form of social control?
    - Is it "justice"?

Works Cited

1. Schwarzschild H. Lethal injection and the death penalty. Hastings Cent Rep. 1980;10(1):4.
2. Sharma BR, Harish D, Sharma A, et al. Injuries to neck structures in deaths due to constriction of neck, with a special reference to hanging. J Forensic Leg Med. 2008;15(5):298-305.
3. Sharma BR, Singh VP, Harish D. Neck structure injuries in Hanging--comparing retrospective and prospective studies. Med Sci Law. 2005;45(4):321-30.
4. Khokhlov VD. Calculation of tension exerted on a ligature in incomplete hanging. Forensic Sci Int. 2001;123(2-3):172-7.
5. Rayes M, Mittal M, Rengachary SS, et al. Hangman's fracture: a historical and biomechanical perspective. J Neurosurg Spine. 2011;14(2):198-208.
6. Ossowski A, Diepenbroek M, Zwolski M, et al. A case study of an unknown mass grave - Hostages killed 70 years ago by a Nazi firing squad identified thanks to genetics. Forensic Sci Int. 2017;278:173-6.
7. Tsai DF, Tsai MK, Ko WJ. Organs by firing squad: the medical and moral implausibility of death penalty organ procurement. Am J Bioeth. 2011;11(10):11-3.
8. Valapour M, Paulson KM, Hilde A. Strengthening protections for human subjects: proposed restrictions on the publication of transplant research involving prisoners. Liver Transpl. 2013;19(4):362-8.
9. Ross LF, Thistlethwaite JR. Prisoners as Living Donors: A Vulnerabilities Analysis. Camb Q Healthc Ethics. 2018;27(1):93-108.
10. No Author Given. The Death Penalty. Available from: https://deathpenaltycurriculum.org/student/c/about/methods/gaschamber.htm.
11. No Author Given. North Korea's Camp No. 22 - update. Digital Globe Analysis Center: 2012.
12. Barnett A. Revealed: the gas chamber horror of North Korea's gulag. The Guardian. 2004.
13. Martschukat J. ["The art of killing by electricity": the sublime and the electric chair]. Amerikastudien. 2000;45(3):325-47.
14. Denno DW. Getting to death: Are executions constitutional? Iowa Law Rev. 1997;82(2):319-464.
15. Kearns TS. The chair, the needle, and the damage done: what the electric chair and the rebirth of the method-of-execution challenge could mean for the future of the Eighth Amendment. Cornell J Law Public Policy. 2005;15(1):197-229.
16. New Jersey State Council of Electrical Contractors Associations I. The Fatal Current 1987. Available from: http://www.physics.ohio-state.edu/~p616/safety/fatal_current.html.
17. Bedau HA. The right to die by firing squad. Hastings Cent Rep. 1977;7(1):5-7.
18. Salk R. Lethal Injection in Uncharted Territory: The Need to Ensure the Humanity of Current Death Penalty Practices. Criminal Justice Ethics. 2015;34(3):284-311.

19. Rogers A. The Shocking Lack of Science Behind Lethal Injections. Wired. 2017.
20. Romanelli F, Whisman T, Fink JL. Issues surrounding lethal injection as a means of capital punishment. Pharmacotherapy. 2008;28(12):1429-36.
21. Reinhold R. Technician Executes Murderer in Texas By Lethal Injection. The New York Times. 1982.
22. Malcom DR, Romanelli F. The Emergence of Second-Generation Lethal Injection Protocols: A Brief History and Review. Pharmacotherapy. 2017;37(10):1249-57.
23. Death Penalty Information Center 2018 [January 12, 2018]. Available from: https://deathpenaltyinfo.org/.
24. Taylor v Crawford, 487 F3d 1072, 8th Circuit(2007).
25. Brown v Beck, No. 5:06-CT-3078-H (ND NC), (April 7, 2006).
26. Ruble JH. The "death" of lethal injection as we know it? The role of chemical execution in the American criminal justice system. J Pain Palliat Care Pharmacother. 2014;28(3):276-81.
27. Bimmerle G. "Truth" Drugs in Interrogation. CIA Historical Review Program. 1993;5(2).
28. Taher Y, Fakhr-el-Islam M, el-Sherif A, et al. The effect of pentothal as a "truth serum". A controlled study. J Egypt Med Assoc. 1969;52(1):75-81.
29. Koniaris LG, Zimmers TA, Lubarsky DA, et al. Inadequate anaesthesia in lethal injection for execution. Lancet. 2005;365(9468):1412-4.
30. Heath MJ, Stanski DR, Pounder DJ. Inadequate anaesthesia in lethal injection for execution. Lancet. 2005;366(9491):1073-4; author reply 4-6.
31. Kas K, Yim R, Traore S, et al. Lethal drugs in capital punishment in USA: History, present, and future perspectives. Res Social Adm Pharm. 2016;12(6):1026-34.
32. Koppel N. Drug Halt Hinders Executions in the US. The Wall Street Journal. 2011 January 22, 2011;Sect. Sunday Business.
33. Zimmers TA, Sheldon J, Lubarsky DA, et al. Lethal injection for execution: chemical asphyxiation? PLoS Med. 2007;4(4):e156.
34. Callahan JC. Ensuring a stillborn: the ethics of fetal lethal injection in late abortion. J Clin Ethics. 1995;6(3):254-63.
35. Spielman B. Certainty and agnosticism about lethal injection in late abortion. J Clin Ethics. 1995;6(3):270-2.
36. Coulibaly B, Piercecchi-Marti MD, Bartoli C, et al. Lethal injection of potassium chloride: first description of the pathological appearance of organs. J Appl Toxicol. 2010;30(4):378-80.
37. Philpott S. Execution by lethal injection: illegal research? Hastings Cent Rep. 2014;44(2):11-2.
38. Mccarthy CR. The Rights of Human Research Subjects and the Necessity of Conducting Animal Research as Illuminated by the Nuremberg-Code and the Declaration-of-Helsinki. Role of the Chimpanzee in Research. 1994:1-6.
39. Shelton JD. How to interpret the federal policy for the protection of human subjects or "Common Rule" (Part A). [for the Working Group of the Human Subjects Research Subcommittee of the National Science and Technology Council]. IRB. 1999;21(6):6-9.
40. Stone TH. Currents in contemporary ethics. Discerning minimal risk in research involving prisoners as human subjects. J Law Med Ethics. 2004;32(3):535-7.
41. Stone TH. Coercion and prisoners as a vulnerable class of human research subjects. Med Health R I. 2000;83(12):380-1.

Essay: Constitutionality and Humaneness of the Lethal Injection

Faithe Elsberry

Capital punishment has been used in the United States since British colonizers arrived in North America, bringing the practice of punishment by death with them. Under the Capital Laws of New England, established in the mid-17th century, there were 15 crimes punishable by death, each backed by a specific verse from the Old Testament of the Bible.[1] Now, after years of reform, murder is the only crime punishable by death, and only in 27 states does the death penalty remain a viable punishment.[2] There are 5 methods of execution that have been used most throughout US history: hanging, firing squad, electrocution, cyanide gas, and lethal injection.[3] Hanging was initially the most common method of execution, but the others have been used or invented as the constitutionality of existing execution methods was questioned. According to the Eighth Amendment of the Constitution, punishment for crime is not to be cruel or unusual.[4] The botching of executions has led to the consensus that some of these methods are indeed cruel or unusual; however, the method with the highest percentage of botched executions in all of US history is the most commonly used method of execution in the US today.

This method is the lethal injection. Lethal injection can be performed by an overdose of a single drug or by 3 drugs administered intravenously in succession. If the single drug method is used, a lethal dose of a short-acting barbiturate, such as pentobarbital or thiopental, is administered.[5] Barbiturates are non-analgesic anesthetics that bring about the depression of the CNS through potentiation of the GABA-A receptor, which, in the case of an overdose, leads to death by respiratory depression.[6] The 3-drug method utilizes thiopental, pancuronium bromide, and potassium chloride.[7] After thiopental is used to induce unconsciousness, pancuronium bromide is administered, paralyzing the skeletal muscle by acting at nicotinic receptors and inhibiting depolarization and therefore muscle contraction.[8] This also results in the slowing of respiration.[9] Finally, a large dose of potassium chloride is administered which causes severe hyperkalemia, resulting in cardiac arrhythmia and eventually cardiac arrest.[10] While death is expected to be the result of the potassium chloride, each of these drugs is administered at a high dose that is intended to have the potential to be lethal.[5] If the procedure goes according to plan, the average time from the beginning of drug administration to death for the 1-drug method is 7–10 minutes and for the 3-drug method is approximately 10 minutes.[11]

While this may seem like a relatively humane death, the steps that precede drug administration have, in some cases, taken up to 2 hours, resulting in what are considered to be botched executions by lethal injection.[12] This prolonged prelude leading up to the execution is usually the result of the and misplacement of the needle or an inability to identify a suitable vein, especially in past drug users.[5] Continuous intravenous drug use may result in collapsed veins, scarring, and chronic vein disease, all of which make intravenous needle penetration difficult.[13] According to data on death penalties administered in the US from 1900–2010, approximately 7.2% of executions by lethal injections were botched.[12] This percentage of mishandled executions is significantly higher than that of the other main methods of execution used in the US.

There is also uncertainty regarding the anesthetic effects and induction of cardiac arrest with the drug doses used in the 3-drug method of lethal injection. Zimmers and colleagues analyzed the doses used in multi-drug lethal injections and concluded that in some cases, the dose of thiopental used may not be great enough to induce unconsciousness.[7] If this is true, the paralyzing, asphyxiating effects of pancuronium bromide and the cardiac arrhythmias and pain caused by the potassium chloride may be consciously experienced. Zimmers and colleagues also found that the doses of potassium chloride used may not always be sufficient to cause cardiac arrest. In the case that thiopental and potassium chloride are administered at sub-optimal doses, the condemned would be paralyzed and aware of his decreasing ability to respire until death.

The most common method of execution in the US today, established for its humaneness in comparison to other methods, is far from humane. Interestingly, it is not yet considered cruel or unusual to repeatedly insert needles into various veins throughout the body as one waits to be put to death. The popularity of this method is also surprising when dosing protocols for the 3-drug lethal injections have not been examined to ensure the efficacy of the anesthetic and the drug expected to induce cardiac arrest. Indeed, more protocols have been established for the quick and painless euthanization of animals by drugs in veterinary practice than for the execution of humans in our justice system.[7] Lethal injection, as it is performed today, should not be upheld as the most constitutional or humane method of execution for the death penalty in the US. Other methods, new or old, should be explored if the death penalty is to remain a part of criminal punishment under the Constitution.

Works Cited

1. The capitall lawes of New-England, as they stand now in force in the Common-wealth. By the court, in the years 1641. 1642 : Capitall lawes, established within the iurisdiction of Massachusetts. London: Printed first in New-England, and re-printed in London for Ben. Allen in Popes-head Allen sic; 1643.
2. No Author Given. Death Penalty Information Center 2018 [January 12, 2018]. Available from: https://deathpenaltyinfo.org/.
3. Methods of Execution 2017 [updated 2022]. Available from: https://deathpenaltyinfo.org/executions/methods-of-execution.
4. ProCon.org. History of the Death Penalty 2013. Available from: https://deathpenalty.procon.org/view.timeline.php?timelineID=000025#1700-bc-1799).
5. Description of Each Execution Method Death Penalty Information Center. Available from: https://deathpenaltyinfo.org/executions/methods-of-execution/description-of-each-method.

6. Loscher W, Rogawski MA. How theories evolved concerning the mechanism of action of barbiturates. Epilepsia. 2012;53 Suppl 8:12-25.
7. Zimmers TA, Sheldon J, Lubarsky DA, et al. Lethal injection for execution: chemical asphyxiation? PLoS Med. 2007;4(4):e156.
8. Das GN, Sharma P, Maani CV. Pancuronium. StatPearls. Treasure Island (FL)2022.
9. Hillman H. The possible pain experienced during execution by different methods. Perception. 1993;22(6):745-53.
10. Saxena K. Clinical features and management of poisoning due to potassium chloride. Med Toxicol Adverse Drug Exp. 1989;4(6):429-43.
11. Romanelli F, Whisman T, Fink JL. Issues surrounding lethal injection as a means of capital punishment. Pharmacotherapy. 2008;28(12):1429-36.
12. Sarat A, Blumstein K, ProQuest. Gruesome spectacles : botched executions and America's death penalty. Stanford, California: Stanford Law Books; 2014.
13. Senbanjo R, Strang J. The needle and the damage done: clinical and behavioural markers of severe femoral vein damage among groin injectors. Drug Alcohol Depend. 2011;119(3):161-5. Epub 20110629.

Essay: The Irony of Investigating Humane Ways to Kill

Lauren Thompson

A drug is a substance used to prevent, diagnose, treat, or relieve symptoms of a disease or condition.[1] This definition facilitates the use of drugs to serve the purpose of therapies, attempting to improve the physical health and quality of life of patients. Though, one combination of drugs is used time and time again to do the exact opposite—execute inmates via lethal injection. The current sequence of drugs first uses sodium thiopental for sedation, then pancuronium bromide for paralysis, and lastly potassium chloride to induce cardiac arrest.[2] Lethal injection is often recognized as the humane route of capital punishment, yet this would be an incredible misconception.

Lethal injection is the most commonly botched execution, with approximately 7.12% of injections going awry.[3] These mishaps are often the result of incorrect dosing or inadequate administration by prison employees.[4] These mistakes can turn a roughly seven-minute death into a two-hour ordeal.[5] And this additional time endured by the inmate is spent in total consciousness, while they experience excruciating pain, panic, and significant respiratory distress.[6] The potentially obvious solution to increasing efficacy would be to implore the assistance of healthcare providers who possess sufficient information regarding dosing and IV insertions. However, this conflicts with the AMA *Code of Medical Ethics,* barring providers from advising or assisting in capital punishment.[7] By permitting physicians to participate in lethal injection, their fundamental intention to sustain life is corrupted, eventually tainting physician-patient relationships.[8]

Without professional input, it is impossible for prison employees to 'perfect' the existing method. Furthermore, there is no way to legitimately explore alternative drugs for execution, as even the current combination has not been tested or approved for this indication. Each lethal injection is merely an uncontrolled human experiment performed by people incapable of learning anything from these trials. Major pharmaceutical companies, such as Pfizer, have caught onto the legal risks and moral controversy surrounding the use of their drugs in this unapproved manner. Pfizer and other

> *"They are opting for a method that they hope will not be torturous over a method that they are certain will be torturous."*
>
> Robert Dunham, Executive Director of the Death Penalty Information Center

pharmaceutical companies began controlling distribution, ultimately limiting the lethal injection drug supply.[9]

This drug shortage forced states to brainstorm other possibilities. Oklahoma presented one of the first substitutes, as they proposed to asphyxiate inmates using nitrogen gas.[10] While nitrogen gas would be inexpensive and accessible, there is a lack of information involving related deaths in humans. Supporters of this method claimed death would occur within minutes and be minimally painful, failing to reference studies that supported this.[11] Even though nitrogen is a known asphyxiant, there is no way to prototype a chamber and prove it would consistently result in a fast and relatively painless death.[12] The absurdity lies within the suggestion that nitrogen gas would be the better option compared to the present drug combination when neither method was evaluated for capital punishment. The arguments only mention basic science to rush the approval of nitrogen gas as access to the standard drugs dwindles.

Seeing that the ongoing shortage of drugs pressures states to discover new options, we must analyze the integrity of these practices before approval. Yet, it may be impossible to establish a system that limits the pain experienced by the inmate without the ability to gather data. Therefore, we cannot determine if any new or current approaches are cruel or unusual. It is clear that assistance from providers obstructs their capacity in healthcare settings, and research regarding 'efficient' death would be a criminal means to misuse talent and resources. Thus, it may be time to entirely reconsider the use of lethal injection or other chemically induced capital punishments in the United States.

Works Cited

1. Dictionary of Cancer Terms. NIH National Cancer Institute. 2021.
2. Zimmers TA, Sheldon J, Lubarsky DA, et al. Lethal injection for execution: chemical asphyxiation? PLoS Med. 2007;4(4):e156.
3. Radelet M. Botched Executions. Death Penalty Information Center. 2022.
4. Denno DW. The lethal injection quandary: how medicine has dismantled the death penalty. Fordham Law Rev. 2007;76(1):49-128.
5. Lethal Injection Drugs. Human Rights Watch. 2006.
6. Silhavy TJ. Death by lethal injection. Science. 1997;278(5340):1085-6.
7. Henry TA. AMA to Supreme Court: Doctor participation in executions unethical. AMA. 2018.
8. Rosoff PM. Perspective roundtable: lethal injection. N Engl J Med. 2008;358(20):2183.
9. Eckholm E. Pfizer Blocks the Use of Its Drugs in Executions. NY Times 2016.
10. Dwyer O. US states consider execution by nitrogen gas as lethal injections grind to a halt. BMJ. 2015.
11. Oklahoma Plans to Use New Execution Method. CNN. 2018.
12. Borron SW, Bebarta VS. Asphyxiants. Emerg Med Clin North Am. 2015;33(1):89-115. Epub 20141115.

Topic: Right (or Wrong) to Die?

In what may appear to be hypocritical opposition to lethal injection and capital punishment, the legal right to die is controversial and permitted, at this time, in 7 states. To be eligible for the right to die in these states, one must be a resident of that state as well as qualify for a euthanasia prescription from a physician, under the auspices of physician-assisted dying laws. Most laws in this regard require the person seeking the end of life to be at least 18 years-of-age, with 6 months left to die, who can petition a physician at least twice orally, at least 15 days apart, and who can write a single written request to die. These US laws are largely based on European laws that predate our country's efforts significantly.[1-5] And, these laws are late for US adults.

We learned very difficult lessons in the cases of Terri Schiavo and Karen Quinlan. For Terri Schiavo, she was suspended in a persistent vegetative state after cardiac arrest and significant brain damage. A feeding tube was inserted and she was provided hydration until her husband, Michael, asked that she be allowed to die. Terri's parents disagreed and a court challenge ensued that lasted 7 years. Terri's parents insisted that she wanted to be kept alive whereas her husband believed she would want to pass away peacefully. Terri was removed from all life-sustaining measures in 2005.

"Euthanasia ... is simply to be able to die with dignity at a moment when life is devoid of it."

Marya Mannes, 20th-century American writer and critic

A second and earlier case involving Karen Quinlan was similar. A young college student, Karen slipped into a coma after consuming benzodiazepines and alcohol. She, too, was diagnosed as being in a persistent vegetative state and placed on life support by the hospital. Her parents petitioned the hospital to allow her to die, but they refused for 9 years to do so. Karen's parents insisted that these medical efforts were "heroic measures" that Karen would not have wanted. The hospital counter-argued that removing the life support measures constituted homicide.[6] These two cases were special because they called for passive euthanasia, without the patient's express consent. Where these cases diverge from current right-to-die controversies is that those now seek the right to end their lives are alive, not passive, but actively petitioning for their lives to end on their terms. The US does not appear to agree that they are deserving of this last gentle gesture.

For instance, in ten US states—Oregon, Washington, Montana, California, Vermont, Colorado, Hawaii, New Jersey, Maine, and New Mexico—and the District of Columbia, the right to die is a legally permitted activity. Then, although legal, there remain obstacles to having this right free and clear. In Oregon, the Oregon Death with Dignity law, made effective in 1997, requires that the patient with a wish to die be an adult, a resident of the state, and make a written request to die that is witnessed by at least two other adults. These witnesses cannot be relatives or people who stand to gain from the death of the patient. Many physicians agree with US lawmakers, too, that wanting to die is suspect and worthy of barriers. Specifically, when a very elderly terminally ill patient requests the right to die via medication-assisted suicide, physicians have been known to recommend lengthy psychiatric evaluations.[7] Indeed, many challenges to receiving aid-in-dying (AID) remain even in states in which this process is declared to be a human right.[8]

"Americans tend to endorse the use of physician-assisted suicide and euthanasia when the question is abstract and hypothetical."

Ezekiel Emanuel, Vice Provost for Global Initiatives and the Diane S. Levy and Robert M. Levy University Professor, Co-Director of the Health Transformation Institute

These medical and legislative outcomes lie in stark contrast with the historical and traditional view in the US that every adult has the right to reduce unwanted medical treatment and that all adults have the right to control his/her own body. The Supreme Court issued the opinion that *"No right is held more sacred, or is more carefully guarded by the common law, than the right of every individual to the possession and control of his own person, free from all restraint or interference of others, unless by clear and unquestionable authority of law."*[9] This idea is borne out by the legality of withholding care at the end of life to hasten the death of terminally ill people and suggests some early agreement on the ability to choose the end of life and the authority to determine if a life is worth living.[10]

However, current options for both physician-assisted suicide and independently conducted euthanasia/suicide are few, and in many states, helping someone to voluntarily end his/her life is a crime punishable by imprisonment.[8] In Alaska, for instance, Statute §11.41.120(a)(2) reads: *"A person commits the crime of manslaughter if the person intentionally aids another person to commit suicide."*[11] In Arkansas, the law is more specific: *"It is unlawful for any physician or health care provider to commit the offense of physician-assisted suicide by prescribing any drug, compound, or substance to a patient with the express purpose of assisting the patient to intentionally end the patient's life or assisting in any medical procedure for the express purpose of assisting a patient to intentionally end the patient's life."*[12, 13]

To prevent the perception that homicide is responsible for a patient's death, AID laws mandate that the patient induce his/her own death, usually by ingesting lethal doses of barbiturates. This often has the unintended consequence of having a patient choose to die earlier to retain independence for the task.[8] Secobarbital and pentobarbital are the only acceptable drugs to use in overdose to hasten death. These drugs, due to their historical use in lethal injection protocols have been restricted by the pharmaceutical companies who manufacture

"My ultimate goal is to make euthanasia a positive experience."

Jack Kevorkian, American pathologist and euthanasia proponent them to prevent their use in this manner. If the drugs can be procured, the sheer amount needed to cause death can be daunting. Approximately 9 grams of secobarbital is required for AID and 10 grams of pentobarbital (liquid) is needed.[14] This is a red flag for a pharmacist who may prevent the prescription from being dispensed and it is an enormous amount of a drug to swallow successfully. Although these very potent and dangerous drugs are not in common use due to their documented ability to kill an adult, they often do not produce the peaceful and rapid death that people may imagine.

Perhaps the right-to-die concept should be more appropriately renamed to "privilege to die," because although it is a socially and medically supported concept to have the choice of bodily autonomy over all other competing ethical principles, we really do not have this right at all.

Writing Prompts

- How is the lethal injection treated in contrast to euthanasia or self-directed suicide at the end of life?
- If a prisoner wants to die and requests that his execution day be moved up, is the state participating in assisted suicide?
- At what point in adulthood do we have the right to live or die
    - Is this right never ours?
    - Always ours?
- Are MDs bastardizing "do no harm"?
    - Almost all residents will kill a patient before becoming an attending, so are they sanctimonious liars?
- Where does patient autonomy end?
    - When it disagrees with the MD
    - Due to religion? Other reasons?

Works Cited

1. Uzych L. End-of-life decision making and developing international law. Pa Med. 1994;97(10):16-8.
2. Lemaire FJ. A law for end of life care in France? Intensive Care Med. 2004;30(11):2120. Epub 20040921.
3. Vincent JL. End-of-life practice in Belgium and the new euthanasia law. Intensive Care Med. 2006;32(11):1908-11. Epub 20060921.
4. Malaquin-Pavan E. [Leonetti Law, care and end of life. Rights, liberties and end of life]. Soins. 2006(708):27.
5. Stork J. [Medical end of life decision making in the Netherlands after the euthanasia law went into effect; four country research]. Ned Tijdschr Geneeskd. 2007;151(38):2130.
6. Heimer C. The Unstable Alliance of Law and Morality. In: Hitlin S, Vaisey S, editors. Handbooks of Sociology and Social Research: Springer; 2012. p. 181–2.
7. Gillick M. Choosing Medical Care in Old Age: What Kind, How Much, When to Stop. Cambridge, MA: Harvard University Press; 1996. 224 p.
8. Buchbinder M. Access to Aid-in-Dying in the United States: Shifting the Debate From Rights to Justice. Am J Public Health. 2018;108(6):754-9. Epub 20180419.
9. Union Pacific Railyard Co. v. Botsford, 141 U.S. 250, 251 (1891).

10. Penders YWH, Bopp M, Zellweger U, et al. Continuing, Withdrawing, and Withholding Medical Treatment at the End of Life and Associated Characteristics: a Mortality Follow-back Study. J Gen Intern Med. 2020;35(1):126-32. Epub 20191025.
11. Alaska Statute § 11.41.120 (a)(2): Current Law Against Assisted Suicide, (2013).
12. Arkansas Code Title 5 - Criminal Offenses, Subtitle 2 - Offenses Against the Person, Chapter 10 - Homicide, § 5-10-104. Manslaughter, (2019).
13. Arkansas Code Title 5 - Criminal Offenses, Subtitle 2 - Offenses Against the Person, Chapter 10 - Homicide, § 5-10-106. Physician-Assisted Suicide, (2019).
14. Worthington A, Finlay I, Regnard C. Efficacy and safety of drugs used for 'assisted dying'. Br Med Bull. 2022;142(1):15-22.

Essay: The Antithesis to the Hippocratic Oath

When is euthanasia or physician-assisted suicide an acceptable way to bring life to a close?

Jason Canizales

Introduction

The extent of one's governance over their own body is a topic that is reminiscent of a plethora of topics in contemporary society. Euthanasia, however, is a far more sensible topic given what is at stake: the irreplaceability of human life. Despite medicine's best efforts and technological achievements, there will always be untreatable illnesses and conditions out of the reach for a medical provider. The Hippocratic oath has been historically taken by physicians as a statement of their loyalty to the ethical and safe practice of medicine.[1,2] However, what is now considered ethical for a patient has drastically changed since its inception in ancient Greece. Particularly sentiments over what is the most humane way to end the agonizing pain of a person (rather than saving it) has been a controversial subject continuing to be debated in medicine and politics across the world.[3,4]

Efforts to Circumvent Assisted Death

Palliative care addresses psychosocial, physical, and spiritual aspects of a severely ill patient's life and remains the chosen course of action in life-prolonging care.[5] Through optimal identification and treatment of new and refractory symptoms, physicians hope to continue to maintain quality of life without recurring to its termination as the only alternative solution. Palliative care has also been positively tied to patient satisfaction, symptom control, and patient understanding of their diagnosis and prognosis in addition to clinician management of a patient's comorbidities.[5,6] Regrettably in some these cases, adequate treatment may not be achievable, available, or overdue and mitigation of symptoms through pain medication may also be powerless to alleviate their afflictions.[7] In these cases, patients may request/implore physicians to consider physician-assisted suicide (PAS) if no therapy or pain-alleviating treatment is available. Unfortunately, some medical societies such as the American Medical Association's House of Delegates and other government bodies may not be subservient to a patient's wishes and deny the privilege over their own life choices.[8]

Worldwide, the Netherlands, Belgium, and Luxemburg along with some US states (e.g., Oregon and Washington) recognize the clinical importance of PAS and have legalized its practice.[9-11] The problem of legalizing PAS relies on the "slippery slope" concept that once it becomes decriminalized, this will ensue in more avenues to justify euthanasia or PAS leading to a fear of an increasing number of fatalities.[12] Some studies have shown that in US states where euthanasia has been approved was associated with a 6.3% increase rate of total suicides.[13] While PAS is legalized in Oregon if diagnosed with a terminal disease and a prognosis of 6 months of life, untreatable agonizing suffering is not sufficient to be eligible given the vagueness of the concept itself. This means that if there are other forms of physical or emotional suffering, a physician is to proceed by recommending palliative care as the only alternative.[12]

Among other miscellaneous concerns, the propagation of high-profile suicidal tendencies may inadvertently lead more people of similar demographics to resort to committing suicide.[14] Given the susceptibility of young audiences who may be suffering from mental stress or depression has raised the concern that ill-exposure to high-profile suicides may lead to spikes in suicides. For example, the airing of certain shows such as Netflix's *13 Reasons Why* was associated with a significant increase in monthly suicides of young people around 10–17 years-of-age in the US.[15] Although non-assisted suicides (NAS) are different from PAS and no data has been acquired to support that increase in NAS correlated to PAS, legalization of PAS has been associated with an increased rate of total suicides but no decrease in NAS.[13] Nevertheless, an expansion on high-profile PAS suicides may result in a homogenous effect to those of NAS in young populations further questioning the role of permissibility as a leading influence in a person's autonomy and decision-making.

Why PAS Matters

The discussion on patient autonomy is paramount for any type of medical procedure because it is the right of competent adults to

"To live is to suffer, to survive is to find some meaning in the suffering."

Friedrich Nietzsche, German philosopher, poet, and philologist

make independent decisions over their own medical care.[4] Even if refusing treatment will be detrimental to a patient's health or contribute to his/her demise, a person still has the right to make such decisions. While arguments inquiring over the legitimacy of patient autonomy over their choices are objectively sound (meaning one's choice is not swayed by other people), seriously/terminally ill patients may likely project their wishes based on the current state of their health. Moreover, efforts to delegitimize a person's decision over their life may inherently undermine their dignity and personal identity.[4] Beyond providing patients with a soothing departure, this would also alleviate their families from suffering in tandem with "quality of death" offering respect to a life that can no longer be saved.[16, 17]

Having purpose drives people to live their lives amid struggles. A purposeless life therefore may also lean people to self-question why they should be enduring the agonizing pain if no inherent good will result from their struggle to hold onto life. However, this also means that not all forms of struggle are irreparable, and the mood of a person with no clear aspirations in life may further intensify their suffering.[18] Although much of a person's struggle may be in part linked to depression, this is something that can be treatable, but those attributed to life-threatening diseases do not have a "second chance" to look forward to. PAS is a humane way to deliver patients "quality of death" but serious considerations as to who is treated and why are also as important to prevent the devaluation of human life.[19]

PAS directly contradicts the Hippocratic oath by allowing the introduction of poison to end one's life. Yet, this form of medical practice also offers patients relief from their pain—also an important part of the Hippocratic oath—which increasingly more physicians have begun to advocate to be the ethical and morally correct choice to alleviate the patient.[1, 14] In addition, PAS can provide a person with a dignified and peaceful death in contrast to other forms of suicide. Regardless of someone's opinion on whether authorization of PAS may lead to an increase in total suicides, the rate of NAS suicides in the US continues to increase regardless of broad PAS legalization.[20] This means that other effective avenues should be contemplated to prevent a further overall increase in suicides; however, attributing PAS legalization exclusively to those individuals who are eligible should not be a considerable reason or factor for the total number of suicides in the US.

Works Cited

1. Greek Medicine National Library of Medicine: NIH; 2002 [updated 2012; cited 2022]. Available from: https://www.nlm.nih.gov/hmd/greek/greek_oath.html#:~:text=The%20Hippocratic%20Oath%20(%CE%9F%CF%81%CE%BA%CE%BF%CF%82)%20is,number%20of%20professional%20ethical%20standards.
2. Van Hooff AJ. Ancient euthanasia: 'good death' and the doctor in the graeco-Roman world. Soc Sci Med. 2004;58(5):975-85.
3. Cohen J, Van Landeghem P, Carpentier N, et al. Different trends in euthanasia acceptance across Europe. A study of 13 western and 10 central and eastern European countries, 1981-2008. Eur J Public Health. 2013;23(3):378-80. Epub 20121229.
4. Fontalis A, Prousali E, Kulkarni K. Euthanasia and assisted dying: what is the current position and what are the key arguments informing the debate? J R Soc Med. 2018;111(11):407-13.
5. Teoli D, Kalish VB. Palliative Care. StatPearls. Treasure Island (FL)2022.
6. Shin SH, Hui D, Chisholm GB, et al. Characteristics and outcomes of patients admitted to the acute palliative care unit from the emergency center. J Pain Symptom Manage. 2014;47(6):1028-34. Epub 20131115.
7. Hawley P. Barriers to Access to Palliative Care. Palliat Care. 2017;10:1178224216688887. Epub 20170220.
8. Frieden J. Physician-Assisted Suicide Once Again Divides AMA Members MedPage Today2019 [cited 2022]. Available from: https://www.medpagetoday.com/meetingcoverage/ama/80384.
9. Deliens L, van der Wal G. The euthanasia law in Belgium and the Netherlands. Lancet. 2003;362(9391):1239-40.
10. Steinbrook R. Physician-assisted death--from Oregon to Washington State. N Engl J Med. 2008;359(24):2513-5.
11. Watson R. Luxembourg is to allow euthanasia from 1 April. BMJ. 2009;338:b1248. Epub 20090324.
12. Pereira J. Legalizing euthanasia or assisted suicide: the illusion of safeguards and controls. Curr Oncol. 2011;18(2):e38-45.
13. Jones DA, Paton D. How Does Legalization of Physician-Assisted Suicide Affect Rates of Suicide? South Med J. 2015;108(10):599-604.
14. Dugdale LS, Callahan D. Assisted Death and the Public Good. South Med J. 2017;110(9):559-61.

15. Bridge JA, Greenhouse JB, Ruch D, et al. Association Between the Release of Netflix's 13 Reasons Why and Suicide Rates in the United States: An Interrupted Time Series Analysis. J Am Acad Child Adolesc Psychiatry. 2020;59(2):236-43. Epub 20190428.
16. Hendry M, Pasterfield D, Lewis R, et al. Why do we want the right to die? A systematic review of the international literature on the views of patients, carers and the public on assisted dying. Palliat Med. 2013;27(1):13-26. Epub 20121105.
17. Schuklenk U, van Delden JJ, Downie J, et al. End-of-life decision-making in Canada: the report by the Royal Society of Canada expert panel on end-of-life decision-making. Bioethics. 2011;25 Suppl 1(Suppl 1):1-73.
18. Svenaeus F. Phenomenological bioethics: Medical technologies, human suffering, and the meaning of being alive: Routledge; 2017.
19. Taylor C. Sources of the self: The making of the modern identity: Harvard University Press; 1992.
20. Martinez-Ales G, Hernandez-Calle D, Khauli N, et al. Why Are Suicide Rates Increasing in the United States? Towards a Multilevel Reimagination of Suicide Prevention. Curr Top Behav Neurosci. 2020;46:1-23.

Topic: The Journey of Ru-486— The Much-Maligned Mifepristone

In 1980, Ru38486 was synthesized in France by chemist Georges Teutsch.[1] Because this was the 38,486th new chemical entity for the innovator pharmaceutical company, Roussel Uclaf (now Sanofi), it was named for its order of discovery (shortened to "Ru-486" later).[2,3] Dr. Teutsch was not attempting to create a drug to end a pregnancy; rather, he sought to develop a glucocorticoid receptor antagonist with multiple potential uses. Of the three glucocorticoid antagonists synthesized at that time, Ru-486 stood out for its ability to antagonize progesterone receptors. Ru-486 has been rechristened "mifepristone" and when coupled with a prostaglandin, it can produce a "medical abortion".[4]

Progesterone receptors are found in few tissues (chiefly the uterine corpus luteum and endometrium of the female reproductive tract) and their function is to allow progesterone binding to permit zygote (fertilized cell) implantation after conception and subsequent fetal gestation.[5] Blockade of the prostaglandin receptor with mifepristone prevents implantation of products of conception as well as disrupts any implantation that has already occurred. Thus, Teutsch and colleagues serendipitously created a chemical abortifacient. Tests in animals confirmed that the drug could induce miscarriage, and human applications began to be explored.[1]

"No woman can call herself free until she can choose consciously whether she will or will not be a mother."

Margaret Sanger, American birth control activist, sex educator, writer, and nurse

Because the researchers never intended to create such a product, they had not anticipated the controversy it would generate.[6,7] Specifically, employees of the French pharmaceutical company were threatened and harassed to the degree that the drug was actually withdrawn from the market one month after it was introduced to the public.[7] Such protests in the US, where pregnancy termination is legal and generally safe, prevented the drug from being marketed to women. Beyond the US, the drug was of enormous interest because data from the World Health Organization suggested that almost one-half million women in developing countries die from pregnancy-related events annually and almost one-half of those women die from improperly performed pregnancy terminations.[4] The science is clear: pregnancy and childbirth carry significantly more risk of mortality than pregnancy termination.[8-13]

Even though mifepristone held such initial promise for allowing reproductive choice and saving the lives of women globally, the public began to protest other drugs manufactured by Roussel-Uclaf and its parent company, Hoechst. This pressure was so great that the patent rights for mifepristone were transferred to a new company which severely restricted its sale, limiting it to the UK, Sweden, and France and imposed residency requirements for women wishing to obtain the drug.[3, 14] Thus, each woman had to live in one of the three countries in which the drug was available and none could travel from beyond those locales to receive the drug.[14] To loosen this restriction on mifepristone, the World Health Organization responded with more than 1,000 physician signatures to a declaration that withdrawal of mifepristone would prevent other countries from researching the compound. This was successful in reviving the drug's availability and soon other countries such as China adopted its use. The US approved mifepristone for medical pregnancy termination in 1997.

Since that time, mifepristone is useful for treating other diseases; although, it will likely always be associated with its historical ties to pregnancy termination because it changed the landscape of medical care and the way the public viewed female reproductive rights.[15] And these changes to a woman's ability to plan a family are not insignificant. Data show that annually, more than three million pregnancies are unplanned, and in 1990, only Ortho Pharmaceutical was researching and developing contraceptives.[16] Because of this, US policymakers speculated that mifepristone's availability would increase the number of pregnancy terminations.

Such speculation was further confused by people in positions to wield restrictions against a pregnant woman who had zero scientific or medical training and who often mistakenly conflated the mechanism of action of all contraceptives with mifepristone. Then, with this misinformation, they counseled and confused patients. Pharmacologically, a contraceptive prevents conception, but it cannot reverse the course of conception once it has occurred. A contraceptive also cannot prevent zygote implantation and fetal gestation. Emergency contraception, also known as the "morning-after pill", works in a manner similar to regular contraception, only differing in the dose which is higher than daily contraceptive tablets. In contrast, mifepristone is only effective after conception. Thus, it can also be considered to be a contragestive or a pharmacological agent that prevents gestation by causing the uterine lining to shed and take with it any implanted products of conception.

With such misunderstanding and subsequent confusion, many pro-life and religious organizations were opposed to mifepristone's approval, sale, and use because they feared increased abortions. This did not occur, however. Instead, abortions that were already planned were performed earlier, and these were medically less risky. A surgical abortion, the technique for which medical students are taught—dilation and curettage—cannot be carried out until at least 6 weeks and it is typically not offered after 20 weeks of gestation. Mifepristone, in contrast, allows termination at the moment's notice of conception. It may be important to note that, physiologically, a "pregnancy" cannot occur without implantation.

Also, after conception, several days—and as many as a few weeks—may elapse after the biological fusion that creates a zygote occurs and conception proceeds to implantation. Once implanted for growth and development, the zygote signals for a hormonal cascade to support gestation. Thus, it may be said that a "termination" occurring as early as conception is confirmed may not truly be defined as an "abortion". Data show that miscarriage, or early pregnancy loss which is defined as occurring before 20 weeks, occurs in up to 15% of pregnancies and that most (80%) occur in the first 12 weeks due to fetal non-viability due to genetic problems (fetal-lethal genomes), trauma, infections, maternal hormonal or immune problems, physical problems, or uterine/cervical abnormalities. Thus, it is completely feasible that a woman can lose products of conception without ever knowing she has conceived at all. So, numbers for miscarriages may be artificially low due to this lack of reporting. The March of Dimes suggests that up to half of all "pregnancies" end in miscarriage if these other data are included.[17]

"The greatest destroyer of peace is abortion because if a mother can kill her own child, what is left for me to kill you and you to kill me? There is nothing between."

Mother Teresa, Roman Catholic Nun, missionary

Comparatively, mifepristone is safer and simpler than a surgical termination which requires trained medical professionals, the correct surgical setting, instrumentation, as well as local anesthetics, antibiotics, and analgesics. Most importantly, a surgical abortion requires patient travel as the number of termination centers across the US are being shuttered due to extreme viewpoints that a woman is not entitled to dictate her reproductive choices. Too, women have been harassed, threatened, and assaulted when entering termination centers, and it has become necessary for some centers to provide escorts to protect women who require clinic services.[18-22] Thus, surgical termination is vastly more complex than swallowing a tablet or two. A medical solution can be carried out at home, in greater privacy.[3] Paradoxically, healthcare providers have suggested that they prefer offering surgical versus medical terminations because they are not comfortable with patients being trusted to take a drug independently, especially multiple drugs that must be timed in a sequence.

Also, clinics charge for surgical terminations based on gestational age. The more advanced the pregnancy is, the more expensive the procedure will be. Mifepristone, however, is the same price irrespective of the timing at which it is needed. Because women frequently pay cash for pregnancy termination, the price can be highly influential to a woman's choices. Also, because the preponderance of pregnancy terminations is performed at special clinics, mifepristone allows other providers (primary care, obstetricians, gynecologists, for example) to offer this drug outside of a specialty setting. This expands options for all women across the nation as well as allows specialized centers a second treatment option to reduce patient volume and associated costs to the care provider.

The pharmacological controversy over medical pregnancy termination raises excellent questions about how we use science to prevent the existence of other humans, how we restrict such drugs to only certain "worthy" populations, and how gender influences what drugs are available to whom and for what purposes.

Writing Prompts

- Should medical and pharmacy students be able to opt out of learning the pharmacology of mifepristone to give plausible deniability about its use so they can deny it to future patients?
    - What should medical schools do with this type of student?
- Are women treated as fragile by the medical community which is overly paternalistic in suggesting we cannot be trusted with self-care?
- Is the use of mifepristone ethically and morally wrong because a drug, like lethal injection, is sold and dispensed to end a potential human life?
- Should employers be required to cover the cost of this drug for female employees or the female dependents of those employees?
- Does the fact that the drug can be used immediately upon confirmation of pregnancy make it less morally offensive than a surgical termination?
- Does the availability of this drug make termination more "thinkable" for women?
- Does this drug increase the privacy of women making a difficult and personal medical decision?
    - Should all potential fathers of these "products of conception" be told of the impending use of this drug?
    - Should they have a voice at all?
- Do people who oppose this drug's approval really disapprove of women controlling their bodies and their ability to reproduce?
- Does the approval of this drug conflict with the FDA's ethical compass about human harm?
    - The drug is considered "safe" is this ironic?
- Data show that only one person died after using mifepristone, a French woman in poor health.
    - But is that accurate if 100,000 fetuses were terminated? Do they count?
- Is it a disturbing trend that pharmacies are omitted from the distribution so that physicians (who are not drug experts) can prescribe and dispense the drug?
    - Does this set a precedent for undercutting the benefit of drug experts for patients?
- Are the current laws restricting access science-based, political, or religious?
    - Because most lawmakers are men, is this paternalistic and demeaning to women?
- Does telling women about reversal add unnecessary complexity to the counseling aspect of dispensing the drug?
    - Is offering a reversal doing illegal experimental research on a subject (the fetus) who cannot consent?

Works Cited

1. Ulmann A, Teutsch G, Philibert D. Ru 486. Sci Am. 1990;262(6):42-8.
2. Baulieu EE. A novel approach to human fertility control: contragestion by the anti-progesterone RU 486. Eur J Obstet Gynecol Reprod Biol. 1988;28(2):125-9.
3. Rosenfield A. Mifepristone (RU 486) in the United States. What does the future hold? N Engl J Med. 1993;328(21):1560-1.
4. Rosenfield A. RU-486 and the politics of reproduction. Female Patient. 1989;14(3):69, 73-4.

5. Baulieu EE, Seidman DS, Hajri S. Mifepristone (RU486) and voluntary termination of pregnancy: enigmatic variations or anecdotal religion-based attitudes? Hum Reprod. 2001;16(10):2243-4.
6. Schlegelmilch BB. Marketing Ethics: An International Perspective: Cengage Learning EMEA; 1998.
7. RU-486: a continuing saga. Abort Res Notes. 1988;17(3-4):1-2.
8. van Pampus MG, Wolf H, Weijmar Schultz WC, et al. Posttraumatic stress disorder following preeclampsia and HELLP syndrome. J Psychosom Obstet Gynaecol. 2004;25(3-4):183-7.
9. Chervenak JL, Kardon NB. Advancing maternal age: the actual risks. Female Patient. 1991;16(11):17-24.
10. Pyone T, Sorensen BL, Tellier S. Childbirth attendance strategies and their impact on maternal mortality and morbidity in low-income settings: a systematic review. Acta Obstet Gynecol Scand. 2012;91(9):1029-37.
11. Barate P, Temmerman M. Surviving pregnancy and childbirth is a human right: the silent tragedy of maternal mortality. Facts Views Vis Obgyn. 2010;2(1):21-30.
12. Gordon CA. Relation of maternal mortality rates to all deaths associated with childbirth. Am J Obstet Gynecol. 1958;76(1):204-9.
13. Furstenberg N. Maternal mortality; a statistical study of earlier and present prognosis in childbirth. Acta Obstet Gynecol Scand. 1949;28(3-4):103-9.
14. Roussel-Uclaf to transfer RU 486 rights. Reprod Freedom News. 1997;6(7):8.
15. Mackenzie SJ, Yeo S. Pregnancy interruption using mifepristone (RU-486). A new choice for women in the USA. J Nurse Midwifery. 1997;42(2):86-90.
16. Meade V. Contraceptive development lags in U.S. Am Pharm. 1990;NS30(5):22-3.
17. Finer LB, Zolna MR. Unintended pregnancy in the United States: incidence and disparities, 2006. Contraception. 2011;84(5):478-85.
18. United States. Court of Appeals FC. Roe v. Abortion Abolition Society, 9 March 1987. Annu Rev Popul Law. 1987;14:43.
19. Jones BS, Weitz TA. Legal barriers to second-trimester abortion provision and public health consequences. Am J Public Health. 2009;99(4):623-30.
20. Indiana. Supreme C. A Woman's Choice-East Side Women's Clinic v. Newman. North East Rep Second Ser. 1996;671:104-13.
21. Sollom T. Clinic defense, parental involvement focus of state abortion debates. State Reprod Health Monit. 1995;6(1):1-2.
22. President to sign FACE bill aimed at deterring antiabortion violence. Wash Memo Alan Guttmacher Inst. 1994(8):1.

Essay: Ru-486: Undeniable Healthcare

Brianna Hunt

Ru-486, or mifepristone, is a progesterone receptor antagonist that is used to terminate a pregnancy.[1] When followed by a dose of misoprostol, it is both incredibly effective and incredibly safe.[1] It is a safe option for women who are seeking an abortion, and it comes with the additional benefit of being able to take this medication in the privacy of one's own home. However, religious adversaries of a woman's right to choose have transformed Ru-486 (and other abortion procedures) from an issue of healthcare to an issue of morality. They believe it is immoral to terminate a pregnancy because it ends life before it can begin; however, is it not immoral to refuse essential healthcare to a currently living woman? The personhood of an embryo or fetus is questionable, but the personhood of the woman carrying it is undeniable. Therefore, a woman's physical health, mental well-being, and right to bodily autonomy should always come first.

A woman deserves to make informed decisions regarding the termination of a pregnancy because pregnancy and childbirth can be downright dangerous. Pregnancy is a process that can alter a woman's body permanently, not to mention the toll that it can take on her mental health.[2] Although pregnancy complications such as preeclampsia and gestational diabetes typically resolve after delivery, they can place a woman at risk for developing long-term illnesses.[3] Mifepristone is a simple and safe way for women to avoid these detrimental health effects, therefore it is a form of healthcare. Unfortunately, women seeking an abortion may be refused a prescription by their physician due to the doctor's personal beliefs. Some physicians take it a step further and refuse to provide a woman with the resources she would need to access an abortion. Denying women essential healthcare, such as abortions, is sexist and should not be permitted. Women seeking treatment should not have to feel vilified by the physicians who swore an oath to provide care. Therefore, even if the doctor has a personal aversion to providing abortion care, it is his or her responsibility to provide the woman with the resources she needs to get this care elsewhere. A woman's health and well-being should not rely on the religious beliefs of her physician; therefore, it is the physician's responsibility to provide care or refer the woman to someone who can provide care, regardless of their religious beliefs.

Seeking an abortion can be a very traumatic process for women. However, there is a possibility that the entire process can be done privately at home. Through telehealth appointments, a woman can be prescribed mifepristone without having to go to a doctor in person.[4] Then, the prescription can be mailed directly to her home where she can take the medication in complete privacy.[4] This process would be ideal for many women, as it would save them the stress of being accosted by protestors at a clinic or being denied care by their physician. However, there are currently laws in 19 states that either ban the use of telehealth appointments for mifepristone prescriptions outright or require the physical presence of the prescribing clinician.[5] Additionally, six states currently have laws that ban mailing mifepristone.[6] Many states also require ultrasounds and waiting periods for women seeking abortions, which are tactics meant to humiliate and guilt the woman for choosing to seek the care she needs. These laws are immoral, as they create obstacles preventing women from obtaining essential healthcare. It is time for lawmakers to remove these obstacles and ensure that mifepristone can be easily accessed by those who require it.

Works Cited

1. Ulmann A, Teutsch G, Philibert D. Ru 486. Sci Am. 1990;262(6):42-8.
2. Ghahremani T, Magann EF, Phillips A, et al. Women's Mental Health Services and Pregnancy: A Review. Obstet Gynecol Surv. 2022;77(2):122-9.
3. Neiger R. Long-Term Effects of Pregnancy Complications on Maternal Health: A Review. J Clin Med. 2017;6(8). Epub 20170727. PMCID: PMC5575578.
4. Upadhyay UD, Koenig LR, Meckstroth KR. Safety and Efficacy of Telehealth Medication Abortions in the US During the COVID-19 Pandemic. JAMA Netw Open. 2021;4(8):e2122320. Epub 20210802. PMCID: PMC8385590.
5. Anderson E, Salganicoff A, Sobel L. State Restrictions on Telehealth Abortions: Kaiser Family Foundation; 2021 [cited 2022]. Available from: https://www.kff.org/womens-health-policy/slide/state-restrictions-on-telehealth-abortion/.
6. Sobel L, Ramaswamy A, Salganicoff A. The Intersection of State and Federal Policies on Access to Medication Abortion Via Telehealth: Kaiser Family Foundation; 2022 [cited 2022]. Available from: https://www.kff.org/womens-health-policy/issue-brief/the-intersection-of-state-and-federal-policies-on-access-to-medication-abortion-via-telehealth/.
1. Ulmann A, Teutsch G, Philibert D. Ru 486. Sci Am. 1990;262(6):42-8.
2. Ghahremani T, Magann EF, Phillips A, et al. Women's Mental Health Services and Pregnancy: A Review. Obstet Gynecol Surv. 2022;77(2):122-9.
3. Neiger R. Long-Term Effects of Pregnancy Complications on Maternal Health: A Review. J Clin Med. 2017;6(8). Epub 20170727.
4. Upadhyay UD, Koenig LR, Meckstroth KR. Safety and Efficacy of Telehealth Medication Abortions in the US During the COVID-19 Pandemic. JAMA Netw Open. 2021;4(8):e2122320. Epub 20210802.
5. Anderson E, Salganicoff A, Sobel L. State Restrictions on Telehealth Abortions: Kaiser Family Foundation; 2021 [cited 2022]. Available from: https://www.kff.org/womens-health-policy/slide/state-restrictions-on-telehealth-abortion/.
6. Sobel L, Ramaswamy A, Salganicoff A. The Intersection of State and Federal Policies on Access to Medication Abortion Via Telehealth: Kaiser Family Foundation; 2022 [cited 2022]. Available from: https://www.kff.org/womens-health-policy/issue-brief/the-intersection-of-state-and-federal-policies-on-access-to-medication-abortion-via-telehealth/.

Essay: RU-486: The Most Controversial Pharmaceutical Miracle

Sarah Wolff

Very rarely can a drug be classified as safe, reliable, and almost as pharmaceutically flawless as mifepristone. Mifepristone has statistically fewer complications than other widely used medications such as acetaminophen, sildenafil, and alprazolam, with side effects affecting fewer than 2 of 1,000 women who use it.[1] Yet very few drugs have received as much backlash, political opinions, and controversy as mifepristone has. Mifepristone gives women the choice to have noninvasive, safe, and effective abortions in the privacy of their own homes. Regardless of the reason behind the abortion though, people have fought to strip women of this choice, including healthcare providers. At a CVS pharmacy that is just a two-hour drive from the University of Arizona in Peoria, Arizona, a woman was publicly refused her prescription that would allow her to end her pregnancy for her fetus that was deceased.[2] Abortions are a lifesaving medical procedure, and to deny a woman this right as a healthcare provider is unfathomable. When comparing how mifepristone and oral contraceptives for women are treated in medicine and politics to other reproductive care options for men such as erectile dysfunction drugs and condoms, this controversy often feels like an attack directly against women.[3] Women deserve the right to have mifepristone and other reproductive services without healthcare workers and politicians villainizing them or denying them this care.

It is extremely disheartening when politicians start having opinions on what should only occur between a woman and her provider. Often, politicians do not know the science of the healthcare that they are trying to regulate. They tend to make decisions solely from subjective reasoning, and because of this, the public does not fully trust them either. According to a poll conducted by *The 19th*, 70% of a national sample of 20,799 adults do not believe that politicians are informed enough about abortion to create fair policies on it.[4] This became especially prevalent when Roe v. Wade was overturned on June 24th, 2022. Now that states have control, local politicians decide whether Mifepristone is an option for women seeking an abortion. Local politicians decide whether the women in their state have the right to access a lifesaving pill. Local politicians decide whether the women in their state can choose for themselves and their futures, saving their bodies from the horrific trauma of giving birth (which is almost always more harmful than receiving an abortion).[5] Local politicians who are primarily men decide, and it is disgusting. Almost all abortions are banned in at least 13 states, with gestational limit bans in another five including Arizona.[6] Not enough providers have a say on the efficacy, safety, and necessity of this drug, and not enough women have a say on their own bodies and lives.

However, this becomes especially problematic when healthcare workers opt out of not just providing abortions but refusing to give resources on where to get one. Healthcare should never be approached with the lens of subjectivity, and the fear of being uncomfortable should not be catered to. However, healthcare employees may refuse to provide abortions due to their religion, morality, and "injunctions of natural law."[7, 8] When one goes into medicine, he/she makes a vow to do no harm, yet, countless studies have shown that women who were denied an abortion and forced to carry their pregnancies to term have worse long-term outcomes regarding health, financial stability, and the safety of their children. They are four times more likely to live on the poverty line, three times more likely to be unemployed, more likely to suffer from anxiety, stress, and lower self-esteem, and more likely to stay in touch with abusive partners.[9]

Additionally, a common misconception that providers who deny abortions may resort to is that women can regret receiving this procedure. A study was conducted in which a group of women was asked whether or not they regretted their abortions right after their abortion was complete, and again another 5 years after the procedure. Over 95% of these women knew that their abortion was the right call, both immediately following the procedure and half a decade later.[9] It is insulting that healthcare providers may deem they know what is best for their patient who is seeking an abortion as if their patient is incapable of making this decision herself. It becomes even more insulting if they provide no guidance to their patients for solely personal reasons. Politicians and healthcare providers should not be obstacles in getting a safe, non-invasive, and effective abortion via Mifepristone. This is an extremely difficult decision that a woman must make as is, and it is outrageous how many hurdles she has to overcome to get the procedure done.

Works Cited

1. Mifepristone is a Safe Choice Pro Choice America 2017. Available from: https://www.prochoiceamerica.org/wp-content/uploads/2017/01/2.-Mifepristone-is-a-Safe-Choice.pdf.
2. Associated Press. Pharmacist Denies Woman Abortion Pill Despite Already Dead Fetus. Canoecom. 2018.
3. Beck J. The Different Stakes of Male and Female Birth Control: The Atlantic; 2016 [cited 2022 11/30]. Available from: https://www.theatlantic.com/health/archive/2016/11/the-different-stakes-of-male-and-female-birth-control/506120/.
4. Shali Luthra JM. 70% of Americans Don't Trust Politicians to Make Abortion Policy: The 19th; 2022. Available from: https://19thnews.org/2022/09/poll-americans-abortion-law-politicians/.
5. Ralph LJ, Schwarz EB, Grossman D, et al. Self-reported Physical Health of Women Who Did and Did Not Terminate Pregnancy After Seeking Abortion Services. Annals of Internal Medicine. 2019;171(4):238-47.
6. Allison McCann ASW, Ava Sasani, Taylor Johnston, Larry Buchanan and Jon Huang. Tracking the States Where Abortion is Now Banned: New York Times; 2022. Available from: https://www.nytimes.com/interactive/2022/us/abortion-laws-roe-v-wade.html.
7. Dooley D. Conscientious Refusal to Assist With Abortion. BMJ. 1994.

8. Health Care Workers May Refuse to Perform Treatments Because of Faith-Based Reasons: SHRM; 2019. Available from: https://www.shrm.org/resourcesandtools/legal-and-compliance/employment-law/pages/health-care-workers-faith-based-exemptions.aspx.
9. Singer J. What Happens to Women Who Are Denied Abortion? 2022. Available from: https://www.glamour.com/story/what-happens-to-women-who-are-denied-abortion-here-are-the-stats.

Essay: Ru-486: Take It Like A Woman

Karlie Flader

Pregnancy terminations are not a foreign topic in history and abortion procedures can be found as early as 1550 BC in the Egyptian Ebers Papyrus.[1] Women's needs for contraception and family planning resources have not gone away since then, but the right to access these resources has become more restricted. The right to birth control and abortions has evolved from being a matter of health and safety to a matter of control over women. It seems that today, the often-male population of judges, politicians, pharmacists, and physicians have a far greater say about female reproductive rights than women do.

Ru-486, or mifepristone, has been used as a safe and effective way to terminate a pregnancy since its FDA approval in the United States in 2000.[2-4] When used in a two-drug combination, mifepristone blocks progesterone which blocks implantation of the zygote, and misoprostol causes uterine contractions that expel the products of conception.[3, 5] The advent of Ru-486 has also lowered the cost of women receiving medical abortions.[6] Due to the effectiveness, minimal health risks, and low cost associated with mifepristone, medical abortions can replace invasive surgical procedures, increase privacy, and allow for the patient to emotionally recover on their terms. Thus, mifepristone has become the preferred choice for terminating a pregnancy.

Making mifepristone available over the counter is essential in maintaining women's mental and physical health. Medical abortions made possible by mifepristone allow women to undergo a personal and emotional procedure in the privacy of their own homes. This is a critical aspect of preserving mental health for women. Women may already feel guilt, fear, or sorrow while obtaining their prescription from the pharmacy and this process would be made easier if they get their prescription swiftly and without complications or opposition every time. Pharmacists have the legal ability to refuse the distribution of oral contraceptives on the grounds of their own religious or moral beliefs, regardless of the patient's needs or wants.[7, 8] For a physician to refuse care for anyone based on his/her personal beliefs is incredibly immoral and is an abuse of power that risks patients' health and unfairly targets women. Healthcare professionals should not allow their personal beliefs to interfere with or influence the way that they care for patients, and a patient's care and well-being should always come first, regardless of the physician's personal beliefs. Additionally, women are at a greater risk of experiencing mental health disorders after receiving an abortion.[9] Terminating a pregnancy may not be a patient's original plan of action, so the refusal of a prescription by a pharmacist is frustrating and embarrassing. Women and uterus-owning individuals should be able to make decisions about their bodies without any false information or guilt-tripping from providers, especially when it comes to pregnancy termination. If they are denied care by pharmacists or physicians, their emotional and physical safety is at risk: 20-40% of the deaths resulting from pregnancy-related matters are due to unsafe or illegal abortions.[10] Therefore, providing women with a safe space to take care of their medical needs in private also reduces the risk factors associated with abortion.

Decriminalizing abortion would allow for the safe practice of abortion and would prevent the fining or incarceration of those seeking or providing pregnancy terminations. Mifepristone has been approved for years, yet its right to be used has been stripped away by federal law. Regardless of the written law, women are going to seek termination if they find that they are not fit for or not prepared to have a child. Ironically, those providing safe abortions are being punished when it is unsafe and illegal abortions that cause death and injury.[11] Criminalizing abortion even in cases of rape, incest, or fetal health will cause more injuries, deaths, and mental health risks.[11] Women deserve the right to privacy and the state should avoid making decisions on a woman's body on behalf of her and her physician. Abortion is an individual decision, and no law should remove or restrict that choice.

Ultimately, women should have unrestricted access to contraception and mifepristone because, without barriers, women are more likely to use these safer methods of termination, and both physical and mental health risks are reduced for those seeking terminations or prevention of pregnancies. Women deserve to have their needs met with the same amount of attention and care as others and allowing those in power to push back against—or outrightly neglect—women's healthcare is only perpetuating the stigma and inattention surrounding women's health.

Works Cited

1. Potts M. History of Contraception 2009; 6:27.
2. Sarrut B, Doreau C. Procedures on handling mifepristone (RU 486) in France. Hosp Pharm. 1990;25(7):655-8.
3. Baulieu EE, Seidman DS, Hajri S. Mifepristone (RU486) and voluntary termination of pregnancy: enigmatic variations or anecdotal religion-based attitudes? Hum Reprod. 2001;16(10):2243-4.
4. FDA panel finds mifepristone safe and effective. Reprod Freedom News. 1996;5(13):7-8.
5. Allen R. Uses of Misoprostol in Obstetrics and Gynecology2009. PMCID: PMC2760893.
6. Jannet D, Aflak N, Abankwa A, et al. Termination of 2nd and 3rd trimester pregnancies with mifepristone and misoprostol. Eur J Obstet Gynecol Reprod Biol. 1996;70(2):159-63.
7. Wernow JR, Grant DG. Dispensing with conscience: a legal and ethical assessment. Ann Pharmacother. 2008;42(11):1669-78.
8. Stein R. A medical crisis of conscience: faith drives some to refuse patients medication or care. Washington Post. 2006:A1, A6.
9. Reardon DC. The abortion and mental health controversy: A comprehensive literature review of common ground agreements, disagreements, actionable recommendations, and research opportunities. SAGE Open Med. 2018;6:2050312118807624. PMCID: PMC6207970.
10. Rosenfield A. RU-486 and the politics of reproduction. Female Patient. 1989;14(3):69, 73-4.
11. Berer M. Abortion Law and Policy Around the World: In Search of Decriminalization. Health Hum Rights. 2017;19(1):13-27. PMCID: PMC5473035.
1. Potts M. History of Contraception2009;6:27.

2. Sarrut B, Doreau C. Procedures on handling mifepristone (RU 486) in France. Hosp Pharm. 1990;25(7):655-8.
3. Baulieu EE, Seidman DS, Hajri S. Mifepristone (RU486) and voluntary termination of pregnancy: enigmatic variations or anecdotal religion-based attitudes? Hum Reprod. 2001;16(10):2243-4.
4. FDA panel finds mifepristone safe and effective. Reprod Freedom News. 1996;5(13):7-8.
5. Allen R. Uses of Misoprostol in Obstetrics and Gynecology2009.
6. Jannet D, Aflak N, Abankwa A, et al. Termination of 2nd and 3rd trimester pregnancies with mifepristone and misoprostol. Eur J Obstet Gynecol Reprod Biol. 1996;70(2):159-63.
7. Wernow JR, Grant DG. Dispensing with conscience: a legal and ethical assessment. Ann Pharmacother. 2008;42(11):1669-78.
8. Stein R. A medical crisis of conscience: faith drives some to refuse patients medication or care. Washington Post. 2006:A1, A6.
9. Reardon DC. The abortion and mental health controversy: A comprehensive literature review of common ground agreements, disagreements, actionable recommendations, and research opportunities. SAGE Open Med. 2018;6:2050312118807624.
10. Rosenfield A. RU-486 and the politics of reproduction. Female Patient. 1989;14(3):69, 73-4.
11. Berer M. Abortion Law and Policy Around the World: In Search of Decriminalization. Health Hum Rights. 2017;19(1):13-27.

Topic: Conscience Clauses in Medicine—The Right to Deny Patient Care

As diversity increases in the healthcare arena, ethical heterogeneity among healthcare providers and patients also increases. This may give rise to unintended consequences of providing drugs, devices, and services to certain types or classes of patients. That we have products to improve human health and then in the same environment, that we can deny these commodities to people in need is indeed controversial as well as complex and fraught with ethical and religious underpinnings. The consequence of this problem is that the rights of patients often oppose the beliefs and preferences of healthcare workers, and this harsh juxtaposition may require government interference.

"I believe in an American where the separation of church of state is absolute."

John F. Kennedy, 35th US President

However, this problem is not new.
It actually dates back to the Church Amendment of 1973, enacted after pregnancy termination became legal.[1] This amendment protected healthcare workers employed by institutions that received federal dollars in the form of grants, loans, or contracts. Specifically, those providers did not have to perform services or offer information or advice about procedures they found objectionable because they violated their "religious beliefs or moral convictions". These included procedures to end a pregnancy or to perform tubal ligation to prevent pregnancy as well as assisting with family planning, giving information about blood transfusions, and offering vaccine counseling. On the surface, this was a powerful message, but in reality, there were no additional regulations to facilitate the implementation of these laws and there was no formal course of redress for providers who believed that their religious or moral rights were violated on the job.

To address this gap, a few weeks before President George W. Bush left the Oval Office in 2009, he implemented the Provider Refusal rule to protect US healthcare providers from reprisal or penalty for refusing to treat patients or provide services, information, or advice for procedures that they found morally repugnant. Also, healthcare workers were protected even if their refusals were based on terribly misguided information. For instance, some providers refused oral contraception to patients because they were under the erroneous assumption that they were abortifacients—they are not. Perhaps an unintended effect of this type of conscience clause revival was that it was pointedly one-sided: the person with the moral or religious objection was free to impose his/her views on the person who did not have an objection to a procedure, plan, or treatment, and to deny care. However, the less conservative individual could not impose his/her views on anyone or even medically benefit from having those views at all.

To address this inequity, President Barack Obama, upon taking office in 2009, announced he would overturn Bush's rule. He suggested that healthcare providers could refuse to terminate a pregnancy but that they could not expand their conscientious objections to block a woman's right to family planning information and contraceptives, which would prevent the need for an abortion in the first place. This effort was to restore patients' rights and increase care availability, especially in medically underserved areas where choices may be limited to one provider or none at all. Part of Obama's legislation included a clause that failure to abide by these regulations could make the healthcare institution vulnerable, again much like the Bush-era legislation, to loss of federal funds.

Even with this rule reversal, any healthcare worker who encountered unique issues during which they felt their rights were violated were permitted avenues for filing complaints and seeking redress. However, data show that such complaints in this regard were actually few; specifically, from 2008–2016, only 10 claims were filed.[2] This may be interpreted to mean that providers were not especially burdened with objectionable requests or that they were avoiding the issue altogether by denying the drug or service outright. Data regarding patients denied care are not available but historically, when institutions and patients reach disagreements about access to care, courts have rarely ruled that the patient's wishes take precedence over the hospital's policy.[3]

Interestingly, Obama was prescient when he reversed Bush's rule: conscience clauses have been expanded so that healthcare entities (hospitals, physicians, nurses, and insurance plans to name a few) can and have denied care for patients based on who or what they were perceived to be.[4] Thus, any physician, nurse, or pharmacist could deny care to lesbian, gay, bisexual, transgender, queer (LGBTQ) patients; decline to provide contraceptives or *in vitro* fertilization for gay or single women; refuse to treat HIV and AIDS patients, and dispute any patient's right to particular procedures for end-of-life care.[5-10] Moreover, conscience clauses have been extended to medical and other professional healthcare training programs, enabling these students to opt out of learning about alcohol addiction and treatment, sexually transmitted diseases, and how to care for members of the opposite sex or any person from an "objectionable" demographic, all based on the student's personal prejudices.[11,12] Student refusal to fully participate in a medical curriculum can result in educational lapses and real professional deficits that can cause patient discomfort at best, and harm or death at the very worst.

"For too long, governments big and small have treated conscience claims with hostility instead of protection…But change is coming and it begins here and now."

Roger Severino, Head: Office of Civil Rights, US Department of Health and Human Services

In an about-face on this issue, liberties were again curtailed when President Donald Trump restored healthcare conscience clauses and appointed politically conservative leadership in the US Department of Health and Human Services (HHS). With these adjustments, again providers could deny care under the auspices of religious freedom.

Specifically, a new branch exists in the HHS Office of Civil Rights, the Religious and Conscience Division, which is devoted solely to enforcing conscience objections and the "religious freedom" of only some US citizens. At this time, scholars are debating whether this office and its actions violate existing statutes such as the right to privacy which is granted by the 1st, 3rd, 4th, and 5th Amendments to the Constitution as well as the right to equal protection. Also up for debate is whether these reinvigorated conscience clauses violate the Civil Rights Act of 1964 which outlaws discrimination based on race, color, religion, sex, or national origin (but not gender identity or sexual preference). Thus, there may be no legal recourse for LGBTQ persons who are denied care. These facts leave us at a controversial philosophical stand-off that may have no easy answers but which may certainly have devastating and preventable outcomes.

Writing Prompts

- Should healthcare providers be allowed to exert their own preferences while performing services if those preferences contrast with that profession's governing bodies?
- Should healthcare providers dissociate their personal beliefs from their professional duties?
- Should patients be allowed to ask the provider to prove their religion disapproves of a type of care?
- What about misinterpretations in scripture, belief systems, and unorthodox faiths (astrologically based beliefs)?
- Are some beliefs more legitimate than others?
- Should providers be interviewed before being hired to ensure all procedures are covered in a hospital or clinic?
  - Is this discrimination if it occurs?
  - What if confessing beliefs prevents a job offer?
- Should professionals deny their beliefs to get hired and then act on them after being employed?
- If a provider refers a patient to another professional for a drug or procedure that violates their beliefs, is that provider still part of the objectionable action?
- Should outside regulatory bodies or courts place demands on physician-patient relationships that honor patient sovereignty?
  - Would this violate patient confidentiality?
- Should faith-based policy be permitted for medical care?
- Do conscience clauses protect only certain classes of individuals?
- If a professional will not treat an LGBTQ person for being "unholy" can an atheist professional refuse to treat a bigot?
- Would the ultimate exercise of conscience be to REFUSE to enter health care to avoid all chance of violating one's deepest beliefs?
- Should students in scientific disciplines be able to opt out of experiments that violate their morals?
- Should health care professional students be allowed to refuse to learn about drugs and procedures that offend them?
- Should insurance be required to cover procedures and drugs that must be acquired out-of-network due to a refusal from an in-network provider?

- Do these clauses run counter to anti-discrimination laws?
- Do these clauses run counter to a patient's rights to medically appropriate care?
- Should licensing boards indefinitely suspend licensure for any professional who refuses care?
- Should professionals who restrict drugs, devices, or procedures be required to post this in a conspicuous place in the office waiting room/on a website/in any ad the office runs regarding its services?

Works Cited

1. Church Amendment 42 U.S.C. §300a-7(c), (1973).
2. Alonzo-Zaldivar R. New Trump office would protect conscience rights of doctors. Associated Press. 2018.
3. New Jersey. Superior Court CDMC. In re Requena. Atl Report. 1986;517:886-93.
4. Buchanan BL. Bush administration issued, and Obama administration seeks to rescind, 'conscience clause' regulation. WMJ. 2009;108(2):117-8.
5. De Panfilis L, Cattaneo D, Cola L, et al. [Conscience clause in end-of-life care.]. Recenti Prog Med. 2017;108(5):216-20.
6. Cowley C. A Defence of Conscientious Objection in Medicine: A Reply to Schuklenk and Savulescu. Bioethics. 2016;30(5):358-64.
7. Constitutional law -- free exercise clause -- Ninth Circuit rejects strict scrutiny for pharmacy dispensing requirement. -- Stormans, Inc. v. Selecky, 571 F.3d 960 (9th Cir. 2009). Harv Law Rev. 2009;123(2):596-603.
8. Mishtal JZ. Matters of "conscience": the politics of reproductive healthcare in Poland. Med Anthropol Q. 2009;23(2):161-83.
9. Bradley CT. Emergency contraception and physicians' rights of conscience: a review of current legal standards in Wisconsin. WMJ. 2009;108(3):156-60.
10. Wernow JR, Grant DG. Dispensing with conscience: a legal and ethical assessment. Ann Pharmacother. 2008;42(11):1669-78.
11. Strickland SL. Conscientious objection in medical students: a questionnaire survey. J Med Ethics. 2012;38(1):22-5.
12. Williams A. Conscientious objection: a medical student perspective. Virtual Mentor. 2009;11(9):686-9.

Essay: Personal Beliefs vs. Professional Obligations

Gabbi Ciadella

Healthcare professionals are protected by law in refusing to participate in, perform, accommodate, or assist with healthcare services due to conflict with religious or moral beliefs.[1] This legal right for healthcare providers to deny care to patients due to disagreeing moral or religious beliefs stems from the Church Amendment of 1973. More specifically, this amendment protected healthcare providers working for institutions that received funding from the federal government through loans or grants. Initially, conscience clauses primarily surrounded sterilization procedures and abortions, but over time conscience clauses have been exercised against individuals in the LGBTQ community. Additionally, the laws are written in such a broad manner that they could apply to end-of-life care and other healthcare areas.[2] Although this concept of conscientious objection, or conscience clauses, may appeal to most Americans who advocate for freedom, this ruling prioritizes the freedom of healthcare workers over patient autonomy.

Pharmacists are included in the population of healthcare workers protected by conscience clauses. While some may argue that pharmacists are justified in refusing to dispense or counsel patients on medications that are not in agreement with their personal beliefs—this practice is a threat to patient care.[3] Entering the healthcare field, it is understood that as professionals, they will serve patients to the best of their ability and put the interest of their patients above their own.[4] Because of this innate social contract, healthcare has no place for religious or moral beliefs. Patient care trumps all personal beliefs in healthcare. Imagine a fireman refusing to assist in saving a family from their burning home because of that family's religious beliefs or a teacher excluding students in her class who are part of the LGBTQ community. It would be completely unacceptable behavior since they are refusing to perform the essential duties of their job. No exceptions should be made in the field of pharmacy. Pharmacists are responsible for providing patients with medications and information that is critical to their therapy. Pharmacists are not responsible for imposing their own political, religious, or moral beliefs upon their patients.

As time continues, society is growing more polarized due to political beliefs. Healthcare should be guarded from this issue and patient care should not be influenced by the personal beliefs held by a pharmacist. To no surprise, oral contraceptives are a large topic of debate in this matter. Women's health is being jeopardized by pharmacists who view contraceptives as immoral. As conscientious objection in healthcare becomes more politicized, women's access to healthcare becomes more limited.[5] Pharmacists have refused to fill prescriptions for contraceptives, refused to refer patients to other pharmacies and refused to transfer necessary patient records to other facilities [2]. Not only are pharmacists denying patient care in their own pharmacy, but they are also inhibiting patients from receiving care elsewhere. Conscientious objections made by pharmacists can become even more detrimental in rural areas where pharmacies are not as abundant. If a pharmacist were to refuse to dispense medication to a patient in a less urban area, the patient may be forced to travel over 20 miles to access the medication. That is if the denying pharmacist is kind enough to offer an alternative route to access the medication.

In a 2008 study of nearly 2,000 practicing pharmacists in Nevada, pharmacists' willingness to dispense or transfer potentially controversial medications including emergency contraception, medical abortifacients, erectile dysfunction medications, oral contraceptives, and infertility medications was investigated. It was found that almost 6% of the total pharmacists studied indicated that they would refuse to dispense and refuse to transfer at least one of these medications. Medical abortifacients and emergency contraception displayed the greatest amount of objection. with 7.5% of pharmacists unwilling to dispense emergency contraception and 17.2% refusing to dispense medical abortifacients. This reluctance was largely predicted by religious affiliation.[6] These statistics should not exist. When healthcare professionals are on the job, they should not be protected under the law in discriminating against or subjecting their patients to their convictions. Tolerating personal bias in healthcare is entirely inappropriate since it puts the health of patients at risk and contradicts the concept of patient autonomy.

It is inappropriate for a pharmacist, who is trusted by the public to take care of and act in the best interest of patients, to be allowed to jeopardize the health of a patient for any reason. A pharmacist should only refuse to fill and dispense a prescription if it is unlawful, potentially harmful, or if the prescription is not appropriate for the patient's therapy. Examples of things pharmacists may keep an eye out for are drug interactions, patient allergies, or incorrect dosage. Pharmacists should be concerned solely with the health of their patients, not their patient's religion or sexual orientation.

America prides itself on being "the home of the free" however conscience clauses only allow freedom for healthcare professionals at the expense of patients. Allowing healthcare providers to exercise conscientious objection sacrifices the health of patients, enables discrimination in the healthcare industry, and places patients at the mercy of headstrong healthcare providers. Protecting healthcare providers who deny patient care due to personal beliefs should no longer be tolerated. If an individual wants to work as a physician, pharmacist, nurse, or other healthcare professional, they should be required to put their personal beliefs at rest while on the job and prioritize the care of their patients above all else.

Works Cited

1. U.S Department of Health and Human Services Ofiice for Civil Rights. Conscience Protections for Health Care Providers 2021 [November 24, 2022]. Available from: https://www.hhs.gov/conscience/conscience-protections/index.html.
2. Tanne JH. "Conscience" clauses allow US corporate providers to refuse care. BMJ. 2004;329(7464):476.

3. Shanawani H. The Challenges of Conscientious Objection in Health care. J Relig Health. 2016;55(2):384-93.
4. Erstad BL. The Conscience of a Pharmacist. Am J Pharm Educ. 2019;83(2):7301.
5. Querido M. Q. What are conscience clauses, and how do they affect a woman's right to choose? Reprod Freedom News. 1998;7(7):2-3.
6. Davidson LA, Pettis CT, Joiner AJ, et al. Religion and conscientious objection: a survey of pharmacists' willingness to dispense medications. Soc Sci Med. 2010;71(1):161-5. Epub 20100413.

Essay: Conscience Clauses: The Marriage of Medicine and Morality

Lauren Thompson

We live in a time at which technology and advances in medicine are at an all-time high, yet the United States fails to prioritize these objective standards. Conscience clauses protect healthcare professionals' right to let personal opinions regarding religion and morality prevail over standardized healthcare training. This denial of treatment creates unnecessary burdens for patients and assigns ethical connotations to safe and efficacious medical treatment. How is it ethical to enable individuals to interfere with patient health to satisfy their moral obligations?

The first national conscience clause originated as a response to the Supreme Court decision in *Roe v. Wade*.[1] The Supreme Court decided a woman's privacy concerning abortion was a constitutional right, while simultaneously protecting the religious freedom of healthcare workers involved with the Church Amendment. The Church Amendment stated that if performing an abortion or sterilization procedure conflicted with an individual's religious beliefs or moral convictions, they could withhold involvement without penalty.[2] These conscience clauses eventually began to encompass all aspects of healthcare as the groups of protected people expanded under President George W. Bush. This expansion of the terms of conscience clauses protects healthcare providers' right to deny any care or treatment to patients based on morality. Since this has been instated, we have seen the inevitable consequences of such a system that assumes such high moral veracity of its employees.

Some of the most common examples of conscience clauses in action are abortion, oral contraceptives, or hormone prescriptions. One count found 180 reports of refusals to dispense oral contraceptives in six months.[3] Not only are oral contraceptives approved as safe and efficacious drugs but also they can be prescribed for a variety of reasons beyond just pregnancy prevention.[4] For a pharmacist to deny care in the case of oral contraceptives, they are assuming the intention of the patient and promoting their moral high ground.

In another instance, a pharmacist in Minnesota refused to dispense an over-the-counter emergency contraceptive. Because of this, the patient had to drive 100 miles round trip to acquire the drug. He defended this denial by explaining that the use of abortifacients did not align with his religious beliefs.[5] However, emergency contraceptives work by delaying or inhibiting ovulation, which is different from the mechanism of action of abortifacients.[6] Despite the science behind his religious beliefs being inaccurate, this rationalization is still protected by conscience clauses. Pharmacists go through extensive education and training to have adequate and useful drug information for the ultimate benefit of their patients. Even though the basic understanding of a drug as common as emergency contraception was not present, his religious principles were still protected. This is a key example of when subjective attitudes supersede science at the expense of the patient.

Patients who tend to suffer the greatest from conscience clauses have limited access to healthcare begin with. Healthcare in rural areas is often associated with a multitude of barriers that impact access to quality care. Rural populations are already at a disadvantage when it comes to healthcare due to their geographic isolation, socioeconomic factors, and educational shortcomings.[7] These already underserved areas do not have an abundance of resources to fall back on when one healthcare worker denies care because of moral or religious reasons.[8] In the case of reproductive care, rural communities already exhibit some of the highest rates of unplanned pregnancy.[9] By denying treatments and using morally motivated arguments to deny this care, disadvantaged communities are at the mercy of their providers.

Another vulnerable population when it comes to conscience clauses is lesbian, gay, bisexual, transgender, and queer patients. Healthcare professionals can discriminate against these LGBTQ patients under the guise of religious freedom while remaining free from punishment.[10] An area we see this in action is counselors and therapists applying this to mental health services, denying sexual and gender minority individuals based on personal beliefs.[11] These already emotionally vulnerable patients may be forced to continue the search for mental health treatment in an already limited field.

While these are all prevalent issues associated with conscience clauses, practicing healthcare providers are not the only people protected. Conscientious objection is relevant in the environment of medical schools as well. Medical students of the Muslim faith at the University of Rochester argued that performing physical examinations on members of the opposite sex interfered with their religious beliefs.[12] The option for alternative experiences would allow students to adhere to the guidelines of their religion but may also detract from their potential as future clinicians. These educational experiences serve as opportunities to practice professionalism and patient care, increasing students' comfort with these tasks in a low-risk environment. When conscience clauses extend into the education of healthcare professionals, it is difficult to establish what can be replaced without weakening the curriculum.

In conclusion, the ramifications of conscience clauses are real and relevant. Healthcare professionals should be expected to place the well-being of the patient above anything. Whether the reasoning is a genuine obstacle to their religious practice or an easy way to discreetly discriminate against patients, either scenario negatively impacts the patient's overall health and well-being. Through education and training, healthcare professionals learn what they will be encountering as they begin to practice. If an individual has serious concerns with the ethical or religious implications of working in healthcare, it may be prudent to explore other career options. It should be an expectation of healthcare professionals to use their education and experiences as an opportunity to care for patients in the safest and most effective way possible. When we deviate from this approach, this insinuates that established treatments are secondary only to one superior individual's moral compass. Healthcare, which is designed to help patients manage their well-being, has no room for this.

Works Cited

1. Rice CE. Overruling Roe v. Wade: An Analysis of the Proposed Constitutional Arguments. Boston College Law Review. 1973.
2. Church Amendment 42 U.S.C. §300a-7(c), (1973).
3. Moralists at the Pharmacy. New York Times. 2005.
4. Hee L, Kettner LO, Vejtorp M. Continuous use of oral contraceptives: an overview of effects and side-effects. Acta Obstet Gynecol Scand. 2013;92(2):125-36. Epub 20121205.
5. Vile JR. Religious Rights of Pharmacists and Morning-After Pills. Middle Tennessee State University. 2022.
6. Najera DB. Emergency contraception: Focus on the facts. JAAPA. 2016;29(1):20-4; quiz 1.
7. Douthit N, Kiv S, Dwolatzky T, et al. Exposing some important barriers to health care access in the rural USA. Public Health. 2015;129(6):611-20. Epub 20150527.
8. Gostin LO. The "Conscience" Rule: How Will It Affect Patient's Access to Health Services? JAMA Network. 2019.
9. Valentine JA, Delgado LF, Haderxhanaj LT, et al. Improving Sexual Health in U.S. Rural Communities: Reducing the Impact of Stigma. AIDS Behav. 2022;26(Suppl 1):90-9. Epub 20210826.
10. Keeley L. Religious Liberty, Immigration Sanctuary, and Unintended Consequences for Reproductive and LGBTQ Rights. Columbia Journal of Gender and Law. 2019.
11. Grzanka PR. Conscience clauses and sexual and gender minority mental health care: A case study. APA PsycNet. 2020.
12. Card RF. Is there no alternative? Conscientious objection by medical students. J Med Ethics. 2012;38(10):602-4.

Essay: Conscience Clauses–The Weight of Reasoning

Aileen Muñoz

When it comes to the law, the past tends to set precedents. However, when it comes to conscientious objection, a refusal to perform a service based on personal beliefs, the application of the law in different contexts varies.[1] That is likely because of the disorganizing nature of religious beliefs and moral convictions. When it comes to military service, religious beliefs are one of the only ways to have a valid conscientious objection to conscription. Likewise, religious values have given parents the ability to dictate their child's learning. In medicine, the concept of conscientious objection led to the introduction of the church amendments wherein physicians can deny care on moral or religious grounds.[2] Having unequal rules for conscientious objection creates stress for those refusing service and those who have service refused. Until equal rights can be applied in every instance where the idea of conscientious objection is being used, there will be a continued disservice to those who are affected. Conscientious objection creates additional stress for patients and can also affect society. Conscience clauses can also have the reverse effect and create stress for healthcare professionals who may have to withhold care or information due to rules or policies that they must abide by, such as those who may work in facilities supported by Title X funding.

Moral convictions and religious beliefs are tied to an innate sense of conscience, a psychological dimension of the mind, which leads individuals to act according to such principles.[3] The first conscientious objectors in the military refused conscription on religious grounds. In these instances, many men died for their faith as an objection to military service was not well regarded, and religious exemptions were unusual.[4] Accepted exemptions in history typically had to be bought or were only accepted on religious grounds. Any other basis for exemption typically resulted in conscription. Even today, to be granted classification as a conscientious objector in the military is a lengthy process and is not always ensured.[5] It is curious that it is so difficult to avoid a situation where one might have to take a life, but not so difficult to avoid other situations.

The idea of conscientious objection has been around for centuries based on the right to freedom of thought, religion, and conscience, enabling individuals to refuse to partake in actions contradicting their beliefs. In the 19th century, parents were granted this right by being allowed to withdraw their children from religious schooling with the passage of the Elementary Education Act of 1870.[6] This act came about at the beginning of compulsory education to appease those who were obstinate in their want for denominational teachings while also catering to minorities who opposed them. Perhaps a more perfect resolution would have been to leave religious schooling to one's home, but at least this act gave a choice to those who needed it. However, this set a precedent that a parent knows what is best for his child. As medicine has advanced and enabled us to defend our population with vaccines, some fear consequences. Nowadays, several diseases are preventable if parents allow their children to be vaccinated. All states have laws that require vaccination for children, but many also allow exemptions on religious grounds and some even on moral grounds.[7] These exemptions pose dangers for society as outbreaks of preventable diseases have occurred due to parents refusing to vaccinate their children. For some, this refusal stems from a belief that vaccines are against their faith. However, for others, refusing to vaccinate their children stems from a fear of side effects. This outbreak of fear corresponds to the integration of the internet. With so much information available, it becomes difficult to distinguish the truth from fear-mongering, and there are plenty of rabbit holes for fearful parents to fall into. Thus, having a right to conscientious objection allows for freedom, but it can also harm others.

Also, the right to a conscientious objection based on moral and religious convictions creates bias. Since this bias can be discriminatory, it should not be associated with a patient's medical care. The AMA states that it is illegal for a physician to refuse to render services to a patient based on demographics.[8] However, two mothers who were denied care for their newborn have experienced otherwise.[9] In this instance, the pediatrician stated that she felt she could not provide adequate care for their child because she had prayed and deemed it so. Contrary to the statement made by the AMA, the actions of the pediatrician were not illegal, and she was met with no repercussions for her decision. The two mothers were left without a pediatrician despite having selected this one in advance for their newborn and would now have to move forward, knowing they might be rejected again.

Curiously, compared to conscientious objectors to war, where an individual might be asked to kill another, there is no lengthy hearing or case presentation that physicians must make to defend their refusal to care for another. Healthcare professionals do not have to protect themselves in these instances because doing so would require the institution of a tribunal for physicians to prove their case, which would be costly.[10] For many, the cost is not seen as justified because they do not believe a physician would lie about their reason for denying care in the first place. As there is no evidence for the validity of this statement, proposing such an idea seems idealistic, especially in a society that enables discriminatory laws. Those presenting such views fail to consider that minorities have been denied care based on their demographics. Despite having a professional or ethical obligation, physicians who can deny care will deny care if their reasoning is not unbiased. This creates a situation where the physician's beliefs trump the patient's choices. Then, depending on the type of appeal to conscience, even the physician's beliefs can be overturned by external policies.

There are two significant appeals to conscience clauses: negative and positive. The conscience clauses introduced in the 1970s and termed the church amendments due to religious foundations would be classified as negative appeals to conscience.[11] These amendments allow physicians to refuse to perform abortion or sterilization procedures due to religious beliefs or moral convictions and protect them in choosing so.[2] Negative appeals to conscience have been reinforced by the Bush and Trump administrations and create a balance entirely swayed towards providers that object to medical decisions.[12] Ethically, negative appeals to conscience infringe on a patient's autonomy.

Among the AMA's principles of medical ethics, it is written that a physician shall respect patients' rights. Although not a law, upon interpretation, one would think this means that each physician will act as a resource and an ally to their patients, helping them reach their own decisions. However, since the introduction of conscience clauses, patient rights have diminished and are unclear for those facing discrimination. Suppose a female patient is regularly attended to in a particular hospital and has had no issues receiving care, but she comes in asking for tubal ligation. Her physician can deny her care due to his beliefs and may perform a vasectomy for a man in the same step.[13] He is not respecting her autonomy; he respects his own and enables discriminatory practices. Conscience clauses contradict the idea that physicians will respect their patients' autonomy as they decide to withhold care due to their beliefs and are protected in doing so.

There are some ethical arguments for conscientious objection, but many patients must face flawed arguments. In the instance of abortion, a moral idea for the acceptability of conscience clauses might be a refusal based on the patient's health. However, data collected by Ralph and colleagues show that abortion does not harm the long-term physical health of women.[14] Instead, data show that the physical health of women who gave birth tended to be worse when compared to women who had abortions. Giving birth takes an extreme physical toll, and it should be a patient's right to decide if they are prepared to undergo this experience.

Likewise, data compiled by Harris and colleagues show that being denied an abortion can increase perceived stress.[15] So, by prohibiting abortions, physicians can actively add to the stress on their patients by limiting their patients' autonomy. Imagine if you were a woman and became pregnant due to circumstances outside of your control, e.g., rape. Then, due to your mental state or physical health, you sought an abortion and were subsequently denied one. Upwards of 32,000 women every year have to contend with the possibility of such a scenario.[16] In certain states, such as Texas, the treatment of women seeking abortion resembles that of a witch hunt where even those who may seek to help her may face the consequences for their attempt.[17] A physician who denies a patient an abortion would do so solely based on his views and not the patient's health.

Negative appeals to conscience also affect patients seeking end-of-life care. Some states have laws such as Oregon's Death with Dignity Act that allow physicians to assist in suicide if the patient has a terminal illness. In this act, Oregon also enables physicians to choose whether to participate without penalty.[18] However, there are no other stipulations barring the procedure from occurring where it is legal.

Interestingly, even if a physician is comfortable performing a procedure that questions conscience, they may not be allowed to. While there is protection for negative appeals to conscience, there is no protection for positive appeals to conscience. In fact, laws prohibiting specific procedures such as abortion or sterilization create the idea of positive appeals to the conscience. An example of a positive appeal to conscience would be when a patient presents to a physician for care, and the physician cannot in good conscience follow the rules or policies prohibiting him from providing care.[11] This occurs when a physician is comfortable performing a procedure such as abortion but cannot perform them due to facility policies.

Currently, many healthcare facilities receive Title X funding. This funding is meant to provide patients with family planning and preventative care access.[19] However, the grant stipulates that the facility can neither offer abortions nor can clinic employees refer patients to facilities that can perform abortions. For a physician who is comfortable with this procedure and cannot in good conscience comply with this stipulation, there is no protection—this asymmetry in protection for appeals to conscience further decreases patient and physician rights. A physician can not only deny a patient care but also with the introduction of stipulations to funding, a physician is unable to provide care even if willing. Where then is this patient supposed to receive care? A physician that is comfortable with the procedure is unable to even refer the patient elsewhere.

These procedures all go beyond the traditional scope of medicine to save lives, heal disease, and relieve pain. It is only natural that there are continuing debates about procedures that appear to contradict these values.[20] In a perfect world, it would make sense that physicians can deny performing operations that offend them. However, it is unfair due to the imbalance of patient rights caused by the asymmetry in protection for negative vs. positive appeals to conscience.

There is a dilemma created by the institution of conscience clauses and the lack of protection for positive appeals to conscience. For a patient, denial of care stemming from either situation can be a source of stress. For a physician, the lack of protection for positive appeals can be a source of stress. All of this is built on the idea that a physician should be able to exert his views when practicing medicine. Suppose that is the reasoning behind conscience clauses. Then, why are other physicians barred from providing the care they believe in? If we allow physicians to deny care based on their views, we must also enable physicians to allow (legal) care based on their views. If that is seen as unacceptable, it is also unacceptable to allow one and not the other. Doing so grants privileges to some and withholds them from others.

All in all, the consequences of conscientious objections differ in severity. For some, such as physicians and parents, objections are readily granted. For others, such as those being conscripted, the task is lengthy without assurance. For those in the military, denial of protest can have consequences with actions they will be forced to take. For parents, their objections can impact others beyond just their children. For patients and providers, conscientious objection has caused their rights to dimmish. It is a genuine concern that a medical procedure such as abortion can be denied despite the circumstances. Even more concerning is that a physician may be forced to deny such a procedure despite having no personal reservations. Ultimately, if the idea of restraints or allowances for conscientious objections is to be applied, it should be done equally.

Works Cited

1. Shanawani H. The Challenges of Conscientious Objection in Health care. J Relig Health. 2016;55(2):384-93.
2. Conscience Protection for Health Care Providers HHS.gov: Office for Civil Rights; 2021 [cited 2022 April 1]. Available from: https://www.hhs.gov/conscience/conscience-protections/index.html.
3. Giubilini A. Conscience Stanford Encyclopedia of Philosophy2021 [cited 2022]. Available from: https://plato.stanford.edu/entries/conscience/#Bib.
4. Matheson JH. Conscientious Objection to Military Service The First Amendment Encyclopedia2009 [cited 2022]. Available from: https://www.mtsu.edu/first-amendment/article/912/conscientious-objection-to-military-

service#:~:text=Conscientious%20objection%20to%20military%20service%20refers%20to%20the%20position%20taken,%2C%20moral%2C%20or%20ethical%20beliefs.

5. Conscientious objectors: Selective Service System; [cited 2022]. Available from: https://www.sss.gov/conscientious-objectors/.
6. Elementary Education Act of 1870 COVE2020 [cited 2022]. Available from: https://editions.covecollective.org/chronologies/elementary-education-act-1870-0#:~:text=The%20Elementary%20Education%20of%201870,13%20in%20England%20and%20Wales.
7. School Vaccination Requirements and Exemptions CDC2017 [cited 2022]. Available from: https://www.cdc.gov/vaccines/imz-managers/coverage/schoolvaxview/requirements/index.html.
8. Obligation To Provide Services: A Physician-Public Defender Comparison. AMA Journal of Ethics. 2006;8(5):332-4.
9. Baldas T. Pediatrician won't treat baby with 2 moms: Detroit Free Press; 2015 [cited 2022].
10. Deans Z. Might a conscience clause be used for non-moral or prejudiced reasons? Journal of Medical Ethics. 2016;42(2):76-7.
11. Wicclair M. Conscience Clauses and Ideological Bias. Am J Bioeth. 2021;21(8):65-7.
12. Johnson SH. Proposed Regulations Favor Providers' Conscience Rights over Patients' Rights. Hastings Cent Rep. 2018;48(4):3-4.
13. Baker CN. Catholic Hospital Denies Woman a Medically Necessary Sterilization, Putting Her Health and Well-Being at Risk: "It's Wrong and It's Dangerous" Ms.2021 [cited 2021]. Available from: https://msmagazine.com/2021/08/10/catholic-hospital-woman-sterilization-health-care/#:~:text=The%20U.S.%20Conference%20of%20Catholic,their%20direct%20effect%20is%20the.
14. Ralph LJ, Schwarz EB, Grossman D, et al. Self-reported Physical Health of Women Who Did and Did Not Terminate Pregnancy After Seeking Abortion Services. Annals of Internal Medicine. 2019;171(4):238-47.
15. Harris LF, Roberts SC, Biggs MA, et al. Perceived stress and emotional social support among women who are denied or receive abortions in the United States: a prospective cohort study. BMC Womens Health. 2014;14:76. Epub 20140619.
16. Holmes MM, Resnick HS, Kilpatrick DG, et al. Rape-related pregnancy: estimates and descriptive characteristics from a national sample of women. Am J Obstet Gynecol. 1996;175(2):320-4; discussion 4-5.
17. Bill: SB 8 Texas Legislature Online2021 [cited 2022]. Available from: https://capitol.texas.gov/billlookup/History.aspx?LegSess=87R&Bill=SB8.
18. Oregon Revised Statute: Oregon's Death with Dignity Act Oregon.gov: Oregon Health Authority; 2019 [cited 2022 April 3]. Available from: https://www.oregon.gov/oha/ph/providerpartnerresources/evaluationresearch/deathwithdignityact/pages/ors.aspx#top.
19. About Title X Service Grants OASH: Office of Population Affairs; 2021 [cited 2022 April 2]. Available from: https://opa.hhs.gov/grant-programs/title-x-service-grants/about-title-x-service-grants#:~:text=Title%20X%20is%20the%20only,and%20related%20preventive%20health%20services.
20. Davenport ML, Lahl J, Rosa EC. Right of Conscience for Health-Care Providers. Linacre Q. 2012;79(2):169-91. Epub 2012/05/01.

Essay: Conscience Clauses—Discrimination and Stubbornness

Baden Cruickshank

Following the recent overturn of Roe v. Wade, attention has been drawn toward healthcare providers and their rights to deny abortions, contraceptives, and other vital care. This is not a new concept, the idea of a legal right for healthcare providers to deny care to patients based on their personal beliefs originated nearly 50 years ago following the initial ruling in Roe v. Wade.[1] In the following years, conscience clauses have allowed healthcare providers to deny patients care, not only for issues relating to abortion and contraceptive access, but also LGBTQ rights, and anything else with which providers might disagree.

Conscience clauses allow healthcare providers to deny access to abortion, abortifacient drugs, and contraceptives based solely on personal beliefs. There have been many cases across the country of healthcare providers such as nurses and physicians refusing to prescribe oral contraceptives or abortifacient drugs, and of pharmacists refusing to dispense these drugs to patients to whom they have been prescribed.[2,3] Companies such as CVS minute clinic as well as hospitals have acted against these providers who allow their personal beliefs to degrade the quality of their care, but these actions have resulted in lawsuits from some fired or reprimanded employees who believe that their rights are being violated.[4] One major point of concern is that some healthcare providers who deny this care to patients may not even be aware of the intended uses and actions of the drugs they are refusing the prescribe or dispense. Data suggest that an alarming number of physicians surveyed believe that emergency contraceptives (39%), oral contraceptives (6%), and other forms of birth control such as IUDs (16%) act by causing abortions.[5] It is an incredibly scary concept that many physicians who prescribe or have the opportunity to prescribe these contraceptives do not even recognize their intended uses or actions; these are the people who we trust with our health, lives, and livelihoods.

Conscience clauses and denial of care stretch beyond abortifacients and contraceptives to LGBTQ rights. Data reflect a high rate of discrimination and health inequities in healthcare settings against members of the LGBTQ community, something that is well within the rights of healthcare workers because of conscience clause laws.[6,7] This includes denial of gender-affirming treatments, as well as the simple outright refusal of any type of care due to the personal beliefs of healthcare workers. LGBTQ parents have been denied care for their children because they did not match the gender roles their pediatrician preferred, transgender women and men have been denied lifesaving care and left for dead because their healthcare team did not agree with their lifestyle, and countless other LGBTQ youth and adults have been denied care simply because of who they are.[8, 9] No one should ever be denied care for themselves or their children because their healthcare provider does not agree with their sexual orientation or gender. Members of the LGBTQ community face enough discrimination in their lives and thus they should always feel welcome and safe in healthcare settings, and healthcare professionals must create this safe environment, regardless of any personal beliefs.

To put it plainly, there is no place for personal beliefs in healthcare. Having personal beliefs and opinions should not be discouraged, but they should never bleed over into interactions with patients. Healthcare providers should only be focused on the health of their patients, and no personal belief will ever outweigh the importance of providing the best possible health outcome to every patient. If healthcare professional students do not wish to learn about drugs or procedures that disagree with their beliefs, they should not be in healthcare at all. Every healthcare provider, regardless of their beliefs, must be able to provide the highest quality of care to every patient, and avoiding certain topics in their education could potentially prevent them from providing quality care.

Conscience clauses do not belong in healthcare, at least not in the form that they currently exist. If this ability for healthcare providers to deny care to their patients is to continue in any way, some changes must be made. It should at minimum be made very clear to prospective patients what their healthcare provider believes, and what treatments they are unwilling to give, prescribe, or dispense because of these beliefs. Healthcare providers should be treated like public figures, their opinions should be known by any future patients, and no patient should ever again find out that their prescriber is unwilling to prescribe them abortifacient drugs or contraceptives, or that their physician is unwilling to provide treatment due solely to their personal beliefs. Decisions to deny care in any way should only be made with patient safety in mind, for instance, if surgery would be unsafe for a certain patient or a certain medication might negatively interact with another medication. Patient safety and health should be the only concerns in a healthcare environment, no decisions should ever be made based on the beliefs of a healthcare provider, and anyone who disagrees likely does not belong in healthcare.

Works Cited

1. Sulmasy DP. Conscience, tolerance, and pluralism in health care. Theor Med Bioeth. 2019;40(6):507-21.
2. Tanne JH. "Conscience" clauses allow US corporate providers to refuse care. BMJ. 2004;329(7464):476.
3. Ollcapriostein A. Patients face barriers to routine care as doctors warn of ripple effects from broad abortion bans 2022. Available from: https://www.politico.com/news/2022/09/28/abortion-bans-medication-pharmacy-prescriptions-00059228.
4. Diaz O. Nurse practitioner says CVS fired her for refusing to give abortion drugs 2022. Available from: https://www.washingtonpost.com/dc-md-va/2022/09/01/cvs-nurse-fired-abortion-pills/.

5. Laura E.T. Swan ASC, Madison Lands, Nicholas B. Schmuhl, Jenny A. Higgins Physician beliefs about contraceptive methods as abortifacients. American Journal of Obstetrics & Gynecology. 2022.
6. Rowe D, Ng YC, O'Keefe L, et al. Providers' Attitudes and Knowledge of Lesbian, Gay, Bisexual, and Transgender Health. Fed Pract. 2017;34(11):28-34.
7. Medina-Martinez J, Saus-Ortega C, Sanchez-Lorente MM, et al. Health Inequities in LGBT People and Nursing Interventions to Reduce Them: A Systematic Review. Int J Environ Res Public Health. 2021;18(22). Epub 20211110.
8. Bowles S. A Death Robbed of Dignity Mobilizes A Community 1995. Available from: https://www.washingtonpost.com/archive/local/1995/12/10/a-death-robbed-of-dignity-mobilizes-a-community/2ca40566-9d67-47a2-80f2-e5756b2753a6/.
9. Phillip A. Pediatrician refuses to treat baby with lesbian parents and there's nothing illegal about it. The Washington Post. 2015.

Topic: Drug Scheduling—The Government Assigns Risk

In 1970, President Nixon signed into law the Controlled Substances Act which was intended to consolidate more than 200 laws governing drugs in the US that were overlapping and difficult to enforce.[1] This Act also created our drug scheduling or classification scheme. Since this time, much has been learned about the pharmacology of scheduled and unscheduled drugs, but little has changed with regard to how these drugs are regulated. To understand the underlying controversy behind how drugs are scheduled, it is necessary to understand how drugs are classified and regulated in the US and how these regulations are communicated to the public. Once this is understood, it may be obvious that the current drug scheduling system is not fully based on science or emerging pharmacological information. It may also be evident that the current system is inflexible to new scientific and medical evidence that contrasts with what was believed about some drugs in the late 60s. Then, it may be suggested that the system suffocates innovation and scientific research with products incorrectly deemed, by the government, to have no legitimate medical use.

> *"We knew we could not make it illegal to be either against the war or black, but by getting the public to associate the hippies with marijuana and blacks with heroin, and then criminalizing both heavily, we could disrupt those communities...Did we know we were lying about the drugs? Of course we did."*
>
> John Erlichman, past chief advisor to President Nixon when the War on Drugs was announced (1971)

First, drugs are categorized into one of five categories based on their perceived or documented medical value.[2] Drugs with a high abuse potential such as some marijuana, heroin, and hallucinogens are thought by the government to have no medicinal value so they are assigned to Schedule I. The remaining schedules for drugs include substances with documented or past medical value, but with decreasing degrees of abuse liability. For instance, Schedule II drugs include some opioids and opiates, amphetamine, methamphetamine, methylphenidate, and drug combinations including these compounds. This schedule of drugs is thought to have greater abuse potential than drugs in Schedules III–V. Schedule III drugs include sedatives such as barbiturates, and they have recognized medical uses but less abuse potential than Schedule II drugs. Drugs in schedules IV and V have decreasing abuse potential and confirmed medical value. This type of categorization is problematic because when the law to schedule substances was enacted almost 50 years ago, little pharmacology was established for most of the substances. Finally, for anything not scheduled, such as "bath salts", which have been reported to cause grave harm to unsuspecting users of these products, anyone can synthesize and sell them. There is no federal law specifically against them at this time. Rather, there are a few state laws that prohibit the possession and sale of substances that mimic drugs, but such offenses are misdemeanors and difficult to enforce equitably.

So, the current drug scheduling system is inflexible, even though on paper, drugs can be added to the schedule, de-scheduled, and rescheduled as the US Drug Enforcement Agency (DEA) deems appropriate, and ideally, these decisions would be based on new pharmacological data. This information would then be published in the US Federal Register which, according to the Federal Register Act of 1935, was designed to be a single source for all government publications regarding regulations as well as "Proposed Rules", and "Notices".[3] This Register has been refined into a Code of Federal Regulations (CFR) which can be consulted for all final decisions such as those made for scheduled drugs. For instance, in the 21st CFR Part 1308, a group of previously controlled but delisted substances is described.

These drugs, which included esterified estrogens and methyltestosterone, were exempt from coverage under the Anabolic Steroids Control Act of 1990 because they were used to treat menopausal women nonresponsive to traditional hormone therapy. Thus, they were not typical steroid

"Penalties against possession of a drug should not be more damaging to an individual than the use of the drug itself; and where they are, they should be changed. Nowhere is this more clear than in the laws against possession of marijuana in private for personal use."

Jimmy Carter, 39th US President

hormones and their delisting was requested by the pharmaceutical companies that manufactured them.[4] The Attorney General, the DEA, and the Department of Health and Human Services agreed that there was no abuse potential for these particular products and no evidence of trafficking of the products even though, pharmacologically, they were in the same drug class as anabolic steroids. A similar treatment or delisting can be done for any scheduled drug.

Thus, delisting appears to be simple and straightforward and Congress could declassify marijuana or any likewise inappropriately scheduled drug. Interestingly, the authority for this is left to the DEA, which may be an enormous conflict of interest. For instance, the DEA could schedule any drug that the agency believes it can easily confiscate, along with the cash associated with that product's sale and distribution. It is widely known that DEA officers can keep the fruits of their drug busts and use that money to finance more searches and seizures.[5] They can also auction in exchange for cash seized cars, homes, and weapons belonging to people who illegally use, buy, sell, or distribute scheduled compounds. So, it would seem controversial that an agency that can enrich itself on the backs of US citizens' drug use might be able to "select" the drugs they prefer to confiscate via the scheduling apparatus. As an officer from Connecticut succinctly put it, collecting money from drug busts for agency use is "an essential tool to obtain additional revenue and it's above and beyond what the city provides us."[6,7]

The incentive to keep drugs tightly scheduled and subject to seizure is especially high when the law is ambiguous. This allows more people to obtain a scheduled product for personal use, such as marijuana, and more people using means more potential illicit drug busts. Over the last 20 years, pleas to reschedule or de-schedule marijuana have been held up in the courts and ultimately, the DEA has overridden expert scientists who confirmed that marijuana requires scientific study to better elucidate its already well-known and peer-reviewed medical properties. So, in both instances of legal appeals, expert opinion about marijuana was ignored and the DEA refused to consider any scientific data that contradicted their assumptions about the drug.[8, 9]

Another oddity of the current scheduling system is that the DEA, not medicine or science, determines whether a drug can be abused at all. Interestingly, in the 50 years that scheduling has been in place, the idea of "abuse" has never been defined for the purpose of federal drug categorization. So, if in the opinion of non-scientists, the drug can be abused, it is scheduled. Only then is the potential medical value of the compound considered.

"In science it often happens that scientists say, "You know that's a really good argument; my position is mistaken," and then they actually change their minds...I cannot recall the last time something like that happened in politics or religion."

Carl Sagan, American astronomer, cosmologist, astrophysicist, astrobiologist, author, science popularizer and communicator

Data are very compelling that marijuana has proven medical benefits for multiple patient categories, but it remains a Schedule I product. This means that it is highly restricted and difficult to obtain for scientific study, as evidenced by few laboratories having access to marijuana. Moreover, until recently, only one farm was authorized to grow the product. Because of these limitations, a drug maker of a scheduled substance is unlikely to attempt to repurpose that drug for any human use, irrespective of the promise it has to treat disease. Thus, scheduling causes oppressive regulatory hurdles, denies citizens potentially lifesaving therapies, and stifles scientific inquiry.[10] Also, drugs as safe as Schedule III already require US import/export permits, something that would be much more restrictive for substances scheduled II or I.[2]

Moreover, with the current and unscientific scheduling system, the DEA can threaten physicians, hospitals, and pharmacies who attempt to work with patients who seek medical marijuana even though this use has been decriminalized in many states. Physicians can lose their right to prescribe and pharmacists can lose their privilege to dispense if convicted of a drug crime.[11] Then, the irrational scheduling of marijuana keeps banks from giving loans to medical marijuana growers and dispensaries and prevents marijuana businesses from having commercial banking accounts. Thus, people who have a marijuana enterprise must carry large amounts of cash to and from their place of business, creating a dangerous situation for the entrepreneur if the work site is in a criminally risky region.

Perhaps a revamped drug scheduling system that is based on science is in order.[12] This might focus on a drug's potential for abuse, irrespective of any potential medical value. Then, alcohol, tobacco, cocaine and similar stimulants, and opioids would be grouped and each drug's potency or potential lethality could direct specific subcategorization. Data from overdose case reports, toxicology studies, and poison control centers would support these classifications. Because the idea of abuse has never been properly defined in the current scheduling system, this could finally be assessed pharmacologically. We know that a handful of drugs have extraordinarily positively reinforcing effects (methamphetamine, cocaine) due to enormous shifts in neurotransmitters and rapid drug half-lives. In contrast, other drugs do not induce addiction as rapidly (alcohol, tobacco).

This science could be applied to stratify drugs of abuse in a cogent and evidence-based manner, omitting approaches that are based on religion, morality, racism, and shame. Then, marijuana, which has less abuse liability and definite medical utility, would be less restricted and research could progress, allowing scientists to investigate its value. Finally, accepting the published and peer-reviewed science about drugs and eliminating the stigma associated with drug use and abuse would have positive effects on society, reducing secretive drug use and increasing help-seeking for those with drug problems when appropriate.

Writing Prompts

- Should the Controlled Substances Act be repealed and replaced or revised?
- Should federal scheduling be redesigned or scrapped?
  - Why is the concept of abuse never defined in drug scheduling?
  - Technically can any drug be abused?
    - If so, how can scheduling make sense as written?
- Why within one schedule, are substances treated differently?
  - E.g., marijuana is punished less severely.
- Should drug scheduling be done by a scientific body instead of a political body?
- Is the medical evidence compelling that marijuana has medicinal value?
  - What are the risks?
- Should this be heeded, irrespective of Jeff Sessions' personal thoughts?
- Should we abolish the federal law and allow states to set rules based on voting outcomes and collective choice?
- Should minimum sentencing for drug use be abolished?
- By having educational loans rescinded for students, is the Education Department being used as a force in the US "war on drugs"?
- Is punishing a person for possession of a scheduled substance a medical or criminal issue?
- What about issues of human rights, compassion, etc. for substances documented to be less risky?
- Should offenses by students be case-by-case, with the amount, intent, and states of intoxication accounted for (merely HAVING it, but not being on it)?
- If we legalize marijuana, could people turn to that for chronic pain instead of opioids?

Works Cited

1. Sonnenreich MR. The Controlled Dangerous Substances Act of 1969. Bull Parenter Drug Assoc. 1970;24(1):14-22.
2. No Author Given. Schedules of controlled substances: rescheduling of the Food and Drug Administration approved product containing synthetic dronabinol [(-) - [DELTA] less than 9 greater than - (trans)-tetrahydrocannabinol] in sesame oil and encapsulated in soft gelatin

capsules from schedule II to schedule III. Department of Justice (DOJ), Drug Enforcement Administration (DEA). Final rule. Fed Regist. 1999;64(127):35928-30.
3. No Author Given. Panama Refining Co. v. Ryan, 293 US 388 US Printing Office: 1935.
4. Drug Enforcement Administration DoJ. Schedules of controlled substances; exempt anabolic steroid products. Final rule. Fed Regist. 2008;73(52):14178-9.
5. US Department of Justice. The DEA's Handling of Cash Seizures. Washington, DC: 2007.
6. Ingraham C. Since 2007, the DEA has taken $3.2 billion in cash from people not charged with a crime. The Washington Post. 2017 May 29, 2017.
7. WSFB Eyewitness News. What happens to all the money seized in drug busts? 2013. Available from: http://www.wfsb.com/story/22078253/what-happens-to-all-the-money-seized-in-drug-busts.
8. Willingham E. DEA's Hypocritical Marijuana Decision Ignores The Evidence. Forbes. 2016 August 13, 2016.
9. Downs D. The Science behind the DEA's Long War on Marijuana. Scientific American. 2016(April 19, 2016).
10. Cavallito CJ. Effects of scheduling on the economics of drug development. NIDA Res Monogr. 1979;27:17-28.
11. Mirken B. Medical marijuana: legal issues for physicians, others. AIDS Treat News. 1996(No 261):3-4.
12. Caulkins JP, Reuter P, Coulson C. Basing drug scheduling decisions on scientific ranking of harmfulness: false promise from false premises. Addiction. 2011;106(11):1886-90.

Essay: Drug Scheduling: Revision Required

Alena LaBree

For decades there has been a desire to create a system to regulate controlled substances for public safety purposes in the US. The Controlled Substances Act (CSA) of 1970 allowed federal regulation over new and existing controlled substances by scheduling them into five categories based on their safety, abuse potential, and accepted medical utility.[1,2] Having a system to regulate controlled substances is important, as many of these drugs have the potential to harm individuals and society. However, it seems these drugs are being scheduled based on too many criteria, which prevents the scheduling system from effectively categorizing controlled substances. This may interfere with patient care as some drugs, such as marijuana, may provide a medical benefit to certain patients, but because of its current federal scheduling, it is not fully available to do so. Additionally, the Drug Enforcement Agency (DEA) is one of the main agencies in control of scheduling drugs, and scientists who have extensive knowledge of the pharmacology of these drugs are rarely consulted, which has implications.[1] At the time of the CSA implementation, this scheduling system may have made sense because little pharmacology was known about these drugs. However, within the last 50 years, advancements in pharmacology require that the current scheduling be rethought.

The CSA is meant to have flexibility so that new controlled substances can be added, and existing controlled substances can be rescheduled or descheduled. Requests based upon new pharmacologic information of compounds should allow for the alteration of the drug scheduling system in a timely manner; however, this typically hasn't been the case. For example, there have been numerous pleas to reschedule or deschedule marijuana. They took years to review and were all ultimately denied.[3] By definition, a Schedule I drug is a drug that has no accepted medical use and a very high potential for abuse.[1] Marijuana does not seem to fit these criteria, yet it is still classified as a Schedule I drug. Numerous times marijuana has been beneficial in certain conditions, such as cancer and HIV/AIDS wasting syndrome, by being used as an appetite stimulant, antiemetic, and analgesic.[4] Because marijuana is a Schedule I drug, research to further the discovery of its medical utility is difficult. It also results in the data we have regarding the benefits of marijuana being ignored, possibly preventing people from benefiting from it.[3] Since marijuana has been shown to be beneficial in pain management, keeping it in Schedule I halts the idea that marijuana could be a drug people could use for pain management rather than opioids, which can be more dangerous. While marijuana is not devoid of abuse potential or dependency, its positive effects should not be ignored, and its scheduling should be rethought.

Basing the scheduling system on the abuse potential, medical utility, and safety of drugs makes the whole system inconsistent and unclear as these criteria aren't always connected. For example, the current system equates heroin and marijuana as they are both Schedule I drugs. It is well known that heroin is much riskier than marijuana, yet scheduling them together makes it appear otherwise.[3] Additionally, it makes marijuana seem more dangerous than methamphetamine (a Schedule II drug). While methamphetamine may have more medical utility than marijuana, based on abuse potential, it should be scheduled higher than marijuana as it is riskier and likely has more societal and individual consequences associated with its use.[3,5]

If we have a system that is scheduling drugs based on medical utility and abuse potential, it seems odd that alcohol is not included anywhere in the schedule. Alcohol is the most misused substance in the US and has no accepted medical utility.[3,6] Based on the definition of a Schedule I drug, alcohol would fit perfectly, yet it has never been scheduled. Arguing to schedule alcohol would be problematic because of its societal acceptance; however, its absence from the schedule illustrates the irony and hypocrisy of the current system. Additionally, if one of the main purposes of the CSA is to control drugs that have the potential to be abused, it also seems odd that the term abuse is not clearly defined.[3] It does not seem feasible that an accurate categorization for drugs of abuse can be made when the term abuse is broadly defined. For effective changes to be made to the scheduling system, it would make sense first to define what is meant by abuse before selecting certain drugs for inclusion while neglecting others.

Unfortunately, while revisions to the current drug scheduling are needed, the system may be too biased for any real changes to be made. The DEA, which is involved with determining what drugs are scheduled, is also involved with performing searches and seizures for those same drugs. This may drive the incentive to keep certain drugs, such as marijuana, high on the list. Overcoming these concerns may require terms to be more clearly defined and the criteria the scheduling system is based on to be limited to avoid confusion. Also, including scientists in the drug scheduling decision process seems logical as these professionals have extensive knowledge and expertise on the pharmacology and toxicology of drugs and could contribute to a more accurate and effective scheduling system.

Works Cited

1. Ortiz NR, Preuss CV. Controlled Substance Act. StatPearls. Treasure Island (FL)2022.
2. Spillane JF. Debating the Controlled Substances Act. Drug Alcohol Depend. 2004;76(1):17-29.
3. Schnellmann J. PCOL 325 UA Controversies in Healthcare Lecture Series Scheduling Drugs 2022.
4. Capriotti T. Medical Marijuana. Home Health Now. 2016;34(1):10-5.
5. Courtney KE, Ray LA. Methamphetamine: an update on epidemiology, pharmacology, clinical phenomenology, and treatment literature. Drug Alcohol Depend. 2014;143:11-21. Epub 20140817.
6. U.S. Department of Health & Human Services. Alcohol Misuse. Available from: https://www.samhsa.gov/data/taxonomy/term/91.

Essay: Hindered Scheduled Substance Research—The Case of Marijuana

Nanase Toda

The Drug Enforcement Agency (DEA) enforces the Controlled Substances Act (CSA), by which substances regulated under federal law are placed into 1 of 5 schedules based on their medical use, abuse potential, and safety.[1,2] Scheduled substances are faced with barriers, which hinder research of their potential medical use. Because this can prevent possible advancement of the treatment for diseases or chronic conditions, regulations for scheduled substance research should be reviewed.[3]

Marijuana in Drug Scheduling

Marijuana is a Schedule I drug, which indicates that it has high abuse potential with no currently accepted medical use in the US.[4] Although many states have legalized the medicinal or recreational use of marijuana, the federal authority to approve drugs belongs to the FDA and currently, no marijuana product has been approved by the FDA for any indications.[4,5] This categorization of marijuana in Schedule I suggests that marijuana is under the influence of restrictive regulations. Consequently, research focused on its beneficial health effects has been limited in the US.[6]

Medical Value of Marijuana

The efficacy of marijuana is observed in reducing chemotherapy-induced nausea and vomiting.[7] In addition, many other indications are reported including appetite stimulation and refractory epilepsy treatment.[7,8] Most importantly, marijuana can be an efficacious analgesic. Patients taking medical marijuana have reported that its efficacy is the same or even better when compared with opioids for the alleviation of pain. Also, marijuana can reduce some risks associated with opioid use such as dependence and fatal overdose. Therefore, supplying patients with marijuana as a treatment option might aid in providing efficacious pain alleviation with less risk.[9]

Barriers to Scheduled Substance Research in the US

Researchers must undergo a sequence of review processes to study scheduled drugs.[6] These processes usually involve obtaining approval from the Institutional Review Board (IRB) to ensure the protection of the well-being of subjects in the proposed research.[6,10] Then, the National Institute on Drug Abuse (NIDA) is contacted to obtain an administrative Letter of Authorization, which is used to reference chemistry, manufacturing, and control information in an Investigational New Drug Application (IND).[6, 10] The IND must be submitted to the FDA.[6, 10] In addition, by the CSA, registration with the DEA is required to conduct studies using scheduled substances.[6, 10, 11] After the IND is approved, researchers must complete the registration application and submit the research protocol to the DEA.[11, 12] Furthermore, additional documents and approvals may be required by some state governments. Overall, this daunting bureaucracy, which emerged from marijuana's categorization as a Schedule I drug has discouraged many researchers from pursuing their research interests.[13]

In the case of marijuana research, barriers to its supply are another holdback. In the US, marijuana for research use is solely provided through the NIDA Drug Supply Program.[6, 14] Because NIDA's mission is focused on elucidating the causes and harmful consequences of substance use and addiction rather than researching the therapeutic potentials of controlled substances, only around 20% of NIDA-funded marijuana research in 2021 is concerned with the medicinal properties of marijuana.[6, 15-17] In addition, due to the restrictions on marijuana production and the fluctuations in its demand and supply, marijuana produced federally is occasionally stored in a freezer for years after being harvested, which can affect the product quality. In fact, the potency of NIDA-controlled marijuana products is often lower than marijuana products available in markets regulated by states. Also, products available in regulated markets such as edibles and topicals are not regularly supplied by NIDA for research purposes. This leads to insufficient reflection of the products consumed in the real world, which may cause a lack of external validity of studies.[6]

Scheduled substance research might also be hampered by ethical and social obstacles. For instance, society might have uncertainty regarding the efficacy of substances without currently accepted therapeutic use. Also, researchers and IRBs are possibly anxious about affecting their reputations by studying illicit drugs. Moreover, subject recruitment for clinical trials will pose ethical challenges. For example, potential subjects may include people who engage in the use of scheduled drugs currently or have engaged in it formerly as well as those who have never used scheduled drugs. Considering the presence of groups with different drug use statuses might add complexity to the subject recruitment, because of the difficulty to determine if any of these groups are more susceptible to developing an addiction or substance abuse than the others and need special caution.[3]

Conclusion
Marijuana has medical value worthy of further research. However, marijuana research is hampered by its categorization as a Schedule I drug. Similarly, other scheduled substances with potential medical values might be faced with regulatory, ethical, or social obstacles. Regulations and restrictions on scheduled substance research should be reviewed for the potential utilization of controlled substances in the treatment of diseases and chronic conditions.

Works Cited

1. Univeristy of Southern California. Overview of Controlled Substances and Precursor Chemicals. Available from:
https://ehs.usc.edu/research/cspc/chemicals/#:~:text=Controlled%20Substances%20Act%20of%

2. Department of Justice/Drug Enforcement Administration. The Controlled Substances Act 2018. Available from: https://www.dea.gov/drug-information/csa.
3. Andreae MH, Rhodes E, Bourgoise T, et al. An Ethical Exploration of Barriers to Research on Controlled Drugs. Am J Bioeth. 2016;16(4):36-47.
4. Department of Justice/Drug Enforcement Administration. Marijuana/Cannabis 2022. Available from: https://www.getsmartaboutdrugs.gov/sites/default/files/2022-11/Marijuana-Cannabis%202022%20Drug%20Fact%20Sheet_0.pdf.
5. Gabay M. The federal controlled substances act: schedules and pharmacy registration. Hosp Pharm. 2013;48(6):473-4.
6. National Academies of Sciences E, and Medicine; Health and Medicine Division; Board on Population Health and Public Health Practice; Committee on the Health Effects of Marijuana: An Evidence Review and Research Agenda. Challenges and Barriers in Conducting Cannabis Research. The Health Effects of Cannabis and Cannabinoids: The Current State of Evidence and Recommendations for Research: National Academic Press; 2017.
7. Kramer JL. Medical marijuana for cancer. CA Cancer J Clin. 2015;65(2):109-22. Epub 20141210.
8. Hamerle M, Ghaeni L, Kowski A, et al. Cannabis and other illicit drug use in epilepsy patients. Eur J Neurol. 2014;21(1):167-70. Epub 20130111.
9. Reiman A, Welty M, Solomon P. Cannabis as a Substitute for Opioid-Based Pain Medication: Patient Self-Report. Cannabis Cannabinoid Res. 2017;2(1):160-6. Epub 20170601.
10. Fossi AS, J. Cannabis Research Information for Jefferson's Institutional Review Boards.
11. Department of Justice/Drug Enforcement Administration. Researcher's Manual. 2022.
12. Department of Justice/Drug Enforcement Administration. DEA Speeds Up Application Process For Research On Schedule I Drugs 2018. Available from: https://www.dea.gov/press-releases/2018/01/18/dea-speeds-application-process-research-schedule-i-drugs.
13. Nutt DJ, King LA, Nichols DE. Effects of Schedule I drug laws on neuroscience research and treatment innovation. Nat Rev Neurosci. 2013;14(8):577-85.
14. National Institute on Drug Abuse. NIDA's Role in Providing Cannabis for Research 2020. Available from: https://nida.nih.gov/research-topics/marijuana/nidas-role-in-providing-cannabis-research.
15. National Institute on Drug Abuse. NIH Research on Cannabis and Cannabinoids 2020. Available from: https://nida.nih.gov/research-topics/marijuana/nih-research-cannabis-cannabinoids.
16. National Institutes of Health. Estimates of Funding for Various Research, Condition, and Disease Categories (RCDC) 2022. Available from: https://report.nih.gov/funding/categorical-spending#/.
17. National Institutes of Health. National Institute on Drug Abuse (NIDA) 2022. Available from: https://www.nih.gov/about-nih/what-we-do/nih-almanac/national-institute-drug-abuse-nida.

Essay: Drug Scheduling and Discrimination

Aileen Muñoz

Drug use is not an unfamiliar concept in history. Before promulgating the CSA, previous measures had been taken to curb the growing use of drugs such as opium.[1] This attempt to curb drug use stemmed from the country's religious foundations that spurred many movements. It was believed that drug use led people astray and would result in amoral individuals.[2,3] This ideology was pronounced in the prohibition era following the ratification of the 18th amendment in 1919 and lasted until 1933 when the 21st amendment overturned the 18th amendment. However, even before prohibition, acts to tax and regulate morphine, opium, opiates, and cocaine had been passed. Lastly, a marihuana tax was passed in 1933 on the sale of cannabis products.[4]

The marihuana tax of 1933 was only the beginning of a history of discrimination. In his "War on Drugs," the Nixon administration spread stereotypes about marijuana and its users. Since the beginning of the 20th century, marijuana was purveyed as a drug that induced violence, led to sexual interactions, and addiction. This view was continually upheld despite being disproved by a report by the Mayor of New York Fiorello LaGuardia in 1944.[5] Then, at Nixon's discretion, a commission headed by Raymond P. Shafer, the governor of Pennsylvania, was tasked with creating a report that would demonize marijuana and its use. Shafer came back with results that contradicted what the Nixon administration wanted and instead reinforced the findings of LaGuardia.[6]

Despite research contradicting the stigmatized view of marijuana, the Nixon administration continued to push these skewed beliefs. Ultimately, the Nixon administration got its wish, and Marijuana was classified the same as heroin as a Schedule I drug defined as having no medicinal use and a high potential for abuse.[1] Five drugs are routinely tested for in the workplace: cannabinoids, cocaine, amphetamines, opiates, and phencyclidine. These drugs are tested for because they reportedly have a high potential for abuse and are *the NIDA 5*.[7] Curiously, not all the drugs tested for are classified as Schedule I drugs.

When a drug is classified as a Schedule I drug, it hinders research on the potential medicinal effects of the substance. In the case of marijuana, despite having similar addictive effects as alcohol and nicotine, it is scheduled with heroin and termed a gateway drug.[8] This creates a catch-22 in which the DEA can continue to deny the rescheduling of cannabis because there is no proper research that documents the medicinal effects of cannabis.[9] However, that has not stopped researchers and physicians from attempting to establish the medicinal properties of marijuana and prescribing it to those in need. For example, there are studies where researchers have found that marijuana can have therapeutic effects such as alleviating chronic non-cancer pain and abating nausea and vomiting caused by chemotherapy.[10] Many people suffer from chronic pain, resulting in desperation for relief. Despite legality, desperate individuals will seek relief from where they can find it. In many cases, this results in the use of illicit substances obtained off the street and can lead to harmful, if not lethal, effects. If drugs such as marijuana and heroin were more thoroughly researched and made available based on physician discretion, as is the case in the U.K., perhaps fewer people would turn to potentially dangerous alternatives.[9]

Some states have decided that the scheduling of drugs is unfair and have taken measures to mitigate the harm done by the CSA. Marijuana is commonly used amongst both African American and white populations. However, African Americans have been four times more likely to be incarcerated than their white counterparts.[11] One of the first steps 18 states have taken to diminish these effects is decriminalizing marijuana. For some of these states, this makes it so that, at least at the state level, there are diminished repercussions for possession (within limits). In addition, many states have begun to create avenues through which those convicted of marijuana possession can apply for expungement.[12] Oregon even went as far as to decriminalize possession of small amounts of previously criminalized drugs such as cocaine. Now, instead of possession resulting in an arrest, citizens will receive a fine. Although this will still result in a criminal record, the punishment is far less severe. This step was to diminish racial and ethnic disparities in drug convictions and arrests.[13] Depending on skin color, the drug someone has in possession can determine the consequences of the possession. Data show that white people tend to choose heroin as their drug of choice, whereas African American people tend to choose marijuana.[11] Despite the differences in lethality and addictiveness between the two drugs, African Americans are still more likely to be incarcerated than white people.[14] Hence, Oregon's move to impose fines is meant to diminish such incarcerations.

Although the CSA was passed with the intention of reducing drug abuse, its enforcement has not been unbiased, and its classification system based on abuse is inconsistent. Since the implementation of the CSA, politicians have held sway over how drugs are scheduled and not the people who will prescribe or research said drugs. Scheduling that is not based on research hinders future research. Drug schedules should be based on science and not political goals. The hindrance of drug research and the targeting of minorities needs to end.

Works Cited

1. Drug Scheduling United States Drug Enforcement Administration DEA; [cited 2022]. Available from: https://www.dea.gov/drug-information/drug-scheduling#:~:text=Drugs%2C%20substances%2C%20and%20certain%20chemicals,drug's%20abuse%20or%20dependency%20potential.
2. Cornelio J, Medina E. Christianity and Duterte's War on Drugs in the Philippines. Politics, Religion & Ideology. 2019;20(2):151-69.
3. Frendreis J, Tatalovich R. "A Hundred Miles of Dry": Religion and the Persistence of Prohibition in the U.S. States. State Politics & Policy Quarterly. 2010;10(3):302-19.
4. Editors. War on Drugs History2017 [cited 2022]. Available from: https://www.history.com/topics/crime/the-war-on-drugs.

5. LaGuardia F. The Marihuana Problem in the City of New York. The Laguardia Committee Report: New York Academy of Medicine, 1944.
6. Nahas GG, Greenwood A. The first report of the National Commission on marihuana (1972): signal of misunderstanding or exercise in ambiguity. Bulletin of the New York Academy of Medicine. 1974;50(1):55-75.
7. Staff CB. NIDA 5 Drug Test Confirm Biosciences2016 [cited 2022]. Available from: https://www.confirmbiosciences.com/knowledge/terminology/nida-5/.
8. NIDA. Is marijuana a gateway drug? National Institue on Drug Abuse: 2021.
9. Andreae MH, Rhodes E, Bourgoise T, et al. An Ethical Exploration of Barriers to Research on Controlled Drugs. The American journal of bioethics : AJOB. 2016;16(4):36-47.
10. Clark PA, Capuzzi K, Fick C. Medical marijuana: medical necessity versus political agenda. Med Sci Monit. 2011;17(12):RA249-RA61.
11. Rosenberg A, Groves AK, Blankenship KM. Comparing Black and White Drug Offenders: Implications for Racial Disparities in Criminal Justice and Reentry Policy and Programming. J Drug Issues. 2017;47(1):132-42. Epub 2016/12/21.
12. Hartman M. Cannabis Overview National Conference of State Legislatures2021 [cited 2022]. Available from: https://www.ncsl.org/research/civil-and-criminal-justice/marijuana-overview.aspx.
13. Westervelt E. Oregon's Pioneering Drug Decriminalization Experiment Is Now Facing The Hard Test NPR2021 [cited 2022]. Available from: https://www.npr.org/2021/06/18/1007022652/oregons-pioneering-drug-decriminalization-experiment-is-now-facing-the-hard-test.
14. author N. Heroin Overdose Data CDC2021 [cited 2022]. Available from: https://www.cdc.gov/drugoverdose/deaths/heroin/index.html.

Essay: Drug Scheduling and Marijuana

Baden Cruickshank

Drug scheduling is an area of heated debate in both the scientific and non-scientific communities, and for good reason. It has been regulated by the same laws for over 50 years, and despite vast medical and scientific developments and improvements, these laws have remained nearly identical. Marijuana can often be seen at the center of this debate, with many arguing that it is too tightly regulated and with some states voting to "legalize" the drug for recreational or medical purposes.

Some scheduling decisions may seem illogical and unscientific, such as marijuana being placed in schedule I along with heroin and LSD and higher than cocaine and many opioids in schedule II, all of which are inherently riskier than marijuana.[1,2] The Controlled Substances Act (CSA) also overlooks some substances with high abuse potential that are known to be harmful, such as alcohol and tobacco, both of which have never been scheduled.[3,4] There is no scientific comparison made to determine how drugs are scheduled, likely because no scientists are making these decisions; instead, they are made largely by lawyers and law enforcement personnel, with zero scientific consultation. The head of the DEA is a lawyer who reports to the United States attorney general, both of whom have no scientific training.[5] Additionally, most DEA employees likely do not have scientific training as they are not required to possess a college degree and mostly come from law enforcement and military backgrounds.[6] The DEA would likely make more logical and scientific decisions if this drug scheduling power was shifted from lawyers and law enforcement to scientists.

Drug scheduling can cause profound harm to students and their educations. Students who are convicted of drug-related felonies at the state or federal level can be made ineligible for federal financial aid for 1–2 years or even indefinitely depending on the number of offenses.[7] In comparison, violent felons convicted of burglary or rape are still eligible for federal financial aid.[8] This contrast of punishment severity is illogical and simply unfair to students who are charged with simple possession of a controlled substance. Controlled substance use is common in college; many students use amphetamines in a misguided attempt to improve academically, and marijuana use is commonly used by many students. Students convicted for simple possession and use should not lose their financial aid in addition to any criminal charges they already receive, and certainly should not be punished more harshly than violent offenders.

The debate surrounding marijuana legalization, decriminalization, and prosecution has become more common in the past decade, appearing on ballots across the country for citizens to vote on legalization at a state level. Colorado and Washington were the first states to legalize recreational marijuana use through ballot measures in 2012, and Vermont was the first state to legalize it through their legislature in 2016, with many other states following since then.[9] These votes come in addition to states that had already legalized marijuana medically but not recreationally.

The scheduling of marijuana, while it may or may not have originated from racism, has had pronounced race-based effects resulting from its criminalization. Data suggest that people of color have been arrested for marijuana possession at much higher rates than whites, despite having a very similar prevalence of marijuana use.[10] State-based legalization and decriminalization of marijuana possession has led to a significant decrease in marijuana-related arrests for all races.[10, 11] Previous stringent marijuana criminalization has unfairly affected people of color, and the decriminalization and legalization of marijuana at a state level is only the first step in combatting this racial discrimination.

Marijuana's placement in schedule I has also hampered any efforts to research potential medical uses, as the CSA severely limits research on substances in Schedule I.[4] Only the University of Mississippi is federally approved to grow marijuana for research purposes, which severely limits researchers' access in addition to the numerous bureaucratic hoops that must be jumped through to even begin marijuana research at all.[12, 13] Despite this, research has uncovered potential medicinal value of marijuana, citing potential benefits for anxiety, chronic pain, depression, PTSD, sleep, and inflammation, as well as potential for treatment of epilepsy, chemotherapy-induced nausea and anorexia, schizophrenia and other psychoses, and other diseases and conditions.[14, 15] Potential adverse effects of marijuana use include risk of addiction, negative effects on adolescent brain development and school performance, potential relations to mental illnesses, and potential risks of cancers or other negative health effects.[16, 17] Research to this point has been severely limited by marijuana's status as a Schedule I substance, and thus these potential medical benefits and adverse effects can not be fully verified. It is also possible that there are additional medical or severe adverse effects that have not been discovered, but this cannot be determined without additional research which is made incredibly difficult by the current federal regulation of marijuana.

It is apparent that some aspects of drug scheduling need to be addressed, and scientists should be involved in the scheduling process in some way. The process of scheduling drugs should be much more scientific and involve much more research than it currently does. There appears to be no rhyme or reason as to why some substances such as marijuana are scheduled restrictively, and why some substances are not scheduled at all, and it feels like such decisions are more political than scientific. I am not suggesting that all scheduled substances should be legalized nationwide, but rather that there should be significantly more scientific consideration incorporated into this decision-making process. Drugs should be scheduled based truly on their potential for harm and medical utility, and these decisions should not be political in any way.

Works Cited

1. Mead A. Legal and Regulatory Issues Governing Cannabis and Cannabis-Derived Products in the United States. Front Plant Sci. 2019;10:697. Epub 20190614.
2. O'Connor SM, Lietzan E. The Surprising Reach of FDA Regulation of Cannabis, Even After Descheduling. Am Univ Law Rev. 2019;68(3):823-925.
3. Keane H. Facing addiction in America: The Surgeon General's Report on Alcohol, Drugs, and Health US DHHS, Office of the Surgeon General, Washington, DC, USA: U.S. Department of Health and Human Services, 2016 382 pp. online (grey literature): https://addiction.surgeongeneral.gov. Drug Alcohol Rev. 2018;37(2):282-3.
4. Ortiz NR, Preuss CV. Controlled Substance Act. StatPearls. Treasure Island (FL)2022.
5. No Author Given. DEA Leadership 2022. Available from: https://www.dea.gov/about/dea-leadership.
6. No Author Given. DEA Qualifications US Government: US Department of Justice; 2018. Available from: https://www.dea.gov/careers/agent/deaqualifications.html.
7. No Author Given. Drug Related Convictions - FAFSA 2022. Available from: https://www.ndsu.edu/fileadmin/onestop/finaid/other/Drug-Related_Convictions_FAFSA_Facts.pdf.
8. Moore LD, Elkavich A. Who's using and who's doing time: incarceration, the war on drugs, and public health. Am J Public Health. 2008;98(9 Suppl):S176-80.
9. Perlman AI, McLeod HM, Ventresca EC, et al. Medical Cannabis State and Federal Regulations: Implications for United States Health Care Entities. Mayo Clin Proc. 2021;96(10):2671-81.
10. Gunadi C, Shi Y. Cannabis decriminalization and racial disparity in arrests for cannabis possession. Soc Sci Med. 2022;293:114672. Epub 20211222.
11. Sheehan BE, Grucza RA, Plunk AD. Association of Racial Disparity of Cannabis Possession Arrests Among Adults and Youths With Statewide Cannabis Decriminalization and Legalization. JAMA Health Forum. 2021;2(10):e213435. Epub 20211029.
12. No Author Given. Challenges and Barriers in Conducting Cannabis Research. The Health Effects of Cannabis and Cannabinoids: The Current State of Evidence and Recommendations for Research. Washington (DC)2017.
13. Solomon R. Racism and Its Effect on Cannabis Research. Cannabis Cannabinoid Res. 2020;5(1):2-5. Epub 20200227.
14. No Author Given. Therapeutic Effects of Cannabis and Cannabinoids. The Health Effects of Cannabis and Cannabinoids: The Current State of Evidence and Recommendations for Research. Washington (DC)2017.
15. Vickery AW, Finch PM. Cannabis: are there any benefits? Intern Med J. 2020;50(11):1326-32.
16. Volkow ND, Baler RD, Compton WM, et al. Adverse health effects of marijuana use. N Engl J Med. 2014;370(23):2219-27.
17. Memedovich KA, Dowsett LE, Spackman E, et al. The adverse health effects and harms related to marijuana use: an overview review. CMAJ Open. 2018;6(3):E339-E46.

Topic: Addiction: A Fiction?

It may be common sense that the concept of addiction to drugs and alcohol (or gambling, sex, or shopping) would be considered a human disease if it appeared to be beyond a person's voluntary control and if the continuation of such was evidently harmful to the person engaging in the behavior. However, understanding how addiction is defined by scientists—and understanding what *is not* an addiction—may be essential for determining whether addiction is a true disease amenable to therapy, or whether addiction is a manifestation of poor choices that can be curtailed by merely choosing differently.

First, all addictions to any abusable substance begin as initial personal choices. Then, if those choices are made repeatedly, and the substance is used continually and one derives pleasure from it, it may be considered to be a ritual or a habit.

"We may think there is willpower involved, but more likely…change is due to want power. Wanting the new addiction more than the old one. Wanting the new me in preference to the person I am now."

George Sheehan, formal medical editor of Runner's World, author, runner

If the habit is not healthful or if it is viewed by society as morally objectionable, it may be assigned the title of proclivity or compulsion. With continued use of substances that can change brain neurochemistry or neurocircuitry, the body and brain may become accustomed to the presence of the substance. Then, in the absence of that substance, craving may occur. Craving and noticing the absence of a substance, however, is not evidence of addiction. In some instances, tolerance to a habit may be felt, and this is evidenced by the need for more of that activity, substance, drug, or compound to achieve the same altered or enhanced state of consciousness, pleasure, or loss of inhibition. Even still, craving and tolerance do not rise to the level of addiction and they are not, as yet, evidence of disease.

Over time, with continued use of a particular substance, forced abstention from the habit or behavior may produce sensations of unpleasantness, a preoccupation with the habitual activity, and substance-seeking behavior. However, once again, this would not be evidence of addiction or disease. Rather, this is the definition of withdrawal. Contrary to popular medical scare tactics, not all withdrawals are dangerous or require medical attention or supervision. Thus, for an activity to qualify as an addiction, the habit must meet the previous criteria of tolerance and withdrawal. Then, there must be a pursuit of the activity or substance to stave off that withdrawal (typically) or to once again alter consciousness (less likely). Finally, this pursuit must be risky to health, home, occupation, self, or others. This critical aspect of addiction is often ignored or not understood by most of society, and this lack of understanding is detrimental to college-age adults. Young adults are the most frequently and carelessly categorized as having addictive behaviors, perhaps due to greater access to abusable substances, less parental oversight, diminished peer networks as they transition to new locations for college or work, and feelings of stress arising from academic and professional competition.[1] As such, adults in their early 20s are the most frequently targeted population for addiction educational information, but if the message is not delivered with accuracy and tact, they are unlikely to hear it.[2]

Indeed, people who lack the requisite training in addiction science are often the fastest to pronounce the need for a daily coffee as a caffeine addiction; the desire to make unnecessary purchases as a shopping addiction; or the need to purchase a weekly lottery ticket into a gambling addiction. The problem with the lay public incorrectly labeling others as having addictions for mere compulsions or bad habits causes shame and may have the unintended consequence of hampering help-seeking by the one encumbered by the socially unacceptable activity. Moreover, such carelessness suggests that all substances are immediately dangerous for all people and that we are helpless to do anything about it, and this is patently false.

Science suggests that addiction, specifically drug addiction, was not considered a disease until approximately 40 years ago; although some would suggest that this concept has been controversial in medicine and science for 200 years.[3] The idea that addiction could be a disease changed the perception of many who viewed addicts as immoral, lazy, or unprincipled. It also ostensibly removed the stigma associated with having an addiction; after all, a disease is an illness, not a choice. This reframing of addiction as a disease also permitted a revenue stream that had not existed before: faith, medical, and secular rehabilitation, detoxification, recovery programs, addiction medicine therapeutic specialties, and insurance coverage to pay for these options. However, if we analyze addiction as a disease using the typical disease model of medicine, there may be some unanswered questions.

> *"What is addiction, really? It is a sign, a signal, a symptom of distress. It is a language that tells us about a plight that must be understood."*
>
> Alice Miller (Alicija Englard), Swiss psychologist, psychoanalyst, and philosopher

First, if a disease is a state of abnormal function of the body, what is the infectious agent that caused this disease? What initiated the addiction? For alcoholics, it would be the choice to have that first drink. For drug addicts, it would be that first willingness to ingest, insufflate (snort), or inject a drug. Next, what is the pathology underlying the disease? Diabetes is characterized by insulin insensitivity and an inability to regulate glucose, which can become sufficiently high as to damage cells of the eye and kidney and delay wound healing. There appears to be no similar pathology that causes addiction. Excessive worry, poor coping skills, depression, or a desire to have an altered sensorium could be considered triggers for addictive behaviors, but these attributes may be chiefly symptoms arising from human intersections with emotionally significant events. This may be why when asked, college students attributed substance abuse disorders as being tied to emotional instability, personal problems, low self-esteem, and rebelliousness, among other less desirable personal attributes.[1]

Thus, if addiction is not a disease, it does not necessarily require treatment. Indeed, we have data to suggest that addiction may not require intervention from surveys of military servicemen who returned from Vietnam. There, many soldiers abused drugs due to boredom, fear, or recreation. Studies show that most of the men who engaged in those drugging behaviors ceased using drugs with no assistance and resumed normal lives once they returned from the Pacific.[4] Along these lines, scientists have suggested that the condition of drug addiction is merely accelerated learning facilitated by powerful neurotransmitters that constantly reinforce drug use in the face of associated risks.[5] If this is true, then the potential for "unlearning" may be real.

Also, if we consider addiction a disease, are we essentially telling someone that they are "sick" and that no choice they make after the fact will reverse their situation without treatment? Often, the idea that addiction is a disease is emphasized with imaging data from brain scans that compare addicts to non-addicts. The purpose of these colorful scans is to suggest that these brain changes are permanent. Specifically, once drug use changes the brain, there can be no more autonomy over refusing to use drugs again. This "altered-brain" model of disease may reduce some of the disapproval felt for the addicted which shames addicts for their issues and discourages them from seeking treatment. However, this model also simultaneously removes any hope for self-directed course correction by the addict.[2] Fortunately, the National Institute of Drug Abuse and Addiction suggests that quite the opposite is true: that the "modified" brains in the scans appear different from non-drugged brains because of the actual presence of the addictive substance. Thus, these scans are not evidence of permanent damage and they may not prove much at all.

In fact, differences in brain imaging between drug users and non-users may always be different, but this is not evidence of impairment for either group. The observed differences could have been present before drug use; images may have been taken after drug use, or images may have been procured after a lengthy addiction and recovery and the brain is changing positively, unlearning something it once depended upon.[6] An example that appears to support the concept of addiction as a choice can be seen with disordered eating (overeating) which science suggests is not a disease or an addiction but a repeated choice to overindulge.[7] The fact that images of brains of overweight teens who were fed sweet foods resemble the brains of drug addicts is strong evidence for this; brain pleasure centers showed increased activity. This indicated that a reward was interpreted for the behavior, not that the person could not control eating or engaged in drug use.[8]

Furthermore, differences in the brains of addicts and nonusers that exist well before drug use begins cannot easily be measured because this would require guessing who would be likely to abuse drugs and imaging them—and we cannot make such predictions. Then, predicting drug <u>use</u> may not predict <u>abuse</u>. Because medical reports using such brain images are not likely to explain these important distinctions to non-scientifically trained readers, the images can only be said to provoke and prejudice people who do not understand what they are seeing and cannot understand how a brain behaves under the influence of drugs.[9] Also, brains imaged in a lab do not, by definition, tell us much about brain function in daily (non-laboratory conditions) life. Indeed, brain images of professors and artists are most certainly different, but this does not mean that one group is damaged.

Moreover, animal studies of human drug abuse are often not terribly representative of what individuals do with illicit substances. For example, animal data for dopamine receptor studies indicate damage after methamphetamine use but this did not mimic human-use patterns. This was because massive doses of methamphetamine were given to the animals, and this is not how humans abuse methamphetamine.[10-12] Rather, humans use small amounts of drugs (such as methamphetamine) and increase the dose as tolerance accumulates. Animal studies that more accurately modeled this type of human use did not show brain damage, so purveyors of scientific studies of addiction should examine the methods cautiously to be sure that dosing patterns reflect human use.[10]

Next, the idea that addictive behaviors are driven by genetics is popular among the lay public. This concept supports the notion that there is an aspect of uncontrollability of addiction; that it may be heritable and thus unavoidable.[1] Indeed, scientists are aligning data to show that a multiplicity of factors may encourage repeated drug use after initial exposure, but again, the environment matters. Thus, there may be a propensity to abuse drugs embedded in one's DNA, but without that first choice of exposure, this propensity is meaningless. Then, we must also thoroughly analyze all of the genetic influences that drive healthy and self-preserving behaviors and weigh those in the balance of so-called genes for addiction to determine which ones predominate. Finally, we must categorically study all organ systems that are either highly susceptible to drug use or which paradoxically appear to withstand ravaging addictive behaviors to learn what human idiosyncrasies are protective or risky for drug use, abuse, and perhaps addiction. Without examining all of these influences *in toto*, we will be left with a lopsided and incomplete picture of genetic influences over addiction.

So, we have a controversy: addiction, if defined as a disease, suggests that human choices are not important, that the body or mind is sick, and that it requires treatment or intervention. Then, there must also be payment for this treatment. This view of addiction is that it is a medical problem. In contrast, if abusing drugs, especially illegal ones, is a poor choice that addicts are continuously making, then the morality and legality of this action are important. In this view, drug addiction is a legal problem and requires a court of law to determine the addict's fate and perhaps the penal system to punish the addict for his/her transgressions. The answer regarding addiction being a disease is not clear and even with miraculous pharmacological innovations, we have not found a pathway to create exclusively non-addictive substances or therapies to treat addiction permanently.

Writing Prompts

- If addiction is a disease:
  - Is the propensity to have it the cause of it?
  - Does choice or agency matter?
  - Might there be a genetic component?
  - Is there a cure?
  - Is there a treatment?
    - If so, should it work for all people with that disease?
    - Antibiotics work against the same organisms, so would this not be similar?
    - Does this suggest you cannot do anything to improve it without intervention?

- Is craving in the face of known harm a "relapse"?
  - Is lack of craving proof of cure?
- Do heritable characteristics exist or do children make choices they see parents making?
  - Does this suggest learning and environment?
- What does the statement "once an addict always an addict" mean?
  - Will they never "get better"?
  - Will they always be addicted to something?
- Is this a way to guarantee a need to pay for medical services?
  - Can you see the financial incentive for healthcare professionals to promote this idea?
- If addiction is a choice:
  - Is it something you can "not choose"?
    - Does this suggest personal responsibility?
    - Does that suggest blame?
    - Does this suggest guilt?
    - Does personal experience influence how we "define" addiction?
- Why might NA, AA, and other faith-based group therapies be effective or ineffective for some populations?

Works Cited

1. Martin JK, Pescosolido BA, Tuch SA. Of fear and loathing: The role of 'disturbing behavior,' labels, and causal attributions in shaping public attitudes toward people with mental illness. J Health Soc Behav. 2000;41(2):208-23.
2. Henderson NL, Dressler WW. Medical Disease or Moral Defect? Stigma Attribution and Cultural Models of Addiction Causality in a University Population. Cult Med Psychiatry. 2017;41(4):480-98.
3. Meyer RE. The disease called addiction: emerging evidence in a 200-year debate. Lancet. 1996;347(8995):162-6.
4. Evans LNC. Substance Abuse in the Theater: The Big Story. In: Camp NM, editor. US Army Psychiatry in the Vietnam War: New Challenges in Extended Counterinsurgency Warfare. Washington, DC: Government Printing Office; 2015. p. 322-71.
5. Dagher A. Addiction as aberrant learning-evidence from Parkinson's disease. Addiction. 2012;107(2):248-50.
6. Filbey FM, Aslan S, Calhoun VD, et al. Long-term effects of marijuana use on the brain. Proc Natl Acad Sci U S A. 2014;111(47):16913-8.
7. Finlayson G. Food addiction and obesity: unnecessary medicalization of hedonic overeating. Nat Rev Endocrinol. 2017;13(8):493-8.
8. Feldstein Ewing SW, Claus ED, Hudson KA, et al. Overweight adolescents' brain response to sweetened beverages mirrors addiction pathways. Brain Imaging Behav. 2017;11(4):925-35.
9. Petri G, Expert P, Turkheimer F, et al. Homological scaffolds of brain functional networks. J R Soc Interface. 2014;11(101):20140873.
10. Johanson CE, Frey KA, Lundahl LH, et al. Cognitive function and nigrostriatal markers in abstinent methamphetamine abusers. Psychopharmacology (Berl). 2006;185(3):327-38.
11. Woolverton WL, Cervo L, Johanson CE. Effects of repeated methamphetamine administration on methamphetamine self-administration in rhesus monkeys. Pharmacol Biochem Behav. 1984;21(5):737-41.
12. Johanson CE, Balster RL, Bonese K. Self-administration of psychomotor stimulant drugs: the effects of unlimited access. Pharmacol Biochem Behav. 1976;4(1):45-51.

Essay: The Changing Etiology of Addiction

What criminalizes a potential substance of abuse? A matter of perspective

Jason Canizales

The topic of addiction has led medical professionals and politicians to argue about the implications of categorizing addicts as deliberate criminals or unfortunate victims of substance abuse. Although not all substances carry the same risk for dependency, illicit behavior, or harm to one's health, some scientists tend to approach the controversy of addiction as a chronic disease that can be treated to reduce dependency.[1,2] Meanwhile, other scientists and political figures incline towards a conglomerate of societal and economic factors as the causative explanation for addiction.[3-5] Regardless of its suggested causes, previous narcotic substances that were once considered illegal/publicly frowned upon (e.g., marijuana) can be deemed "acceptable" for public use and vice-versa. To understand these shifts in perspective, the characterization of what is understood to be an addiction in addition to its concerns in healthcare and the political landscape should be evaluated.

Unclear Definitions and Implications

The use of psychoactive substances has been a recurrent practice throughout recorded history. Whether their intended purpose was directed towards religious, medicinal, or recreational use, the growing understanding of the negative behavioral and health effects of substance abuse began to be a cause for concern.[6] Addiction, even in science, is a term that has slightly different meanings across different disciplines. The American Psychological Association defines it as a state of psychological or physical dependence.[7] The National Institute on Drug Abuse considers it a relapsing brain disorder due to its involvement in rewiring the reward, stress, and self-control neuronal pathways.[8] While some research claims it to be a neurological disease, hesitancy in its definition is still questioned.[9,10] Because substance abuse can be subject to self-regulation without the necessity of a cure, the idea of addiction as a form of disease does not seem to fit the treatment protocol of any other pathological disease. Nonetheless, the lack of agreement in the scientific community attributes to the complexity of the underlying implications of how to address the multiple convoluted factors encompassing addiction.

A person is not born an addict but through time one can grow accustomed to a substance's pleasant stimulating effects. This means that a spectrum of addiction exists in which the severity of dependence can vary but is not as easily quantified. Although addiction and dependence may sometimes intertwine in literature, these terms should be treated differently, and it matters.

Misdiagnosing an individual with an addictive disorder rather than a physiologic dependence on a substance can evoke undue medical and criminal scrutiny.[11] For instance, if the neurologic effects of sugar are compared to those of opiates, similarities can be observed: cravings, withdrawal symptoms, overdosing/overeating, dopamine receptor and expression effects, including other neurologic effects.[12, 13] Both, if taken at higher recommended doses can lead to serious health complications or even death. However, these can also be moderately taken without overdose concerns. Therefore, careful consideration should be given to "labeling" individuals as addicts given the extent of exposure to a substance.

Politicians are concerned with addiction linked to illicit activity. The perceived danger given to some substances of abuse more than others is attributed to the extent of physical or physiological harm caused to an individual. Especially when psychoactive substances may alter an individual's actions that may prove dangerous to the community. The "war on drugs" starting in the 1970s hoped to fight illicit drug use through incarceration to combat the opioid epidemic that remains an issue to this day.[14] However, the intended solution did not provide the expected results. Because addiction to these illicit drugs spread with ineffective intervention efforts, a proportionally larger number of imprisonments than in any other industrialized county ensued. Thus, in 2005 an incarceration ratio of 1:136 US adults resulted in excessive funds expended to solve a problem that would only exacerbate in due time.[15, 16] Since the threat of incarceration proved to be an ineffective method to reduce drug abuse, harm reduction policies began to be implemented as cost-effective medical treatments to ease the spread of addiction.[17] This meant that alternative solutions could be presented to individuals who struggle to fight addiction, but consequently disrupting the standardization of what constitutes a criminal and a victim to one's body a harder task to classify.

The Severity Spectrum of Addiction
Speaking of addiction in healthcare or the court of law tends to have a negative connotation which can lead to misconceptions about someone who is not necessarily dangerous. Perhaps, in pursuit of managing the magnitude and severity of substance fixation, individuals that tend to comply with rehabilitation, withdrawal, or reduction have shifted the perspective of milder cases of addiction to a more "positive" status. Therefore attributing to the difference between dependence and addiction status as previously discussed.[11] Regardless of how "bad" or "good" a substance is in comparison to others, failure to manage a severe form of addiction can be dangerous as any other. Criminalization of a potential substance of abuse does not imply that only those categorized as such are toxic or promote high-risk behavior. For this reason, science has had an important impact on shaping policy and public opinion through objective rationale that has helped expose logical inconsistencies of some addictions in relation to others.

Alcohol
Although some contemporary legal and leisurely used substances may not be at a glance an immediate concern for a population's safety, situational and chronic dependence factors should be taken into consideration when evaluating their underlying hazards. Despite its prevalence of consumption, alcohol is responsible for many hospitalizations and deaths globally. In the US, about 95,000 people die from alcohol-related causes (e.g., cirrhosis) making it the third leading-preventable cause of death below tobacco use and overweight-related complications.[18]

Furthermore, alcohol can have concerning interactions with many drugs which—unknowingly to most people—put their life at risk. Intoxication may result if alcohol is conjointly used with amphetamines, severe respiratory depression with barbiturates, and cardiac death using cocaine.[19]

Another important aspect of serious alcohol dependence can lead to dangerous effects on behavior. Individual risk factors of alcohol abuse include temperament, impaired cognitive function, attention deficit, and lack of self-control, among others which can extend and negatively impact close relationships.[19] In addition, alcohol use can also be associated with criminal activity. In 2011, 73% of recorded homicides in the US were related to alcohol use, and between 2006–2010 a reported estimate of 7,756 homicides related to excessive alcohol abuse each year.[20-22] Aggressive behaviors can also be expected to lead to domestic abuse that may victimize both a child and/or parent. For cases of aggravated assault, more than a quarter are linked to heavy drinkers.[23]

Since antiquity, Aristotle had noted in alcohol-related research its grim withdrawal effects and dangers of consumption in pregnant women.[24] Today, the detrimental effects of fetal alcohol spectrum disorders are well understood making alcohol abuse a risk factor for pregnancy. Aside from potential renal and cardiovascular problems, a baby may suffer later in life from poor reasoning, judgment, learning, impaired cognition, and abnormal hyperactivity for which no minimum threshold for safety consumption exists during pregnancy. Moreover, failure to comply with public health recommendations for women's behavior during pregnancy can have lawful repercussions.[25-27]

Marijuana
Cannabis has recently surged from the blacklist of illicit drugs as a potential therapeutic for treating certain illnesses. FDA-approved analogs of marijuana have served to treat a range of conditions: severe forms of epilepsy, syndromes, some forms of anorexia, refractory chemotherapy-induced nausea, neuropathic pain, and an increase in appetite for some disorders to name a few.[28] Contrary to alcohol which has been in circulation for a long time, population studies on marijuana consumption are limited but expected to increase as its legalization allows for more robust data to be collected. THC, the psychoactive component of marijuana modulates the CNS as both a stimulant and depressant similar to alcohol, thus an expectation for violent tendencies and psychosis are expected but have been loosely associated.[28-30]

Relative to other inhaled addictive substances, tobacco has ample evidence surrounding its carcinogenic potential relative to cannabis. Being the number 1 risk factor for lung cancer and linked to 80–90% of related deaths, the danger of cigarette smoking is attributed to a mix of more than 7,000 chemicals of which at least 70 are known to be carcinogenic.[31] In comparison, marijuana has more than 400 chemicals of which 60 are cannabinoids and limited evidence of carcinogenic toxicity is known. Few uncontrolled studies have suggestive evidence of marijuana smoking as indicative of a higher risk of lung cancer while well-designed population studies do not.[32, 33] Even if a substantial amount of data supported that the majority of compounds found in marijuana are carcinogenic, these would only constitute approximately 6% of the total amount found in tobacco. While better documentation of the carcinogenic potential of marijuana is needed, chronic use of marijuana can have undesirable health effects. Periodontal disease and premature births have been associated with long-term use in addition to cannabinoid hyperemesis syndrome.[34, 35] Among the milder forms of adverse effects, one can expect panic attacks, increase heart rate, seizures (if ingested with cocaine), respiratory depression, and coma (in some cases).[28, 36, 37]

At a glance, cannabinoids may not seem to be a serious issue, but given enough time, a better understanding of its overuse may uncover more serious health concerns. Although sound arguments about the dangers of marijuana usage can be a cause for concern, given a similar profile to other legal substances with no current inclination for greater deleterious effects should be placed into perspective when the recreational use of marijuana is not excessive.

Opioids
Medical use of opioids is important for acute and chronic pain treatment for a variety of different conditions. Ranging from mild injuries to severe post-surgical pain, their high analgesic effects in contrast to other drugs have made them highly desirable. Unfortunately, long-term exposure to opioids can lead to the development of tolerance which can progressively bring people closer to toxic doses. The US has been facing a surging opioid crisis that has tripled in the number of cases and quadrupled in prescriptions since 1999.[38, 39] This is particularly dangerous because unlike alcohol or other substances of abuse, some opioids can have extremely low therapeutic windows that typically result in severe respiratory depression. Fentanyl which is 50–100 times more potent than morphine can be fatal if more than 100 µg are administered; an amount barely visible to the naked eye.[40] For this reason, the use of fentanyl is strictly reserved for medical applications when severe pain is experienced. Nevertheless, patients may become dependent on prescription opioids posing a risk of tolerance among a population that requires them for their intended use.

To reduce the risk of opioid dependence, less potent alternative medications have been used as a gateway to control addiction. Methadone, an FDA-approved drug for detoxification and opioid use disorder treatment has been shown to improve mortality rates of opioid abusers while the best results are obtained when used in long-term therapy.[41] Although methadone is an effective opioid to reduce cravings and withdrawal symptoms, similar side effects to other opioids and overdose can still occur.

Naloxone, an increasingly accessible drug used to counteract a fatal opioid overdose has been highly efficacious as an opioid receptor antagonist. Public health and political officials have considered broadening naloxone availability to the public similar to nebulizers for treating asthma to reduce the number of overdose fatalities. Despite government, clinical, and research intentions to reduce opioid-related fatalities, the treatment prospect may have inadvertently encouraged further opioid misuse. Addicts who survive naloxone treatment tend to continue their use of opioids, and spreading knowledge about its life-saving potential tends to create a misguided sense of security.[42] Because of this, the prescription of naloxone has become scrutinized in certain states; however, more data is required to establish a relationship between the higher risk of opioid use and naloxone.

Misuse of any opioid—regardless of its potency—can lead to the development of addiction. Yet, their practical use in the medical field is of great importance for a patient's acute and chronic quality of life for pain treatment. Until better opioid variants or another group of analgesics are "discovered" to reduce dependency, the best course of action should be to reduce the number of prescriptions in favor of NSAIDs whenever possible. Opioid addiction in many cases is not the result of deliberate ill intention. Rather, it is the struggle to live a normal life held hostage by incessant pain.

Evaluation of the Severity Spectrum

Understanding the hazardous effects of any substance is important to comprehend the extent of complexity that encompass their misuse. Though many forms of addiction can place an individual's health at risk, not all of them do so to the same degree. Furthermore, concerns about illicit behavior do not seem to be parallel across every form of dependence. While excessive alcohol intake has been shown to compromise an individual's health in tandem with impaired cognition and violent tendencies, it is rather the consequences/actions of intoxication that are criminalized rather than its consumption. In comparison, the consumption of cannabis was deemed illegal despite not enough evidence documented that proves a dissimilar or more excessive danger profile to alcohol. Moreover, its carcinogenic and addictive potential has been largely omitted in contrast to tobacco smoke. Regardless of the severity of their respective abuse, low to moderate consumption of each can be much more manageable. Thereby reducing negative health effects and tendencies for criminal activity.

Opioid dependence can be different from other substances because many people may not have the luxury of choice when it comes to alleviating their condition. Even so, opioids can be far more fatal than both alcohol and marijuana, albeit this does not necessarily make all its users more prone to dangerous behavior. For this reason, prescriptions have limited the circulation of opioids without excessive legal scrutiny as a way to protect the public. Though efforts to reduce opioid dependence have yet to be particularly effective, giving healthcare professionals agency on determining what is best for a patient appears to be a reason why policies around previously illegal substances have slowly shifted the perspective of public officials. After all, all forms of addiction are not the same and many can be managed with appropriate therapy.

Substance fixation is a byproduct of an individual's conditioned stimuli to the pleasant effects of a drug. Due to an inaccurate understanding of how exactly this conditioned stimulus works in situations where dependence does not occur, it is therefore not reasonable to assume that all substances of abuse are addictive. A true disease is transmissible, autoimmune, or degenerative and results in death if left untreated. Although treatments exist to reduce cravings and overdose, cessation of intake would not be expected to result in a person's death. The lack of a clear quantifiable rubric to compare the varying severities of substance dependence is an indication of the volatile nature of how danger is classified. Thus, inconsistencies and disagreement in both medicine and legislation are expected to continue to redefine how the dangers of addiction are perceived in the community.

Works Cited

1. Chandler RK, Fletcher BW, Volkow ND. Treating drug abuse and addiction in the criminal justice system: improving public health and safety. JAMA. 2009;301(2):183-90.
2. Heyman GM. Addiction and choice: theory and new data. Front Psychiatry. 2013;4:31.

3. Lewis M. The Biology of Desire: Why Addiction is Not a Disease. First ed. United States: PublicAffairs; 2016.
4. Vintiadis E. Scientific American. 2017. [cited 2022]. Available from: https://blogs.scientificamerican.com/observations/is-addiction-a-disease/#.
5. Greenstein M. The Problematic Role of the Judge in Assessing Addiction. American Bar Association. 2018.
6. Crocq MA. Historical and cultural aspects of man's relationship with addictive drugs. Dialogues Clin Neurosci. 2007;9(4):355-61.
7. Substance use, abuse, and addiction. American Psychological Association. 2022.
8. Drug Misuse and Addiction. National Insitute on Drug Abuse. 2020.
9. Leshner AI. Addiction is a brain disease, and it matters. Science. 1997;278(5335):45-7.
10. Berridge KC. Is Addiction a Brain Disease? Neuroethics. 2017;10(1):29-33.
11. Szalavitz M, Rigg KK, Wakeman SE. Drug dependence is not addiction-and it matters. Ann Med. 2021;53(1):1989-92.
12. Avena NM, Rada P, Hoebel BG. Evidence for sugar addiction: behavioral and neurochemical effects of intermittent, excessive sugar intake. Neurosci Biobehav Rev. 2008;32(1):20-39. Epub 20070518.
13. Ting AKR, van der Kooy D. The neurobiology of opiate motivation. Cold Spring Harb Perspect Med. 2012;2(10). Epub 20121001.
14. Polcin DL. Addiction science advocacy: mobilizing political support to influence public policy. Int J Drug Policy. 2014;25(2):329-31. Epub 20131118.
15. Clear TR, Reisig MD, Cole GF. American corrections: Cengage learning; 2018.
16. Grattet R, Petersilia J, Lin J, et al. Parole violations and revocations in California: Analysis and suggestions for action. Fed Probation. 2009;73:2.
17. Rhodes T, Hedrich D. Harm Reduction: Evidence, Impacts, and Challenges2010.
18. Alcohol Use in the United States. National Insitute on Alcohol Abuse and Alcoholism. 2022.
19. Alozai U, Sharma S. Drug and Alcohol Use. StatPearls. Treasure Island (FL)2022.
20. Landberg J, Norstrom T. Alcohol and homicide in Russia and the United States: a comparative analysis. J Stud Alcohol Drugs. 2011;72(5):723-30.
21. Control CfD, Prevention. National Violent Death Reporting System Web Coding Manual. December; 2018.
22. Naimi TS, Xuan Z, Cooper SE, et al. Alcohol Involvement in Homicide Victimization in the United States. Alcohol Clin Exp Res. 2016;40(12):2614-21. Epub 20160927.
23. Galbicsek C. Alcohol-Related Crimes: Recovery Worldwide; 2022 [cited 2022]. Available from: https://www.alcoholrehabguide.org/alcohol/crimes/.
24. O'Brien JM. Alexander and Dionysus: the invisible enemy. Ann Scholarship. 1980;1(83):105.
25. Seiler NK. Alcohol and Pregnancy: CDC's Health Advice and the Legal Rights of Pregnant Women. Public Health Rep. 2016;131(4):623-7.
26. Alcohol Use During Pregnancy: Centers for Disease Control and Prevention; 2021 [cited 2022]. Available from: https://www.cdc.gov/ncbddd/fasd/alcohol-use.html#:~:text=Growth%20and%20central%20nervous%20system,to%20alcohol%20at%20any%20time.
27. Alcohol Use in Pregnancy. In: Prevention CfDCa, editor.
28. Turner AR, Agrawal S. Marijuana. StatPearls. Treasure Island (FL)2022.
29. Murray JB. Marijuana's effects on human cognitive functions, psychomotor functions, and personality. J Gen Psychol. 1986;113(1):23-55.
30. Berenson A. Marijuana Is More Dangerous Than You Think. Mo Med. 2019;116(2):88-9.
31. What Are the Risk Factors for Lung Cancer? Centers for Disease Control and Prevention. 2022.

32. Tashkin DP. Effects of marijuana smoking on the lung. Ann Am Thorac Soc. 2013;10(3):239-47.
33. Atakan Z. Cannabis, a complex plant: different compounds and different effects on individuals. Ther Adv Psychopharmacol. 2012;2(6):241-54.
34. Auer R, Vittinghoff E, Yaffe K, et al. Association Between Lifetime Marijuana Use and Cognitive Function in Middle Age: The Coronary Artery Risk Development in Young Adults (CARDIA) Study. JAMA Intern Med. 2016;176(3):352-61.
35. Lapoint J, Meyer S, Yu CK, et al. Cannabinoid Hyperemesis Syndrome: Public Health Implications and a Novel Model Treatment Guideline. West J Emerg Med. 2018;19(2):380-6.
36. Degenhardt L, Coffey C, Romaniuk H, et al. The persistence of the association between adolescent cannabis use and common mental disorders into young adulthood. Addiction. 2013;108(1):124-33. Epub 20121018.
37. Appelboam A, Oades PJ. Coma due to cannabis toxicity in an infant. Eur J Emerg Med. 2006;13(3):177-9.
38. Hah JM, Bateman BT, Ratliff J, et al. Chronic Opioid Use After Surgery: Implications for Perioperative Management in the Face of the Opioid Epidemic. Anesth Analg. 2017;125(5):1733-40.
39. Rosenblum A, Marsch LA, Joseph H, et al. Opioids and the treatment of chronic pain: controversies, current status, and future directions. Exp Clin Psychopharmacol. 2008;16(5):405-16.
40. Ramos-Matos CF, Bistas KG, Lopez-Ojeda W. Fentanyl. StatPearls. Treasure Island (FL)2022.
41. Toce MS, Chai PR, Burns MM, et al. Pharmacologic Treatment of Opioid Use Disorder: a Review of Pharmacotherapy, Adjuncts, and Toxicity. J Med Toxicol. 2018;14(4):306-22. Epub 20181030.
42. Doleac J. The Moral Hazard of Lifesaving Innovations: Naloxone Access, Opioid Abuse, and Crime. Institute of Labor Economics. 2018.

Essay: How Do We Cure Addiction?

Can it be cured at all and what are potential treatments?

Nanase Toda

Introduction

About 35 million people are affected by drug addiction globally.[1] By the medical community, addiction is widely perceived as a disease characterized by the habitual and compulsive use of substances despite deleterious health consequences, and it is included in the Diagnostic and Statistical Manual of Mental Disorders, or DSM, and other diagnostic manuals and schemas.[2-4] Alternatively, there is also a view in which addiction is depicted as a voluntary choice as well as an outcome affected by various factors such as personal life events, easy access to abusable substances, and underlying mental disorders.[3-5]

Is It a Disease?

First, addiction is self-acquired as its initiation is accompanied by the choice to take an abusable substance.[6] If there is no access to cocaine, one will never develop cocaine addiction. Although some argue that over time, voluntary control over drug use will be compromised and using drugs becomes an uncontrollable behavior, the majority of addicts accomplish the cessation of substance use often without interventions.[3, 5, 7] For instance, some addicts naturally recover from addiction with pressure from others, especially their family or loved ones without treatment.[8] This suggests that addicts can voluntarily "choose" to recover from addiction and that their drug use is not involuntary.[9] Moreover, the behaviors pursued by addicts indeed are associated with potential risks and harmful consequences; however, this is equally true for some common voluntary behaviors such as consuming unhealthy food and driving faster than the speed limit, which indicates that potentially detrimental behaviors are not necessarily involuntary.[5]

Next, a measurable physiologic or anatomical deviation from the norm, which is presumed to be correlated with addiction such as the increased amount of dopamine in the brain, is common to many other pleasing experiences including exercise.[5] Also, some argue that addicts have distinct neuronal activities and functions from those of non-addicts, and this indicates that addiction is linked to functional alterations in the brain, which renders it a disease. However, any sustained behavior change is likely associated with alterations in the brain because the brain regulates behavior.[9] Interestingly, even instantaneous social behavior can result in reversible changes in the brain.[10] If any structural or functional alterations in the brain render a particular behavior or condition a disease, engaging in seemingly healthy activities such as reading books should also be considered a disease because it can cause changes in the brain.[9, 11] Overall, addiction is not a disease, rather, it is a maladaptive strategy made to respond to undesirable personal situations such as emotional instability or underlying mental disorders including depression.[6]

Can It Be Cured?
Interventions for those seeking them entail changing their habit or behavior so that they will be able to inhibit themselves from making poor choices, namely, using drugs. Unfortunately, changing habits or behavior is an unstable process, and frequent relapses occur. Data show that nearly 70% of individuals who have succeeded in discontinuing the use of addictive substances revert to their old habits and behaviors within a year.[12] In addition, heterogeneity in the recovery process of addicts creates complexity and variation in addiction treatment.[2] Therefore, it cannot be ethically claimed that a cure is available for addiction, or that therapies can always amend it. To maximize the effects of treatment for those in need and increase the chance of recovery, the personal situations, personalities, and underlying mental health conditions of addicts should be considered when creating treatment plans.

Detoxification
Often, addiction treatment begins with detoxification, which involves the clearing of substances of abuse from individuals suffering from acute intoxication, and the assistance of safe withdrawal.[13, 14] As needed, medications are utilized to ease withdrawal symptoms.[14] In addition, successful detoxification involves linkage to the subsequent treatment. Detoxification and the introduction to the appropriate following treatment are crucial as they lead to an increased chance of recovery.[13]

Inpatient Treatment
Inpatient treatment entails residing in licensed, substance-free facilities where around-the-clock medical care and therapeutic support are offered.[7, 14] Generally, the objective to be achieved at these facilities is to adopt a lifestyle free from substances of abuse and crime. The settings of inpatient treatment include shorter-term residential treatment, therapeutic communities, and recovery housing. In shorter-term residential treatment, detoxification and initial counseling are typically provided, which prepares addicts for treatment in a community-based setting. In therapeutic communities where addicts stay at a treatment facility typically for 6–12 months, their attitudes and behaviors associated with substance use are aimed to be positively influenced. Often following other types of inpatient treatment is recovery housing, which provides short-term housing with supervision. In this treatment setting, service providers aid people in transitioning to independent life by providing them opportunities to learn finance management and seek employment.[7]

Inpatient treatment may be a great option for individuals dealing with severe, chronic addiction as well as those suffering from co-occurring mental disorders.[14] Also, it may be suitable for those living alone as a lack of supervision at home might challenge their recovery process. Furthermore, addicts having family issues might benefit from this type of treatment as well because stress or mental instability caused at home might facilitate the continuation of drug use and create difficulty in its cessation.

Outpatient Treatment

Outpatient treatment allows addicts to remain at home during the recovery process, which enables them to continue caring for their families and working.[14] Behavioral therapies are offered in most programs to modify attitudes and behaviors related to substance use and increase healthy living skills. In the beginning, addicts usually attend multiple outpatient sessions each week and then transition to attending less frequent, shorter sessions for the sustainment of their improvement.[7]

Because outpatient treatment does not sequester addicts from their surroundings, triggers that challenge their recovery is encountered more than in inpatient treatment. Thus, outpatient treatment programs might be a great option for individuals battling mild forms of addiction.[14] In addition, because recovered addicts tend to attribute their cessation of drug use to financial and family concerns, this type of treatment may be suitable for addicts living with others and having healthy relationships with them. In this case, the presence of others can positively reinforce their commitment to recovery and provide oversight.[9] Outpatient treatment is also a great program to participate in after inpatient treatment to sustain recovery.[14]

Faith-Based Treatment

A spiritual approach to addiction might be preferred by followers of a religion. In faith-based treatment, specialized programs, which incorporate teachings and values from a particular religion are provided.[15] This allows addicts in recovery to interact with individuals of like mind who are also seeking guidance from a higher power.[14]

Conclusion

Addiction is not a disease, but a choice made to respond to undesirable personal situations. Although interventions are not necessarily required for recovery, personal situations, personalities, and underlying mental health conditions should be taken into consideration when creating treatment plans for people in need. Some common addiction treatments include inpatient, outpatient, and faith-based treatment. Each treatment has distinct properties and would be suitable for different situations.

Works Cited

1. World Health Organization. Drugs (psychoactive) [cited 2022 November 15]. Available from: https://www.who.int/health-topics/drugs-psychoactive#tab=tab_3.
2. Zou Z, Wang H, d'Oleire Uquillas F, et al. Definition of Substance and Non-substance Addiction. Adv Exp Med Biol. 2017;1010:21-41.
3. Leyton M. Are addictions diseases or choices? J Psychiatry Neurosci. 2013;38(4):219-21.
4. Lamb RJ, Maguire DR, Ginsburg BC, et al. Determinants of choice, and vulnerability and recovery in addiction. Behav Processes. 2016;127:35-42. Epub 20160412.
5. Henden E, Melberg HO, Rogeberg OJ. Addiction: choice or compulsion? Front Psychiatry. 2013;4:77. Epub 20130807.
6. Holden T. Addiction is not a disease. CMAJ. 2012;184(6):679.
7. National Institute on Drug Abuse. Treatment Approaches for Drug Addiction DrugFacts: National Institute on Drug Abuse; 2019 [cited 2022 November 7]. Available from: https://nida.nih.gov/publications/drugfacts/treatment-approaches-drug-addiction.
8. Mariezcurrena R. Recovery from addictions without treatment: Literature review. Scandinavian Journal of Behaviour Therapy. 1994;23(3-4):131-54.

9. Branch MN. Drug addiction. Is it a disease or is it based on choice? A review of Gene Heyman's Addiction: A disorder of choice. Journal of the Experimental Analysis of Behavior. 2011;95(2):263-7.
10. Fernald RD. How does Behavior Change the Brain? Multiple Methods to Answer Old Questions. Integr Comp Biol. 2003;43(6):771-9.
11. Berns GS, Blaine K, Prietula MJ, et al. Short- and long-term effects of a novel on connectivity in the brain. Brain Connect. 2013;3(6):590-600. Epub 20131009.
12. Bouton ME. Why behavior change is difficult to sustain. Prev Med. 2014;68:29-36. Epub 20140615.
13. Miller NS, Kipnis SS, Center for Substance Abuse Treatment (U.S.). Detoxification and substance abuse treatment. Rockville, MD: U.S. Dept. of Health and Human Services, Public Health Service, Substance Abuse and Mental Health Services Administration, Center for Substance Abuse Treatment; 2006. xix, 245 p. p.
14. Addiction Center. Treatment: Addiction Center; 2022 [cited 2022 November 7]. Available from: https://www.addictioncenter.com/treatment/.
15. Sharp A. Christian Drug & Alcohol Rehab Centers Near Me 2022 [cited 2022 November 16]. Available from: https://americanaddictioncenters.org/rehab-guide/christian.

Topic: Compassionate Use and Expanded Drug Access—Should the Dying Have the Right to Try?

In the US, drugs are only marketed and made available to the public after a lengthy and formal process of pre-formulation (optimizing the chemistry and dosage form), preclinical (studies in animals), and three to four phases of clinical (studies in humans) trials that take as long as 20 years and millions of dollars to complete.[1-4] However, new ideas are emerging that would give the gravely ill special but limited rights to circumvent this long and expensive process. Specifically, there is interest in allowing dying patients to have access to a drug that has passed pre-formulation, preclinical, and early clinical trial hurdles for safety but has not been trialed in the population it was intended to treat. In fact, ideas for expanded access to experimental drugs existed as early as the 1980s when disenfranchised patients sought to be included in clinical trials for HIV drugs.[5] This led, in the 1980s, to investigational new drug (IND) treatment access as well as compassionate use rules for drugs allowing them to be provided to people who could not gain access to or participate in Phases II or III of a clinical trial. The compassionate access avenue also gave hope to those who had no other therapeutic options for treating a disease or condition that was imminently fatal.[6-9]

"Supporters of this legislation talk as if effective treatments are being withheld from patients....The vast majority of experimental therapies are toxic or ineffective."

Dr. Robert M. Califf, Commissioner of the FDA under President Obama

Even so, current expanded access and treatment IND laws are considered, as they exist now, to be ineffective by many people. Thus, Right-to-Try laws are being unanimously signed across the nation with the purpose of calling attention to the problems faced by the terminally ill and reducing the previously 100-hour paperwork burden of the initial drug inquiry application.[7,10] This lengthy petitioning process was an obstacle to many patients, preventing the timely presentation of investigational therapy when it may have been most useful. Presently, only approximately 1,000 people have been able to receive investigational medications. Through Right-to-Try laws, state leaders and patient advocacy groups seek to increase this number of patients significantly.

And this type of access would represent a significant bump to the front of the line. Clinical trials typically require a preliminary first phase (Phase 0) and in this phase, a small group of healthy subjects is given the drug in small and then escalating doses to assess safety. A preferred dose may be determined from these studies. Then, in Phase I trials, the experimental drug is given to several hundred healthy volunteers. This phase exists to confirm drug safety at a chosen dose and to assess side effects. Usually, the study subjects are randomized to a group that will be given the drug under investigation or assigned to a group that is given an inactive or placebo substance. Typically, in very rigorous trials, neither the study director nor the subject knows if he has been given the active compound or a placebo. For the most detailed studies (and the most lengthy and expensive), a cross-over design may be used in which Phase I subjects are given the drug or placebo for a period. Then they undergo a no-drug period of several days or weeks, called a wash-out. After this wash-out, the groups are switched. Then, the previous placebo recipients are given the active drug, and those who received the active drug get a placebo.

If, and only if, the drug passes this initial rigorous safety review, it is tested in a small group (maybe fewer than 100) of individuals with the symptom, condition, or disease the drug is intended to treat (Phase II). This trial may include a narrower dose range if data from the Phase I study indicate that this is necessary. If the drug appears to work, again compared to a placebo-tested group, it can progress to Phase III which allows the study of the drug in a larger population of subjects who have the disease. These types of studies help scientists to determine true drug effects on a disease or symptom or the efficacy compared to no drug treatment at all. If the data provide overwhelming evidence that the drug does what the manufacturer says it does *and it is safe*, the drug can be approved and placed on the market. Here, the drug undergoes a less publicized Phase IV trial or post-marketing surveillance.

Right-to-Try/compassionate or expanded use would significantly change this multi-phase drug approval approach but for only a few drugs, and for only a few people, a concept that may be greatly misunderstood by the public, and perhaps by people in Congress and some physicians who oppose it. With expanded use, the Phase I healthy volunteer study to establish safety would still occur but it would be considered sufficient evidence for offering the experimental drug to selected desperately ill individuals. In the most positive light, the drug would produce a therapeutic response and extend or save the life of a person who has no more options. It has been incorrectly stated that patients would be exposed to "a potentially toxic drug with no proven benefit," with Right-to-Try laws, but this is merely evidence that a Phase I safety trial is completely misunderstood by those who make these erroneous statements.[11] There can be no exposure to a toxic substance because the Phase I trial, which would still occur, would eliminate that risk. Also, this additional law in no way can compel any pharmaceutical company to give a drug to anyone. People who assume this simply do not understand how drugs are approved.

Also, although many argue that Right-to-Try laws would endanger patients by weakening or circumventing FDA protective measures of informed consent and institutional review boards to oversee human subject research, this logic is again horribly flawed. First, the FDA has nothing to do with expanded access or compassionate use. Rather, physicians, patients, and pharmaceutical companies create a partnership to determine whether access to an investigational substance is prudent.[9] This access can be made available to a single patient. Also, applications for several individual patients who are resistant, unresponsive, or unable to acquire a particular, but less effective standard of care for their disease can be bundled to create a small group for expanded access.[12] Such laborious and detailed form-filling indicates the height of informed consent for all involved and a willingness to move forward with an experimental but safe therapy. Also, the patient (the most important person in this discussion) and his physician (who is a consultant, not a gatekeeper nor an experimental drug expert) make these decisions regarding a solitary drug. Access to one drug is too limited to be considered undermining the FDA. The FDA will still move forward with Phase II and III trials if they are appropriate. The sick person is merely getting the documented-safe drug earlier. And again, no drug company has to comply with the request.

Thus, patients and physicians only complete the paperwork and submit it if approval is imminent. This buried statistic is how the FDA can comfortably say to the public that virtually all applications for expanded access are approved. This statistic, however, does not address those applications that were never submitted due to paperwork challenges, any forms that went unfinished due to the death of the patient, the refusal of the physician to cooperate in the petitioning process, or the rejection by the drug company of the request before the paperwork is even initiated. Pharmaceutical companies have the first right of refusal for all such expanded access requests. Also, although pharmaceutical companies truly cannot profit from expanded use, they can pass on drug research, synthesis, and handling costs; thus, the right to try an experimental drug may not be free to the patient. It goes without saying that any "hit" on an experimental drug to save a dying person would be a media-drenched event that would catapult the drug under approval to a fast-tracked status and have patients lining up to purchase it before the first tablets were pressed.

So, much of the opposition to Right-to-Try lies in mischaracterizations of what terminally ill patients actually face. First, most frequently, the drug is ineffective and rarely, it may actually hasten death. Also, stopping a trial at safety and holding off efficacy studies for a later date to give the drug to one or a few terminally ill persons effectively diminishes the pool of potential Phase II and III subjects for later investigations. This could be exacerbated by the premature departure of enrolled study subjects who would reduce the study subject numbers below critical statistical thresholds for accurately measuring drug effects. Because statistical data are required to demonstrate proof of a good drug candidate, ideally the drug is tested in as many sick persons as possible. Large subject samples lend "power" to data interpretation and the more people who have a positive outcome, the more likely the drug is to be approved.

Then, people anticipating that a compassionate use protocol would be granted to allow them to have the drug after safety has been demonstrated may be dissuaded from even inquiring about other phases of clinical trial enrollment. If the drug is then never offered for expanded use—again, only a few are—then the patient has missed every opportunity to receive the experimental therapy. Because all clinical trial protocols are written before a trial can be initiated, drug approval studies cannot be modified once they begin. Thus, no additional patients can be added and no patient criteria can be altered to accommodate others not originally included in the study design. So people interested in a specific drug under investigation are better served by expressing interest early and often and not waiting for an individual exception to access to be granted.

Also, there can be no premature stop of a trial, no artificial trial extension, and no switching of any assigned patient groups to other categories of therapy. Only in this way can scientists know what worked, how well, and for whom. This may mean that to save the lives of many with an approved drug, the health or lives of a few may be sacrificed for a time. This is an acceptable burden for those who believe that patients should never have access to unapproved experimental therapies at all and that physicians and pharmaceutical companies can rightfully withhold such treatments and deny access to anyone.[10]

Also, if the petition to the pharmaceutical company takes too long to complete, the subject may be too ill for any intervention. Timing is a continual threat to drug approval. For those who do acquire expanded access, their data are still collected as part of the drug approval portfolio. So, subjects who die sooner after treatment or who have side effects due to the drug which may be solely attributed to their poor health and not the therapy must be documented. These data, although they apply to one or a few very ill person(s), may be sufficient to trigger a denial of drug approval. This would eliminate the drug as a potential therapy for thousands of people who could have been treated in earlier stages of the disease and perhaps saved.

"In this great country of ours, I am allowed to take my own life, in some states, but I ca not try an experimental treatment that may save me."

Matt Bellina, a 32-year-old former Navy fighter pilot diagnosed with ALS in 2012

It is difficult to disagree with the underlying intent of compassionate and expanded use protocols, but it is critical that people know that rarely does access to an unapproved drug stop the progress of a serious disease and less frequently is a life actually extended or improved through expanded access. However, during these last-ditch maneuvers, emotions understandably rule human actions and the rigor and truth-seeking nature of science are of little importance to those who want just a little more time on this planet.[13] Likely, to see the positive outcomes we desire from Right-to-Try, we need to facilitate the process (not obstruct it) and allow more patients to try earlier in their disease. This may give us sufficient numbers of successes from which we can learn.

Because not all countries offer this type of forward-thinking solution for the sickest patients, it is natural for a rift to form between poor and wealthy nations. Such a chasm occurred previously when European medical personnel suggested that a US drug company was not as generous with expanded access to a new HIV drug as they were in their own domestic market.[14] Such perceptions have sparked conversations to create a non-US, global drug rationing process such that all countries have equitable access to life-saving medications.[14] Of course, because the US shoulders most of the research and development burden and US citizens pay the highest prices for new prescription medications, the real cost of this type of access may not be realized by countries beyond the US that benefit from drug pricing negotiations and more open drug markets. So, financing such a noble effort may be impossible or it may again fall to the US to organize and support financially.

We are facing a crossroads in pharmacology: pharmaceutical companies want to focus efforts where the money is, in chronic conditions for which a patient will take a drug for a long time or a lifetime. There is less interest in developing a drug that will be used by few or used once or for a short time. Incentivizing innovation will be a goal for pharmacologists moving forward, but we must remember that our efforts are for one cause—patient health and well-being—not profits and headlines.[15]

Writing Prompts

- Just because we approve drugs this way, is this an excuse to keep doing it the same way?
- Should all drug companies that make life-altering drugs be obligated to create expanded use protocols for any person or group of people requesting such?
- Should all expanded use patient data be exempt from approval documentation (few participants, participants are sicker)?
- If the expanded access data are hopeful, should this be used to accelerate any ongoing formal clinical trial?
- Should we be able to cherry-pick data this way
- For those with confirmed terminal illnesses, should ANY drug with ANY glimmer of hope be allowed?
    - Who pays for follow-up care if the drug harms the patient?
    - Should lawsuits be prohibited if the drug hastens the death of the patient?
    - What remedy (if any) does the family get?
- Should children be restricted from expanded access due to their unique pharmacology?
    - What limitations for children—if any—should be imposed?
- How does expanded use complicate clinical trials?
- Should expanded use data be available for potential trial participants even if it causes them to decline to participate in a clinical trial?
- Would withholding such data violate the concept of informed consent or are the data considered proprietary information owned by the drug company?
    - What compromise might be reached?
- Should patients with potentially fatal diseases who are current clinical trials but in placebo arms be allowed to leave the trial and petition for expanded access for the active form of the drug?
- Is a placebo arm suddenly unethical for sick people?
    - Why or why not?
- Is expanded access a cruel joke because no company HAS to comply?
- If a compassionate use is successful, is that a free pre-marketing advertisement/endorsement for the drug company?
    - Do these programs cause false hope for our sickest patients?
- Should we revamp our clinical trial system and only do preliminary safety (but not efficacy) testing to drastically reduce approval time?
- If patient can be charged for drug, how might this affect future pricing for us?
- Should the price "charged" be public information?
- If the approved drug is thousands of dollars but free for expanded care, should insurance companies lobby for price breaks?
    - What about patients with no insurance?
    - Should this be rolled into current pharmaceutical patient drug assistance programs?
    - Should patients never have to pay for expanded access?

- Because of the expertise required and the cost associated with submitting an expanded use application, are poorer, rural patients unfairly disenfranchised?
- Should trial subjects who were instrumental in helping the drug company obtain positive data and drug approval be given access to the drug for free?
  - Should crowdsourcing drive science?
- Does the trial process inherently violate civil rights of patients by denying them life-saving drugs?
- Is access to a drug at any stage of approval a constitutional right?
  - Where in the constitution is this guaranteed?
- Does denial of right to try laws deprive citizens of self-preservation?
- Should patients be the sole arbiter of their risk:reward thresholds for trying experimental drugs?
  - Are all patients sufficiently competent in this regard?
- Are sicker patients worse at risk assessment?
- Is it paternalistic for the government to make these decisions for the gravely ill/dying patient?

Work Cited

1. Pinto EM, Willan AR, O'Brien BJ. Cost-effectiveness analysis for multinational clinical trials. Stat Med. 2005;24(13):1965-82.
2. Shaya FT, Samant N. Cost studies in clinical trials. Expert Rev Pharmacoecon Outcomes Res. 2004;4(6):591-4.
3. Conti CR. Clinical trials and the cost of medical care. Clin Cardiol. 1999;22(9):549-50.
4. Are clinical trials cost-effective? JAMA. 1990;263(11):1491-2.
5. Buhles WC. Compassionate use: a story of ethics and science in the development of a new drug. Perspect Biol Med. 2011;54(3):304-15.
6. Raus K. An analysis of common ethical justifications for compassionate use programs for experimental drugs. BMC Med Ethics. 2016;17(1):60.
7. Hoerger M. Right-to-try laws and individual patient "compassionate use" of experimental oncology medications: A call for improved provider-patient communication. Death Stud. 2016;40(2):113-20.
8. Miller D. Expanded Access Allows for Compassionate Use of Investigational Cancer Drugs. ONS Connect. 2015;30(2):47.
9. Jarow JP, Lurie P, Ikenberry SC, et al. Overview of FDA's Expanded Access Program for Investigational Drugs. Ther Innov Regul Sci. 2017;51(2):177-9.
10. Simmons Z. Right-to-Try Investigational Therapies for Incurable Disorders. Continuum (Minneap Minn). 2017;23(5, Peripheral Nerve and Motor Neuron Disorders):1451-7.
11. Brower V. Food and Drug Administration responds to pressure for expanded drug access. J Natl Cancer Inst. 2014;106(6):dju171.
12. Smart T. Expanded access and expanded trials. GMHC Treat Issues. 1996;10(1):8.
13. Servick K. Patient advocacy. 'Right to Try' laws bypass FDA for last-ditch treatments. Science. 2014;344(6190):1329.
14. Alcorn K, Nary G, Pernet AG, et al. Europeans outraged over expanded access. J Int Assoc Physicians AIDS Care. 1996;2(4):48-51.
15. Jung E, Zettler PJ, Kesselheim AS. Prevalence of Publicly Available Expanded Access Policies. Clin Pharmacol Ther. 2017.

Essay: The Uncompassionate Truth About Compassionate Use

Hannah Ducasse

A patient's life is drastically affected when their physician reduces their future down to a couple of months or weeks due to the effects of a severe medical condition. Whether caused by fear of death or determination to live, poignant desperation sinks in and this patient is frantic to find a solution. For some it may be simple: modern medicine provides an abundance of sufficient FDA-approved treatments for thousands of diseases. However, not all are afforded that luxury; If the severe medical condition has no readily available treatments on the market, what is the patient expected to do?

Compassionate Use, or Expanded Access, is a law that allows terminally ill patients to have early access to investigational drugs, bypassing the tedious Food and Drug Administration approval process—that every new molecular entity is required to endure. Although compassionate use is a gracious and humane law, some pharmaceutical companies find it to be unrealistic regarding the logistics of these requests. The controversy that surrounds this topic is a war of morality: compassion versus rigidity.

For a subject to be granted the benefit of compassionate use, they must be diagnosed with a severe condition that medical professionals deem irreversible even with the administration of current FDA-approved drugs and treatments.[1] They must have expended all FDA-approved treatment options with no luck and concluded to be unsuitable for any ongoing clinical trials before resorting to the Compassionate Use Program. In the years 2010–2014, over 9,000 applications have been sent with 99% of them being approved.[2] All these patients have experienced similar conversations with MDs assessing their declining health, having no options to offer. Physicians do not have a fool-proof method of calculating life expectancy and when a physician says you have 6 months left to live, they may be overshooting or undershooting. For these patients, the opportunity to try an experimental drug dictates which side of the life expectancy line they could fall on.

Although Expanded Access grants severely ill patients the chance to try a new drug, in no way does this opportunity warrant that the drug will be effective. There are a variety of factors that contribute to whether the treatment will work and allowing severely ill patients to try drugs that have, at most, passed Phase I trials, gives them false hope. The odds are stacked against them. Treatments that have merely been deemed safe for human ingestion are not very promising in becoming a life-saving miracle drug made just in time. Drugs at this stage in the clinical trial process generally have sufficient safety data and barely any efficacy data. More than 90% of drugs entering Phase I trials are eventually deemed unacceptable and those that do pass exhibit, at the most, minor improvements rather than life-saving cures[3]. Pharmaceutical companies may disfavor the Expanded Access law due to its requirement that all adverse events must be reported to the FDA regardless of whether it occurred in a clinical trial subject or an Expanded Access subject.[4] If a subject dies while on the non-approved treatment, this event could derail all efforts made towards approving the drug and releasing it onto the market. Even if the non-approved treatment were to have 100% efficacy—which is not possible, but for the sake of the example—in treating a specific condition, one major adverse event in an Expanded Access subject could condemn that company from exploring all future advancements. Because the FDA approval process takes anywhere from 10–20 years to complete, attending to a Compassionate Use subject may be a risk drug companies are not willing to take.

There are miracle stories where an experimental drug is administered to a desperately ill patient and works successfully in minimizing their condition or lengthening their life expectancy. People need to understand that these are truly miracles, rarities. Even when a Compassionate Use subject is administered a drug that exhibits significant improvements, it is not guaranteed that the manufacturer will provide this drug to the subject following the trials. The 21st Century Cures Act requires manufacturers to publicly state all needed information regarding expanded access opportunities, eligibility, and processes; however, it does not require that the manufacturer provide access to the investigational drug once the trial has been completed.[4] This omission raises major questions concerning the intentions of the Expanded Access program. The 21st Century Cures Act does promote awareness of compassionate use opportunities for many investigational drugs, yet it does not specify whether the drug itself should be provided following initial trials. Such situations have happened where the company ceases distribution as trials end and sudden discontinuation of the non-approved drug causes the subject's condition to revert back to its original state.[5] In these cases, families have turned to sharing this injustice on social media and news outlets in attempts of getting access to the drug again.

When put under the scrutiny of the public eye, pharmaceutical companies are often successfully coerced into releasing the drug. The distinction between a patient and a subject is a concept essential to understanding the seemingly harsh guidelines set by drug companies. A "patient" receives medical care from an MD whose goal is to rectify and alleviate the patient's condition whereas a "subject" is monitored by an MD whose goal is to obtain data for the treatment being tested.[6] Expanded access blurs the line between these terms, causing the dynamic between a clinical trial participant and a drug company to be misunderstood. It is not the company's responsibility to handle the subject's aftercare and their priority is strictly the approval of their drug. As miracle stories gain traction on social media, a certain detrimental mindset is fostered within the public: that access to all investigational drugs is a human right. The frequent occurrence of terminally ill patients using online petitions or social media campaigns engenders these warped mindsets.[7]

There are multiple reasons why a drug manufacturer would refrain from providing access of an experimental drug to a compassionate use participant. Because the drug is expensively synthesized to undergo clinical trials, manufacturers make small quantities of them and clinical trial subjects will always take priority over expanded access patients in consideration of the drug's FDA approval progress.[4] An unapproved drug is less likely to be covered by insurance companies and smaller drug companies may not have the financial capacity to provide access to the drug for a discounted price if the patient cannot pay for it. A special protocol must be made apart from the clinical trial format to accommodate the terminally ill subject and that may take hours—of which the drug company may not have. Such circumstances lead to expanded access applicants being rejected by the drug companies even prior to asking the FDA for permission.

The Compassionate Use Program has weak foundations and hypocritical regulations that counteract its intended purpose. No pharmaceutical company is required to comply with Expanded Access participants and a majority of them don't. If families must resort to social media awareness for gaining access to a drug that was effective in significantly improving life quality, then the Expanded Access Program is not accomplishing much. The current system is not beneficial enough to outweigh the emotional trauma caused by giving these dying people false hope. A terminally ill patient should have the right to try eligible experimental drugs; however, if the professedly humane Compassionate Use Law is substantially misleading desperate people through omitted information and loopholes, then that terminally ill patient would be better off living their last days with loved ones in peace.

Works Cited

1. Meyerson D. Medical Negligence Determinations, the "Right to Try," and Expanded Access to Innovative Treatments. J Bioeth Inq. 2017;14(3):385-400.
2. Walker S. Expanded Access Versus Right-to-Try. Hosp Pharm. 2020;55(2):79-81. Epub 20191025.
3. Gesme D. Should terminally ill patients have the right to take drugs that pass phase I testing? No. BMJ. 2007;335(7618):479.
4. Finkelstein PE. Expanded Access to Investigational Drugs: What Physicians and the Public Need to Know about FDA and Corporate Processes. AMA J Ethics. 2015;17(12):1142-6.
5. Goodman M. Twitter storm forces Chimerix's hand in compassionate use request. Nat Biotechnol. 2014;32(6):503-4.
6. Caplan AL, Bateman-House A. Should patients in need be given access to experimental drugs? Expert Opin Pharmacother. 2015;16(9):1275-9.
7. Mackey TK, Schoenfeld VJ. Going "social" to access experimental and potentially life-saving treatment: an assessment of the policy and online patient advocacy environment for expanded access. BMC Med. 2016;14:17.

Essay: How Compassionate is Compassionate Use?

Alena LaBree

The development and approval of a new drug is a lengthy process. On average, it takes 10–15 years for a drug to complete preclinical and clinical testing.[1] Then, the drug must be FDA approved before it can be marketed and used in patients. This lengthy timeline raises concerns for patients who are terminally ill and need treatment now as they may pass away before sufficient treatment becomes available to them. These patients cannot always enroll in clinical trials for the treatment they wish to receive because patients who are terminally ill usually do not meet the inclusion criteria.[2] Additionally, even if they were able to enroll in a clinical trial because of standard clinical trial designs, there could be only a 50% chance they will receive the new treatment. To combat these issues of clinical trial enrollment for a terminally ill patient, compassionate use (or expanded access) programs are offered. Compassionate use allows for seriously or terminally ill patients to be granted access to experimental new drugs currently in phase II or phase III clinical trials.[2] Compassionate use has become a popular idea and has gained much public support in recent years from social media. It is thought that compassionate use will benefit the terminally ill patient; however, this may not be the case and is possibly providing false hope.

On the surface, compassionate use seems like a great idea. If a treatment could potentially save someone's life, it seems cruel to refuse someone the ability to use it, especially when they provide consent for its use. However, while the patient must be fully informed of the unpredictable outcomes and possible risks of an experimental treatment and voluntarily consent to receive it, these patients are likely to underestimate the risks associated with an unapproved treatment.[3] Since the experimental treatments given under compassionate use typically have only gone through phase I clinical testing, there is likely

> "Expanded access is not drug development. The understanding of the safety and efficacy of experimental medicines is constantly evolving, and there are no guarantees that the drug will have the desired effect without undesired side effects."
>
> ─ Kenneth I. Moch

minimal safety data and relatively no efficacy data for the experimental treatment; thus, there is the potential that the drug given could be unsafe and inefficacious.[4] This can be especially harmful when given to a terminally ill patient with a very different physiology from the healthy individuals used to demonstrate the safety of the experimental drug in phase I trials. Additionally, many drugs that make it to phase III clinical trials fail to get approved because of failed efficacy or risky side effects, and even the drugs that do get approved do not work for everyone.[2] Therefore, the administration of experimental drugs to terminally ill patients is a bit of a guessing game as there is not a sure way to know if it will be efficacious and not cause more harm via side effects.

There is a significant difference between the use of an experimental drug in clinical trials versus in a compassionate use program. For clinical trials, the experimental drug is being administered for drug development research; however, for compassionate use programs, the purpose of administration is clinical treatment.[2] Therefore, while in both cases, a potentially unsafe and inefficacious drug is given, there are likely differences in the mindsets of individuals consenting to receive an experimental drug. Patients in need of compassionate use are commonly unable to be treated by current therapies on the market, so an unapproved drug is most likely their last resort; thus, patients may be more willing to consent to receive an experimental drug.[2,4] Furthermore, terminally ill patients may overestimate the benefits of the experimental drug, which could result in false hope as they may believe that a drug with potentially minimal efficacy data will be efficacious.[2,3]

Since pharmaceutical companies have control over their experimental drug, this could make it difficult for fair allocation of experimental drugs to terminally ill patients. Pharmaceutical companies do not have to provide their drug outside of clinical trials (many don't); when they do, they can allocate the drug in any way they prefer.[2] Because there is no widely-used system that drug companies use to grant compassionate use to terminally ill patients, this can complicate fair enrollment in compassionate use programs. Many patients may be unaware of the programs or may not have access to them, putting them at a disadvantage.

For patients who can access these programs, pharmaceutical companies commonly produce a limited supply, so decisions must be made as to which terminally ill patient is more qualified to receive the drug. Certain patients may be more social media savvy than others, making it easy for them to gain public support, which could influence a pharmaceutical company's decision. Unstandardized allocation of experimental drugs may also result in the exploitation of the terminally ill patient. Some pharmaceutical companies may require terminally ill patients in a compassionate use program to pay for an experimental drug, resulting in financial benefit for the pharmaceutical company.[2] For some patients, this may be another added financial burden that they are unable to pay for, potentially making less financially fortunate people unable to qualify for compassionate use programs.

Compassionate use programs have the potential to slow or even halt the drug development and approval process for an experimental drug.[4] Terminally ill patients using experimental drugs in compassionate use programs may have to report adverse effects to pharmaceutical companies.[4] While the FDA states these adverse effects will not be used against the pharmaceutical companies for decisions on the approval of the experimental drug, pharmaceutical companies may be skeptical and are reluctant to provide their experimental drugs for compassionate use.[4] If these compassionate use programs negatively affect the drug development of an experimental drug, this could prevent potentially lifesaving drugs from being approved and available to terminally ill patients who might benefit from them in the future.

As with most ethical issues, there is no one solution in determining if compassionate use is something that should continue. Experimental drugs indeed have the potential to benefit a terminally ill patient, but overall, the risks of an unapproved drug being used to treat a terminally ill patient seem to outweigh the benefits. Outside of clinical trials, patients who are not terminally ill would not be given the option to receive an experimental drug from which they could benefit due to an experimental drug's potentially unsafe and inefficacious nature. Therefore, terminally ill patients should not be regarded any differently in a treatment setting. Even though this experimental treatment may be their last resort, there is no guarantee that this drug will be lifesaving, and it could end up inflicting more harm through unpredictable side effects. The bottom line is that an unapproved drug has not yet demonstrated sufficient safety or efficacy data, and therefore, should probably not be used in patients outside of clinical trials. While the drug development and approval process are long, it is necessary to ensure a drug is safe and efficacious for clinical practice. Furthermore, it is important to protect the drug development process to ensure that potentially efficacious drugs can be available for future patients in need.

Works Cited

1. Williams CT. Food and Drug Administration Drug Approval Process: A History and Overview. Nurs Clin North Am. 2016;51(1):1-11. Epub 20160113.
2. Raus K. An analysis of common ethical justifications for compassionate use programs for experimental drugs. BMC Med Ethics. 2016;17(1):60.
3. Borysowski J, Gorski A. Compassionate use of unauthorized drugs: Legal regulations and ethical challenges. Eur J Intern Med. 2019;65:12-6. Epub 20190426.
4. Caplan AL, Bateman-House A. Should patients in need be given access to experimental drugs? Expert Opin Pharmacother. 2015;16(9):1275-9.

Essay: Compassionate Use of Drugs

Ines Studer

As of April 2022, there are more than 400,000 ongoing clinical trials globally. Of these trials, approximately 133,000 are US-based, a significant portion of which are interventional studies.[1-3] The time it takes for experimental drugs to be approved and become available in the United States is often a 10–15 year process, although there are significant variations.[4] The time-consuming aspect of the drug approval process is a controversial topic because there are many patients with terminal illnesses who are not approved for clinical trials, which is often their last hope. As a result, the Expanded Access Program, often referred to as "compassionate use", was created in addition to the more recent implementation of Right-to-Try laws. This allows some patients to take experimental drugs without enrolling in a clinical trial.[5-8]

Before clinical trials can begin, preclinical in vitro and in vivo studies must be conducted.[9] The primary objective is to determine if the drug has a favorable safety profile sufficient to justify human studies. Additionally, the pharmacokinetics, pharmacodynamics, and appropriate doses of the drug are investigated.[10, 11] If the data show that the drug is "reasonably safe," an investigational new drug application is submitted to the FDA. If the FDA approves the drug for human studies, a clinical trial ensues.[12] Clinical trials consist of four phases, and the trial can be terminated at any phase pending the data gathered. The main objective of the first phase is to determine if the drug is safe for human use and to obtain a dose-toxicity profile. This is often accomplished by administering the drug to 20–80 healthy subjects.[13, 14]

The second phase of the trial is intended to expand the drug's safety profile and investigate its efficacy in the population of interest.[15, 16] Phase three trials are generally much larger than the previous trials, ranging from 300 to 3,000 subjects. This phase is useful for further investigations of drug efficacy and for documenting common adverse events. At this time the drug is compared to the standard of care to determine its utility.[10, 17] Lastly, phase four trials occur after the FDA has approved the drug, and it is widely accessible. These are observational studies that are not always required; the researchers use the data gathered to document infrequent adverse events and further evaluate drug efficacy.[10, 18]

The Right-to-Try laws expanded on the compassionate use program. To be approved for the experimental therapy both programs require that the seriously or terminally patient must have exhausted the standard of care treatment options, be ineligible for clinical trials, and have a physician sponsor them.[12, 19, 20] A significant difference between the programs is that through Right-to-Try laws the patient, with physician oversight, is requesting access to the experimental drug directly from the manufacturer, without FDA involvement. Access to the experimental drug, for both programs, is dependent on manufacturer approval.[21]

As a result of this difficulty, some believe that a drug should be approved for open access following the determination of a favorable safety profile. While this desire is understandable, because for many it is the last glimmer of hope, it would not be an advisable decision. Knowing the efficacy of the drug is exceedingly important as there is a significant possibility that the drug will have no therapeutic effect on the disease or illness. This is evidenced by the lack of drug efficacy resulting in the termination of 52% of clinical trials from 2013 to 2015.[22] Additionally, while drugs may be considered safe, they will have undesired adverse events, resulting in the possibility of patients suffering from a drug that may have no therapeutic effect.[23]

Another point of controversy is whether patients can properly assess the risk-to-reward ratio of taking experimental drugs. While gaining access to these drugs requires a physician's support, there is the question of if the patient understands the high probability that the drug will be inefficacious and cause undesired adverse events. To combat this problem, a patient should attend a meeting in which someone verbally explains to them the probability that the drug will have no therapeutic effect, in addition to how severe the adverse events may be before they can gain access to the drug.

The cost of treatment is an important aspect to consider as well. Through clinical trials, if the subject enrolled has an insurance provider, their routine healthcare costs are covered by the Affordable Care Act.[24] However, under Right-to-Try laws, the patients must cover the cost of manufacturing and shipping, as there is no incentive for insurance companies to cover the costs associated with the treatment. Patients risk losing some health care coverage, their right to hospice care, and more.[25-29] This is a concern because the use of these experimental drugs increases the already heavy burden felt by these patients and their relatives. This also brings into question if patients with lesser means have equal access to experimental drugs. Unfortunately, it appears that they are not provided the same benefits as wealthy patients. This is because they likely cannot afford the high cost associated with these treatments or have comparable insurance coverage. It is not uncommon for people to have difficulty paying medical bills, but this should not be the deciding factor on whether someone receives the treatment or not.[30, 31]

Some argue that pharmaceutical companies should be obligated to provide the experimental drug to all terminal and seriously ill patients who request it. One of the reasons the manufacturer may not be willing to do this is the potential of a negative association with the drug if the patient dies or experiences a severe adverse event. Another consideration is that the price for access to the drug through this program may lead to speculation by others about the price set after the clinical trial. Finally, the lack of clarity regarding how the expanded access data will be used is a serious concern.[21, 25, 32] Regardless, the current system in which the company determines who has access to the drug seems to be the only logical option.

While allowing the ill to take the experimental drug may be seen as an act of compassion and reflect well on the company, it is not something that should be required. This is because it is a drug that the company developed financing it with its resources and it is its property. In the case that the government did not contribute financially to the research and development of the drug, it should not have a say on who is given access to the drug. The government's role is to grant permission to conduct clinical trials and to oversee the safety components of the research and clinical trials. However, if the manufacturer received government funding, the government should be able to participate in the decisions regarding which patients can take the drug. In the case that there was no government funding, there should be some sort of incentive to encourage manufacturers to allow patients to take the experimental drugs.

An additional concern is whether subjects who participated in clinical trials that yielded positive results should be provided the approved drug at no cost. While this is an understandable desire, I do not believe that they should receive the drug for free. However, if the insurance will not pay for the drug, they should be able to purchase it at the manufacturing cost. The subjects assumed the risk regardless of the outcome, furthering knowledge of how efficacious treatment is. Because of this, they deserve to be able to purchase the drug at a significantly reduced cost.

Works Cited

1. Trends, Charts, and Maps 2022 [4/12/2022]. Available from: https://clinicaltrials.gov/ct2/resources/trends.
2. Glossary of Common Site Terms 2022 [4/12/2022]. Available from: https://clinicaltrials.gov/ct2/about-studies/glossary.
3. Interventional Versus Observational Studies: What's the Difference? [4/14/2022]. Available from: https://www.cff.org/interventional-versus-observational-studies-whats-difference.
4. How long a new drug takes to go through clinical trials [4/12/2022]. Available from: https://www.cancerresearchuk.org/about-cancer/find-a-clinical-trial/how-clinical-trials-are-planned-and-organised/how-long-it-takes-for-a-new-drug-to-go-through-clinical-trials.
5. Investigational New Drug (IND) Application [4/12/2022]. Available from: https://www.fda.gov/drugs/types-applications/investigational-new-drug-ind-application.
6. Right to Try [4/12/2022]. Available from: https://www.fda.gov/patients/learn-about-expanded-access-and-other-treatment-options/right-try.
7. Borysowski J, Gorski A. Compassionate use of unauthorized drugs: Legal regulations and ethical challenges. Eur J Intern Med. 2019;65:12-6. Epub 20190426.
8. Jarow JP, Lurie P, Ikenberry SC, et al. Overview of FDA's Expanded Access Program for Investigational Drugs. Ther Innov Regul Sci. 2017;51(2):177-9.
9. Farrington P, Miller E. Clinical trials. Methods Mol Med. 2003;87:335-52.
10. Umscheid CA, Margolis DJ, Grossman CE. Key concepts of clinical trials: a narrative review. Postgrad Med. 2011;123(5):194-204.
11. Rich K. An overview of clinical trials. J Vasc Nurs. 2004;22(1):32-4.
12. Expanded Access [4/12/2022]. Available from: https://www.fda.gov/news-events/public-health-focus/expanded-access.

13. Ivy SP, Siu LL, Garrett-Mayer E, et al. Approaches to phase 1 clinical trial design focused on safety, efficiency, and selected patient populations: a report from the clinical trial design task force of the national cancer institute investigational drug steering committee. Clin Cancer Res. 2010;16(6):1726-36. Epub 20100309.
14. Diez Pascual C. Clinical Drug Trials: The Path to the Patient. Methods Mol Biol. 2021;2296:411-21.
15. Torres-Saavedra PA, Winter KA. An Overview of Phase 2 Clinical Trial Designs. Int J Radiat Oncol Biol Phys. 2022;112(1):22-9. Epub 20210804.
16. Winter K, Pugh SL. An investigator's introduction to statistical considerations in clinical trials. Urol Oncol. 2019;37(5):305-12. Epub 20190326.
17. Buyse M. Phase III design: principles. Chin Clin Oncol. 2016;5(1):10.
18. Cesana BM, Biganzoli EM. Phase IV Studies: Some Insights, Clarifications, and Issues. Curr Clin Pharmacol. 2018;13(1):14-20.
19. Brown B, Ortiz C, Dube K. Assessment of the Right-to-Try Law: The Pros and the Cons. J Nucl Med. 2018;59(10):1492-3. Epub 20180810.
20. Compassionate Drug Use [4/12/2022]. Available from: https://www.cancer.org/treatment/treatments-and-side-effects/clinical-trials/compassionate-drug-use.html.
21. Walker S. Expanded Access Versus Right-to-Try. Hosp Pharm. 2020;55(2):79-81. Epub 20191025.
22. Harrison RK. Phase II and phase III failures: 2013-2015. Nat Rev Drug Discov. 2016;15(12):817-8. Epub 20161104.
23. Finding and Learning about Side Effects (adverse reactions) [4/12/2022]. Available from: https://www.fda.gov/drugs/information-consumers-and-patients-drugs/finding-and-learning-about-side-effects-adverse-reactions.
24. Martin PJ, Davenport-Ennis N, Petrelli NJ, et al. Responsibility for costs associated with clinical trials. J Clin Oncol. 2014;32(30):3357-9. Epub 20140915.
25. Gabay M. RxLegal: A Rapid Review of Right-To-Try. Hosp Pharm. 2018;53(4):234-5. Epub 20180620.
26. Bateman-House A, Robertson CT. The Federal Right to Try Act of 2017-A Wrong Turn for Access to Investigational Drugs and the Path Forward. JAMA Intern Med. 2018;178(3):321-2.
27. Right to Try - Unapproved Drugs or Biologics [4/12/2022]. Available from: https://research.uci.edu/human-research-protections/clinical-research/drugs-and-biologics-used-in-clinical-research/right-to-try-drugs-biologics/.
28. Be Ready for Patient Questions about Right-to-Try and Expanded Access to Investigational Therapies With ASCO FAQ [4/12/2022]. Available from: https://connection.asco.org/magazine/features/be-ready-patient-questions-about-right-try-and-expanded-access-investigational#:~:text=Under%20expanded%20access%2C%20insurance%20companies,not%20provide%20these%20patient%20protections.
29. Corieri C. Everyone Deserves the Right to Try: Empowering the Terminally Ill to Take Control of their Treatment [4/12/2022]. Available from: http://goldwaterinstitute.org/wp-content/uploads/cms_page_media/2015/1/28/Right%20To%20Try.pdf.
30. Lee J, Cagle JG. A conceptual framework for understanding financial burden during serious illness. Nurs Inq. 2021:e12451. Epub 20210812.
31. Bielenberg JE, Futrell M, Stover B, et al. Presence of Any Medical Debt Associated With Two Additional Years of Homelessness in a Seattle Sample. Inquiry. 2020;57:46958020923535.
32. Klein R. Right to Try Legislation Should Focus on Patients, Not Politics. P T. 2018;43(3):147-8.

Topic: Medicating Others for Our Needs—Acceptable or Abuse?

The concept of social medication or the drugging of specific populations—notably pediatric and geriatric individuals—without their knowledge and/or consent is a real and current problem. Because these two populations are uniquely vulnerable in the context of awareness, their frequent inability to give informed consent, and the absolute differences in how drugs behave in each group compared to the general healthy adult population, this issue is highly controversial. Thus, the legal consequences of medicating these individuals for the benefit of others can be severe. The term for such drugging of individuals for purposes other than their direct benefit is "social medication" and although it is not uncommon, it is also not well studied in the scientific literature.

"...You need to have the compassion and caring for helping to protect vulnerable people."

Ellen Sauerbrey, former Head, US Department of State's Bureau of Population, Refugees, and Migration

Therefore, when the lay public is reminded of this issue, the cases presented in the media are often over-the-top egregious and malicious, obviously abusive, or arising from the most profound ignorance on the part of the perpetrators. When the media sensationalize these situations, they inflame the public's perception of the issue but fail to capitalize on the moment to educate their audience about the appropriate treatment of children and the elderly and why these special populations are unique. This is a missed opportunity to inform the public about critical aspects of pharmacology and it allows the cycle of social medication to continue. Until we engage in more responsible and science-based reporting, this trend will likely not change. When pediatric or elderly populations are medicated for reasons not tied to their safety, several areas of concern emerged in the context of social medication: consent or patient autonomy, pharmacokinetic differences in the populations treated, and incorrectly placed rationales given for drugging another person to make them more pliable and less problematic.

An extreme example of social medication was documented in the scientific literature in 2014 and involved kindergarten teachers in China. They administered antivirals to their small students to control hand-foot-mouth disease, a highly contagious illness that targets pediatric populations. Parents were outraged at this mistreatment and were not impressed that the drugging was to boost attendance by decreasing absences due to illness. Antivirals such as those used for hand-foot-mouth disease are prescription but they are inexpensive and available over-the-counter in China. So, adults can easily obtain sufficient amounts to treat entire classrooms, as is what occurred here.[1] Adults must give consent for children to be medically treated, and no consent was ever supplied. One acceptable area in which medication can be used on a child or adolescent to control his/her behavior is in the context of chemical restraint of a hospitalized person.[2] This is used if the individual is at risk of self-harm, but again parental consent is usually obtained prior to drugging. Only when a lifesaving procedure is being implemented is parental (or adult patient) consent expressly implied.

Likewise for many older adults lacking the ability to make medical decisions, treating them with drugs can be problematic to illegal because the elderly do have rights.[3] This does not seem to be accepted by the medical community who tends to ask for informed consent in a manner disproportionate to the patient's age—the younger elderly are asked permission for treatment but older elderly are less likely to be asked.[3] This is a concern because the elderly have the most chronic illnesses of any patient population and they require information about their diseases so that they can be included in treatment decisions. And the converse is true, too. The elderly have every right to refuse any treatment and they often do in a manner proportional to the number of co-morbidities that they have.[4-8] Therefore, the sicker an elderly patient is, the more likely that person is to request being the sole decision maker for care and then to refuse all treatments.

Not all social medication of children is to prevent communicable diseases. Reports appeared on television and in US newspapers describing daycare workers who administered melatonin to children to "calm them down" before their nap time.[9] Another center gave children the same supplement to induce sleep so that a worker could attend a tanning session.[10] The idea that melatonin, a non-drug supplement, may be safer than an actual pharmaceutical preparation is beyond the point. Daycare workers are required to have a high school diploma at most, so they are completely unqualified to prescribe or dispense drugs or supplements. Appropriately, daycare workers caught drugging children have been charged with first-degree criminal mistreatment.

Sadly, those daycare workers did not think that drugging the children in their care was inappropriate. They claimed that the medication was over-the-counter, so it must be safe.[9] Over-the-counter medications can cause disability and death, even though many laypersons do not consider them risky and as such, may overuse them to a dangerous degree.[11, 12] Severe toxicities have been caused by over-the-counter cold and cough medications, which have never been approved for children under six years-of-age. This is evidenced by emergency room visits after such drug administration to children.[13] Thus, parents may be ignorant of the potential severity of drug outcomes in non-adult individuals. Worse, when non-family individuals administer drugs to children whose medical history is unknown to them, and for whom they have no rights to treat at all, the risks increase exponentially. Then, there is little to no possibility that the drugging will be reported. So, if the child is harmed, she/he will likely not receive timely medical assistance.

Sometimes, social medication efforts occur in plain sight: on airplanes or on other forms of transportation when parents exploit the sedative effects of over-the-counter drugs to induce sleep in their children. Nursing homes, too, have been documented to use antipsychotic medication on non-psychotic patients to induce calm and compliant behavior. While the justification for these approaches appears to center on child and elderly "safety" and agreeableness, the fact remains that the purpose of

"The way the elderly are treated, and in some cases warehoused and medicated, rather than nurtured and listened to, is distressing."

🎗 Bill Nighy, award-winning British character actor

drugs is to treat or mitigate illness, not to control individuals. Thus, drugs are intended to benefit the treated person, not an untreated bystander, but this is how the drugs are being used every day. When parents of small children have been interviewed about medications used to sedate or reduce irritating behavior in their offspring, the drugs they used and their rationales for using them were misguided. Specifically, the reasons behind their use directly contradicted the actually indicated uses and the drugs given to the children never possessed the pharmacological properties the parents claimed they had.[14] This type of ignorance can cause organ failure or death of small children, so parents should be cautioned against drugging children with compounds they do not understand.

Finally, the small and the elderly are considered special patient populations by pharmacologists. Children are not small adults, so their bodies do not respond to medications in a manner similar to adults. Also, there are very few FDA-approved medications for pediatric purposes and this severely limits the variety of drugs that have known safety profiles for children. Adults who administer medications without pediatric approval to children are risking the health and life of the child as well as their status as legal guardians. Parents have been jailed for causing drug-induced accidents from the inappropriate medication of children. Child abuse allegations for parents who mistreat children with drugs may result in legal charges, penalties, and jail. Parents have virtually total control over minor children in their care, but this control does not include drugging children into stuporous submission.

Drugging the elderly appears to be concentrated on medicating problematic dementia patients, with Alzheimer's subjects being the most commonly mistreated. The combative behaviors exhibited by those with dementia stem from severe confusion and agitation and often elder care centers administer antipsychotic drugs with hopes that this will prevent the hitting, biting, and kicking common to aggressive demented patients.[15-18] Data show, however, that antipsychotics are never to be used in this manner.[19, 20] These drugs exacerbate dementia symptoms and can cause death. Antidepressants are also not to be used in the severely demented either.[20, 21] Having a cognitive disease is not the same as being depressed. Virtually no antidepressant has been approved to lift the mood of those with dementia, so using neurotransmitter-modulating drugs is malpractice and can have deadly consequences.[22] Finally, demented elderly people frequently act out because they have uncomfortable medical problems such as undiagnosed urinary tract infections, broken bones, painful feet, and bed sores.[23-25] Drugging them into compliance or sedation does not address the immediate cause of their aggression and it may even make it worse. In short, unnecessarily sedating the elderly is elder abuse.[26, 27]

Writing Prompts

- Should drugging "certain" patients be ok if they are disruptive to others?
  - What criteria should we apply?
- If you can consent to refuse care/medication, can this consent be labile (one day you are competent; the next day you are not)?
  - What diseases may cause this unusual fluctuating competency and ability to consent?
- Should religious objections be respected when they can result in a patient's death, especially if the religion has few adherents?
  - What if the "religion" is not one that the health care provider recognizes?
  - Could not people "make up" or invent this objection? How would we know?
- If a parent is caught socially medicating a child, should he/she be fined, imprisoned, or lose custody?
  - In what cases might these punishments be appropriate?
- If a parent presents to the ER with an obviously drugged child and the drugging points to the parents, should the police/social services be called?
  - Should all new parent classes include the topic of social drugging?
    - Could this be a role for medical and pharmacy students, to talk to parent groups?
- Should staff who drug the elderly be fired? Fined? Jailed?
  - Should the family of the elderly person be notified in writing about what occurred?
    - Often, they are the last to know what is being done to their loved one.
- Should social drugging education be offered to families with incompetent elders in care?
  - Should the competency evaluation for those elders be tied to the gravity of their situation?
  - Would a competency evaluation disenfranchise the illiterate, the scientifically illiterate, the uneducated, or the foreigner who may not share Western medicine's values?

Works Cited

1. Parry J. China to investigate widespread drugging of kindergarten children. BMJ. 2014;348:g2457.
2. Libal G, Plener PL, Fegert JM, et al. [Chemical restraint: management of aggressive behaviours in inpatient treatment--theory and clinical practice]. Prax Kinderpsychol Kinderpsychiatr. 2006;55(10):783-801.
3. Perez-Carceles MD, Lorenzo MD, Luna A, et al. Elderly patients also have rights. J Med Ethics. 2007;33(12):712-6.
4. Requarth JA. Informed Consent Challenges in Frail, Delirious, Demented, and Do-Not-Resuscitate Adult Patients. J Vasc Interv Radiol. 2015;26(11):1647-51.
5. Weinberger LE, Sreenivasan S, Garrick T. End-of-life mental health assessments for older aged, medically ill persons with expressed desire to die. J Am Acad Psychiatry Law. 2014;42(3):350-61.
6. Plawecki LH, Amrhein DW. When "no" means no: elderly patients' right to refuse treatment. J Gerontol Nurs. 2009;35(8):16-8.
7. Smith GP, 2nd. "Just say no!": the right to refuse psychotropic medication in long-term care facilities. Ann Health Law. 2004;13(1):1-35, table of contents.
8. Annas GJ, Glantz LH. The right of elderly patients to refuse life-sustaining treatment. Milbank Q. 1986;64(Suppl. 2):95-162.

9. Wilusz L. Des Plaines day care teachers charged with drugging kids with sleep aid. Chicago Sun Times. 2018.
10. Elizalde E. Oregon day care owner who drugged, abandoned kids to go tanning gets 21 years in prison Daily News. 2018.
11. Jones A. Over-the-counter analgesics: a toxicology perspective. Am J Ther. 2002;9(3):245-57.
12. Gunn VL, Taha SH, Liebelt EL, et al. Toxicity of over-the-counter cough and cold medications. Pediatrics. 2001;108(3):E52.
13. Goldman RD, Canadian Paediatric Society DT, Hazardous Substances C. Treating cough and cold: Guidance for caregivers of children and youth. Paediatr Child Health. 2011;16(9):564-9.
14. Allotey P, Reidpath DD, Elisha D. "Social medication" and the control of children: a qualitative study of over-the-counter medication among Australian children. Pediatrics. 2004;114(3):e378-83.
15. Koopmans RT, van der Molen M, Raats M, et al. Neuropsychiatric symptoms and quality of life in patients in the final phase of dementia. Int J Geriatr Psychiatry. 2009;24(1):25-32.
16. Rabinowitz J, Katz I, De Deyn PP, et al. Treating behavioral and psychological symptoms in patients with psychosis of Alzheimer's disease using risperidone. Int Psychogeriatr. 2007;19(2):227-40.
17. Rabinowitz J, Davidson M, De Deyn PP, et al. Factor analysis of the Cohen-Mansfield Agitation Inventory in three large samples of nursing home patients with dementia and behavioral disturbance. Am J Geriatr Psychiatry. 2005;13(11):991-8.
18. Rabinowitz J, Katz IR, De Deyn PP, et al. Behavioral and psychological symptoms in patients with dementia as a target for pharmacotherapy with risperidone. J Clin Psychiatry. 2004;65(10):1329-34.
19. Somers M, Rose E, Simmonds D, et al. Quality use of medicines in residential aged care. Aust Fam Physician. 2010;39(6):413-6.
20. Alexopoulos GS, Streim J, Carpenter D, et al. Using antipsychotic agents in older patients. J Clin Psychiatry. 2004;65 Suppl 2:5-99; discussion 100-2; quiz 3-4.
21. Drach LM. [Drug treatment of dementia with Lewy bodies and Parkinson's disease dementia--common features and differences]. Med Monatsschr Pharm. 2011;34(2):47-52; quiz 3-4.
22. Desai AK, Grossberg GT. Buspirone in Alzheimer's disease. Expert Rev Neurother. 2003;3(1):19-28.
23. Brodaty H, Ames D, Snowdon J, et al. A randomized placebo-controlled trial of risperidone for the treatment of aggression, agitation, and psychosis of dementia. J Clin Psychiatry. 2003;64(2):134-43.
24. Di Giulio P, Toscani F, Villani D, et al. Dying with advanced dementia in long-term care geriatric institutions: a retrospective study. J Palliat Med. 2008;11(7):1023-8.
25. Nicholson PW, Leeman AL, O'Neill CJ, et al. Pressure sores: effect of Parkinson's disease and cognitive function on spontaneous movement in bed. Age Ageing. 1988;17(2):111-5.
26. Ralph SJ, Espinet AJ. Use of antipsychotics and benzodiazepines for dementia: Time for action? What will be required before global de-prescribing? Dementia (London). 2017:1471301217746769.
27. Amad A, Geoffroy PA, Vaiva G, et al. [Personality and personality disorders in the elderly: diagnostic, course and management]. Encephale. 2013;39(5):374-82.

Essay: Use of Antipsychotics in Nursing Homes

Brianna Hunt

In nursing homes across the country, a troubling practice is occurring: care staff are sedating patients with antipsychotic medications to make them more "manageable." The caretakers are drugging patients for their own benefit, to the detriment of the patients who are already in a fragile state. As a result, residents of these nursing homes have become like zombies, unable to enjoy the remaining time they have with their families. There needs to be more harsh punishment in place for nursing home staff members that recklessly medicate their patients for their own personal gain.

It is no surprise that as we grow older, our bodies change and can become more fragile. Aging also changes the way the body interacts with drugs. Both the clearance rate of drugs and the distribution of drugs can be altered with aging.[1] Since most medications are tested in younger populations, using them to treat patients with a different pharmacokinetic profile (such as older patients) can result in unforeseen consequences.[1] Therefore, the creation of dosing regimens for elderly patients requires extra attention and care. Many nursing home staff members seem to ignore this, and instead, give elderly patients doses large enough to sedate them for hours at a time. Recklessly giving medication is also especially dangerous in these patients because most elderly patients have several comorbid conditions, and as a result, are taking multitudes of additional medications. There is a high potential for drug-drug interactions in these cases, which means extra care must be taken when prescribing new drugs to protect the patient's safety.[2] Unfortunately, the safety of these patients does not seem to be of concern to some staff members.

Antipsychotic drugs are indicated to treat schizophrenia and related disorders, yet they are being prescribed to elderly patients who do not have this condition.[3] This is because care staff are exploiting the drug for its side effect of sedation to control patients' behavior.[4] Patients with dementia do not benefit from receiving this medication, and it may cause severe adverse effects, even increasing the risk of death.[5] Although patients with dementia can sometimes be agitated or aggressive, this is no excuse for nurses to give them potentially dangerous medication simply so they will not have to deal with this behavior.

In almost every other healthcare setting, patients must consent to the treatment they are receiving. Why should elderly patients be treated any differently? The right to bodily autonomy does not just disappear once a person becomes old, so giving these patients these medications is violating their right to control what happens to their own body. If patients do not or cannot consent to being drugged, they should not be drugged. It seems so simple, yet care staff still value their own comfort and convenience over the very lives of the ones they supposedly care for.

Simply put, care providers must do what they signed up for. By taking this job, they agreed to provide care to these patients. Providing care means that they must treat their patients like people, rather than inconveniences that they must deal with. If they cannot handle "caring" for these people without sedating them for hours at a time, then they need to find a new profession. Patients with dementia can be agitated at times, especially if they are in an unfamiliar environment like a nursing home surrounded by strangers. The correct response is to treat these patients with compassion, not drug them so they cannot do or feel anything. There are plenty of nonpharmacological treatment options available, so these drugs are not necessary in these patients.[6]

Even after the FDA issued a black-box warning on certain antipsychotics indicating the dangers of prescribing them to dementia patients, in recent years the Centers for Medicare and Medicaid Services estimated that 16 percent of nursing home residents are being given off-label prescriptions for antipsychotic medications.[7] This is unacceptable. Currently, nursing homes only face modest consequences for these actions. They usually only have to pay a fine, and then they are allowed to continue with business as usual. In order to protect elderly patients, much more severe consequences must be put into place. Nurses who drug patients for their own convenience should, at the very least, be terminated and blacklisted from the industry. They have proven they cannot provide adequate care to patients, so they should no longer be permitted to work in a healthcare setting. More preferably, they should be jailed for essentially poisoning their patients. Elderly patients in nursing homes deserve to receive quality care, and we need to make sure healthcare professionals who violate this face real consequences.

Works Cited

1. Ishizawa Y, Yasui-Furukori N, Takahata T, et al. The effect of aging on the relationship between the cytochrome P450 2C19 genotype and omeprazole pharmacokinetics. Clin Pharmacokinet. 2005;44(11):1179-89.
2. Sinha A, Mukherjee S, Tripathi S, et al. Issues and challenges of polypharmacy in the elderly: A review of contemporary Indian literature. J Family Med Prim Care. 2021;10(10):3544-7. Epub 20211105.
3. Christian R, Saavedra L, Gaynes BN, et al. Future Research Needs for First- and Second-Generation Antipsychotics for Children and Young Adults. Rockville (MD)2012.
4. Dyer AH, Murphy C, Lawlor B, et al. Sedative Load in Community-Dwelling Older Adults with Mild-Moderate Alzheimer's Disease: Longitudinal Relationships with Adverse Events, Delirium and Falls. Drugs Aging. 2020;37(11):829-37. Epub 20200914.
5. Muhlbauer V, Mohler R, Dichter MN, et al. Antipsychotics for agitation and psychosis in people with Alzheimer's disease and vascular dementia. Cochrane Database Syst Rev. 2021;12:CD013304. Epub 20211217.
6. Kalisch Ellett LM, Lim R. We need to do better: most people with dementia living in aged care facilities use antipsychotics for too long, for off-label indications and without documented consent. Int Psychogeriatr. 2020;32(3):299-302.

7. Introcaso D. The Never-Ending Misuse of Antipsychotics In Nursing Homes: Health Affairs; 2018 [cited 2022].

Essay: The Dangers of Moving Towards Treatment

Aileen Muñoz

It is strange to exist in a body with little to no knowledge of its functions. After all, not everyone is an expert in physiology and anatomy. So, it can be worrisome when something seems to be amiss, such as an older adult experiencing chest pain. For most in such a situation, the solution is to reach out to a physician for care. In some cases, the physician may have an answer, such as medication or surgery. In other cases, the physician may have no fast solution, which is unlikely to be what the patient wants to hear. In either case, a need for treatment has provoked a complex phenomenon of medicalization. Whether it stems from personal gain or a feeling of pressure, physicians recommend treatments that have no benefits and may instead cause harm. Additionally, normal human behaviors and bodily functions are becoming diseases requiring treatment.

When it comes to mental health, there are many blurry lines regarding treatment and even diagnosis. The DSM-V offers criteria for diagnosis, and there are many overlaps between differing diagnoses.[1] Since there are already many medications available to those who do get diagnosed with mental health disorders, the current trend seems to be to expand the indications for the drugs already available for these disorders.[2] Recently, prolonged grief disorder was added to the DSM-V as a disorder that requires treatment.[3] Among the diagnosis criteria, a year after the loss is experiencing intense intrusive thoughts, pangs of severe negative emotions, and maladaptive loss of interest in hobbies.[4]

This classification sets the condition apart from a major depressive disorder. Consequently, investigators have begun researching the efficacy of different treatments for the new condition. Reynolds and colleagues found that nortriptyline, a tricyclic antidepressant, was efficacious in causing remission for prolonged grief disorder and it had an even greater effect when combined with psychotherapy. However, the sample sizes for their treatment groups are small. The largest sample size was the treatment group receiving medication and this group only enrolled 14 subjects.[5] This is worrisome because often, these numbers are overlooked. We should not ignore these numbers because medications cause side effects, especially when combined with other medications. So, it is not in a patient's best interest to place them on drugs that might be unnecessary.

Furthermore, Simon and colleagues researched the effect of antidepressants when combined with two different psychotherapies: targeted psychotherapy for CG (CGT) and interpersonal therapy (IP). The data show that antidepressant use made subjects more likely to complete CGT but had no effect on the completion of IP (in fact, it had the opposite effect).[6] Some might interpret this as support for antidepressant use combined with therapy. However, perhaps the results have less to do with the medication and more with the efficacy of the psychotherapy. Psychotherapies are efficacious in treating mental disorders, and they are more cost-effective when compared to the addition or replacement of medications.[7] We should not be steering towards attempting to medicalize every condition created, and instead, we should try to offer services that will treat the problem at the root, as is the case with psychotherapy.

Is it worse to do nothing or to receive unnecessary treatment? The anxiety over doing nothing compels some people to want whatever treatment is available. For others, a quick google search might cause them to avoid any treatments unless they are necessary. On the one hand, receiving unnecessary treatment does not always result in life-threatening consequences, but they often result in negative drawbacks. For instance, Dr. Atul Gawande recounts an encounter with a patient who was advised she had a lump on her thyroid and the best thing to do would be to remove her thyroid gland entirely. Gawande advised that the lump was unlikely to cause harm and recommended just watching it for any sign of progression. Still, the knowledge of the existence of the lump made the patient anxious and made doing nothing impossible for her. Gawande moved forward with the surgery and found that the lump was benign. Luckily the patient had no adverse reactions to the surgery but would now have to take thyroid replacement for the rest of her life.[8] This was the best-case scenario.

In contrast, there are cases when unnecessary treatments result in death. Dr. David Brown encountered a patient who had recovered from Hodgkin's lymphoma but was left with severe scarring over his lungs that was suffocating him. This patient had experienced difficulties with respiration earlier on and had received treatment at a different hospital. At that hospital, a cardiologist had concluded that his labored breathing stemmed not from the scarring on the lungs caused by lymphoma but instead from a blocked artery. So, the physician implanted a stent for the supposed blocked artery. When this patient arrived was seen by Dr. Brown and received a proper diagnosis, the post-stent medications delayed the appropriate surgery due to the risk of complications. This delay resulted in the patient's death.[9] In either case, the consequences differed in severity, but it turned out worse to receive unnecessary treatment either way.

The two cases present different dilemmas in medicine. In the first case, there is the danger of overdiagnosis. As medical technology progresses, many scans have been made available. This was the case for Dr. Gawande's patient. The patient was not misdiagnosed, but if she had not been diagnosed in the first place, there would have been no harm to her, and she would not be on thyroid medication for the rest of her life. With improved technology, there has been an increase in the detection of cancers, but no decline in interval cancers (which tend to be more aggressive) and possibly an increase in false positives.[10, 11] Interval cancers are cancers that are detected in between two scheduled screenings and tend to be more malignant than those that are detected on screens. An increase in screening has led to the detection of more tumors, but not all tumors are malignant, hence the stability of interval cancers.[11] However, being told that a tumor has been found increases anxiety, even if it is known to be benign, causing many patients to want treatment.[12] There is no completely normal person. So, the various available tests make it easy to find abnormalities. These abnormalities typically cause no harm, but that can be hard to believe for a patient. In these instances, physicians move forward with screenings to reassure themselves and the patient but can end up causing more anxiety in doing so.[13]

In the second case, there is the use of a treatment that has been shown to have no medical benefits. This often happens with revascularization for those who have stable ischemic heart disease. Research shows that when the condition is stable, invasive procedures have no health benefits when compared to simply relying on non-invasive medical therapies.[14, 15] In the instance of Dr. Brown's patient, moving forward with these unnecessary invasive treatments does more harm than good. There are many reasons why a physician might choose to do such a procedure, such as fee-for-service, a dismissal of clinical research, or patient pressure. When there are incentives, people will go after the incentives. For instance, if a physician is paid per service instead of providing improved health, their first option will be to recommend the procedure.[16] This has held for many physicians paid by service when it comes to treatment for carotid stenosis.[17] Also, many physicians tend to move forward with invasive treatments because they believe them to be "bio-plausible," which means that, in theory, the procedure should work. However, many clinical trials have proven otherwise.[9, 15] When combined, the incentives and misguided ideology result in recommended procedures that are unlikely to benefit the patient.

Finally, a physician might move forward with a procedure they do not recommend just to appease a patient. For example, when Dr. Gawande removed his patient's thyroid gland because of her anxiety, he did so because she was adamant in her desire for treatment.[8] Physicians can and have been sued for a failure to provide service, which creates a reasonable fear of undertreatment that could result in a lawsuit.[9] So, when they feel pressured by their patients, some will go against their judgment and prescribe according to the patient's expectations.[18] These are just some of the reasons unnecessary procedures are green-lighted. As a society with access to so much information on a little screen, we should be moving away from such procedures when information opposing any supposed benefits is readily available.

Not every abnormality requires treatment. In fact, most abnormalities do not require treatment. However, our increasing ability to find abnormalities causes anxiety in those who are found to have something abnormal. In this case, technology is a double-edged sword. Physicians should be aware of this and move forward with the intent to educate themselves and their patients about this phenomenon. Also, providing surgery or recommending medication should never be the first suggestion made to a patient, unless and until their symptoms indicate it is the best option.

Works Cited

1. Brus MJ, Solanto MV, Goldberg JF. Adult ADHD vs. bipolar disorder in the DSM-5 era: a challenging differentiation for clinicians. J Psychiatr Pract. 2014;20(6):428-37.
2. Alexander GC, Gallagher SA, Mascola A, et al. Increasing off-label use of antipsychotic medications in the United States, 1995-2008. Pharmacoepidemiol Drug Saf. 2011;20(2):177-84. Epub 20110106.
3. Lombardo L, Lai C, Luciani M, et al. [Bereavement and complicated grief: towards a definition of Prolonged Grief Disorder for DSM-5]. Riv Psichiatr. 2014;49(3):106-14.
4. Horowitz MJ, Siegel B, Holen A, et al. Diagnostic criteria for complicated grief disorder. Am J Psychiatry. 1997;154(7):904-10.

5. Reynolds CF, 3rd, Miller MD, Pasternak RE, et al. Treatment of bereavement-related major depressive episodes in later life: a controlled study of acute and continuation treatment with nortriptyline and interpersonal psychotherapy. Am J Psychiatry. 1999;156(2):202-8.
6. Simon NM, Shear MK, Fagiolini A, et al. Impact of concurrent naturalistic pharmacotherapy on psychotherapy of complicated grief. Psychiatry research. 2008;159(1-2):31-6. Epub 2008/03/12.
7. Myhr G, Payne K. Cost-effectiveness of cognitive-behavioural therapy for mental disorders: implications for public health care funding policy in Canada. Can J Psychiatry. 2006;51(10):662-70.
8. Gawande A. Overkill The New Yorker2015 [cited 2022]. Available from: https://www.newyorker.com/magazine/2015/05/11/overkill-atul-gawande.
9. Epstein D. When Evidence Says No, But Doctors Say Yes ProPublica2017 [cited 2022]. Available from: https://www.propublica.org/article/when-evidence-says-no-but-doctors-say-yes.
10. van Bommel RMG, Weber R, Voogd AC, et al. Interval breast cancer characteristics before, during and after the transition from screen-film to full-field digital screening mammography. BMC cancer. 2017;17(1):315-.
11. Brawley OW, Paller CJ. Overdiagnosis in the Age of Digital Cancer Screening. Journal of the National Cancer Institute. 2021;113(1):1-2.
12. Keyzer-Dekker CMG, van Esch L, de Vries J, et al. An abnormal screening mammogram causes more anxiety than a palpable lump in benign breast disease. Breast cancer research and treatment. 2012;134(1):253-8. Epub 2012/03/21.
13. Gordon M. Why Do Doctors Overtreat? For Many, It's What They're Trained To Do NPR2019 [cited 2022]. Available from: https://www.npr.org/sections/health-shots/2019/04/19/715113208/why-do-doctors-overtreat-for-many-its-what-they-re-trained-to-do.
14. Maron DJ, Hochman JS, O'Brien SM, et al. International Study of Comparative Health Effectiveness with Medical and Invasive Approaches (ISCHEMIA) trial: Rationale and design. Am Heart J. 2018;201:124-35. Epub 20180421.
15. Maron DJ, Hochman JS, Reynolds HR, et al. Initial Invasive or Conservative Strategy for Stable Coronary Disease. The New England journal of medicine. 2020;382(15):1395-407. Epub 2020/03/30.
16. DuBois JM, Chibnall JT, Anderson EE, et al. Exploring unnecessary invasive procedures in the United States: a retrospective mixed-methods analysis of cases from 2008-2016. Patient Saf Surg. 2017;11:30-.
17. Nguyen LL, Smith AD, Scully RE, et al. Provider-Induced Demand in the Treatment of Carotid Artery Stenosis: Variation in Treatment Decisions Between Private Sector Fee-for-Service vs Salary-Based Military Physicians. JAMA Surg. 2017;152(6):565-72.
18. Macfarlane J, Holmes W, Macfarlane R, et al. Influence of patients' expectations on antibiotic management of acute lower respiratory tract illness in general practice: questionnaire study. BMJ (Clinical research ed). 1997;315(7117):1211-4.

Topic: There is A Drug for That!

As pharmaceutical innovation and advances in medical care emerge, society is undergoing a slow but likely irreversible iatrogenesis, or the medicalization of what was once a simple consequence of being human.[1] Indeed, as we move from birth to death, processes that were once deemed acceptable and normal bodily functions are being scrutinized as problems that require interventions. Having a long life or aging is no longer focused on acquiring wisdom and experience but now it is a pathological journey that requires treatment at every juncture. Interestingly, this phenomenon appears to be a chiefly US controversy and it consistently includes medicalization of natural life events, engagement in wish-fulfilling medicine, and the promotion of disease mongering.

The idea of medicalizing something is legitimate, and this term was conceptualized by the World Health Organization in 1946.[2] At this time, however, the concept of medicalization has allowed patients to transition into "clients", thereby shifting their personal responsibilities and expectations to healthcare. For instance, childbirth, once a normal consequence of pregnancy now must be guarded by health professionals because this most natural of human acts is now considered very dangerous for mother and child.[3,4] Never mind that humanity began and flourished without medically assisted birth for centuries; a hospital birth is considered most prudent. Thus, traditional home birth is seen as the height of irresponsibility.[5]

> "Modern medicine is a negation of health. It is not organized to serve human health, but only itself, as an institution. It makes more people sick than it heals."
>
> Ivan Illich, Croatian-Austrian philosopher, Roman Catholic priest, and critic of modern Western cultural institutions

Then, during childhood, conceptual medicalization may occur—a child's tantrum is now categorized as "oppositional defiant disorder" and wanting of intervention. Next, a child who fidgets during a non-stimulating school environment may be drugged to reduce a perceived attention deficit hyperactivity disorder.[6] Then, teens who are shy are suddenly "socially avoidant" and in need of medication.[7] Finally, often, a single candid interaction with medical personnel can create a "diagnosis" that is added to the patient chart as a billable item. Once "documented", this "issue" then transforms a simple personal inquiry while making conversation into a pathology with a permanent label such as alcoholism or obesity.[1]

Other aspects of being human that are being medicalized for dubious purposes include aging and all of the attendant diseases and decrepitude that go with it.[8] That aging medicine is not an official specialty recognized by the American Medical Association is telling: at least some physicians are drawing the line at overreaching medicalization of the straightforward process of getting older. Thus, women fight aging with a host of personal care products, supplements, prescription medications, and experimental hormone therapies all designed to "rebalance" the body as if aging could be cured. Men are not immune to this nonsense either: andropause, the male counterpart to female menopause, is getting attention from cash-only clinics that promise to restore hair, muscular physiques, vigor, and libido with expensive pharmaceutical products, many of which are not FDA-approved for this use.

Interestingly, when a group of men was asked if they were aware of andropause and whether a therapy could be applied to it, few actually knew the term.[9] Thus, marketing for these novel disease states is being created or outright invented, likely for the financial gain of those supplying the tests and treatments. Then, targeting men and woman about life changes that bring the most heartache—the loss of sexual function—clever healthcare providers and Pharma have created an innovative area of care referred to as "couplepause" and expensive treatments that insurance will not cover are suggested.[10]

Next, wish-fulfilling medicine, or the use of drugs to improve non-pathological issues, such as to increase wakefulness, reduce a few vanity pounds, or medicate stressful insomnia, is shifting the landscape of medical care. This pattern creates continual pressure for physicians to listen to self-diagnosed clients who demand a drug they have seen on the television or read about in a popular magazine.[11] An indirect consequence of medicalization of every human wobble in emotional or physical health may be the lifting of personal responsibility for self-care or self-harm to an external locus of control: a physician, clinic, or hospital.

Indeed, if eating too much is not a bad habit but an addiction, then the blame rests not on the person overconsuming food. Rather, these people are victims of an illness for which they should seek and receive treatment, and ideally, insurance should cover it. Other behaviorally induced ills have already been medicalized with an emphasis on drug treatment (costly and potentially risky) instead of a lifestyle intervention (often free with immediate effect) such as high blood pressure, high cholesterol, and type II diabetes.

Finally, the term "disease mongering" is the creation of problems by drug companies so the client feels the need for a drug product to correct the new illness.[12, 13] A better term for this phenomenon may be "treatment expansions" as these are often additional drug uses for lifestyle factors that predispose the individual to a greater risk of future disease.[14] For instance, osteopenia, or less than optimal bone strength, is not a disease. However, pharmaceutical companies market expensive drugs to improve bone strength and to prevent the inevitable (as the patient is led to believe) loss of bone and subsequent osteoporosis, fractures, and death.[15, 16] Likewise, erectile dysfunction, which is chiefly a consequence of poor cardiovascular health, is not a disease. It may not even be a true life-limiting disability that requires medication, but the drugs to treat it are blockbusters (generating more than one billion dollars in revenue). Then, we are beginning to see drugs being promoted to mitigate side effects of *other drugs*, a comical cycle of polypharmacy at its worst. Improved recognition and management of disorders are laudable but commercial interests distort how we define treatable illnesses and burden publicly funded healthare systems.[17] So, physicians should resist these efforts to invent diseases and then suggest expensive therapies.[14]

Interestingly, this medicalization of humanity is a predominantly Western issue. Less industrialized or resource-rich countries are likely unable to meet the demand for services and goods tied to manufactured illnesses. Then, because drugs are the most expensive in the US, artificially expanding markets strains the economy. For countries with barely sufficient resources to treat patients now, inflating the need for health services could create an imbalance as demand outstrips supply.[2] Physicians are already spending little time with truly ill patients. Also, once we begin to medicalize something, reversing this trend is impossible.

Writing Prompts

- Should we keep medicalizing everything that bothers us?
  - E.g., defiant oppositional disorder is really crummy kid behavior!
- Are we disease mongering?
  - We cannot effectively treat current diseases, so let's invent some (social anxiety disorder, female sexual dysfunction, restless legs syndrome, night eating syndrome, extreme exam anxiety).
  - Is this a form of disease sponsorship?
- Is medicalization paternalistic?
  - Here, take this drug (my choice for your behavior).
- Is medicalization suggesting some classes are helpless?
  - E.g., you cannot help but take another (and another and another) bite; take this drug to lose weight!
- Are we using social control by drugging people out of unacceptable behavior?
  - Is someone with kleptomania just being bad?
  - Is an obese person refusing to abide by social body-size constructs?
- Are we moving from a democracy to a "pharmacracy"?
- Should we reverse course and demand people change the habits that cause them to be ill?
  - What carrot or sticks can we use to achieve this?
- Should we stop investing in pharmacological remedies for "social ills"?
  - Diabetes, obesity, depression, ADHD, low libido, alcoholism, drug addiction, smoking.
- Should we instead focus on diseases we cannot control?
  - Alzheimer's, heritable and gene-mediated diseases, childhood diseases.
- Should we restrict drugs to diseases that cause pain and premature death?
- Should we stop treating "incidentalomas"?
- If we continue to pharmacologically treat all human predicaments, should we disallow insurance to cover the disease of choice?
  - Can we make these drugs cost significantly more (social tax)?
- Is medicine being used to pursue health or disease?
  - For example, now we take Botox for wrinkles, Viagra for an erection, Paxil for shyness, Prozac for grief, Rogaine for hair loss, Ritalin for focus, and Buspar for anxiety...are we now seeking happiness from drugs?

- What is the role of "public awareness campaigns" for conditions manufactured by Pharma?

Works Cited

1. Maturo A. Medicalization: current concept and future directions in a bionic society. Mens Sana Monogr. 2012;10(1):122-33.
2. Blasco-Fontecilla H. Medicalization, wish-fulfilling medicine, and disease mongering: toward a brave new world? Rev Clin Esp (Barc). 2014;214(2):104-7.
3. Christiaens W, Van De Velde S, Bracke P. Pregnant women's fear of childbirth in midwife- and obstetrician-led care in Belgium and the Netherlands: test of the medicalization hypothesis. Women Health. 2011;51(3):220-39.
4. Fano V. [The medicalization of delivery and the time of birth]. Epidemiol Prev. 1996;20(2-3):96-8.
5. Shaw JC. The medicalization of birth and midwifery as resistance. Health Care Women Int. 2013;34(6):522-36.
6. Searight HR, McLaren AL. Attention-deficit hyperactivity disorder: The medicalization of misbehavior. J Clin Psychol Med S. 1998;5(4):467-95.
7. Wilberg T. Avoidant personality, cluster A traits and Taijin kyofusho: Deconstructing a treatment resistant socially fearful young man: A commentary on a case by Maruta et al. Personal Ment Health. 2012;6(3):276-8.
8. Gladyshev TV, Gladyshev VN. A Disease or Not a Disease? Aging As a Pathology. Trends Mol Med. 2016;22(12):995-6.
9. Samipoor F, Pakseresht S, Rezasoltani P, et al. Awareness and experience of andropause symptoms in men referring to health centers: a cross-sectional study in Iran. Aging Male. 2017;20(3):153-60.
10. Jannini EA, Nappi RE. Couplepause: A New Paradigm in Treating Sexual Dysfunction During Menopause and Andropause. Sex Med Rev. 2018.
11. Robinson AR, Hohmann KB, Rifkin JI, et al. Direct-to-consumer pharmaceutical advertising: physician and public opinion and potential effects on the physician-patient relationship. Arch Intern Med. 2004;164(4):427-32.
12. Wolinsky H. Disease mongering and drug marketing. Does the pharmaceutical industry manufacture diseases as well as drugs? EMBO Rep. 2005;6(7):612-4.
13. Moynihan R, Heath I, Henry D. Selling sickness: the pharmaceutical industry and disease mongering. BMJ. 2002;324(7342):886-91.
14. Doran E, Henry D. Disease mongering: expanding the boundaries of treatable disease. Intern Med J. 2008;38(11):858-61.
15. Wright J. Marketing disease: is osteoporosis an example of 'disease mongering'? Br J Nurs. 2009;18(17):1064-7.
16. Sambrook P, Stenmark J. The pharmaceutical industry and disease mongering. Authors were incorrect in their comments about Osteoporosis Australia. BMJ. 2002;325(7357):216; author reply
17. Vance MA. Disease mongering and the fear of pandemic influenza. Int J Health Serv. 2011;41(1):95-115.

Essay: Medicalization of Everything

Ines Studer

Health is defined as "a state of complete physical, mental, and social well-being."[1] In the pursuit of good health, more than 20,000 prescription drugs have been approved in the United States.[2] This significant number of drugs were created to combat many diseases, but this begs the question of what warrants a disease being pharmaceutically treated. An example of this is obesity, which is responsible for approximately 400,000 deaths in the US, annually.[3] For this disease prevention is of the utmost importance, as evidenced by successful long-term weight loss occurring in only 20% of obese people.[4] Anti-obesity medications are hardly a cure, as the percent weight loss after one year is approximately 2.9% to 6.8% depending on which of the 6 weight loss drugs is being evaluated.[5] The prevalence of anti-obesity medications and treatments in combination with the high frequency of obesity are evidence that there is a larger emphasis placed on treating a disease as opposed to preventing it. This is likely a result of the treatment of obesity being more profitable than its prevention. In the US alone, $100 billion is spent annually on the treatment of obesity and its adverse effects.[6]

> "The highly successful medical model promises cures for many diagnostic entities. A dilemma is created when this model exceeds its scope and fails to meet its promise ... The pervasiveness of the medical model for solving all our ills is the issue we must confront."
>
> Ed Jones, PhD, senior VP for the Institute for Health and Productivity Management

Pharmaceutical interventions are commonplace, with 131 million US adults taking prescription drugs.[7] Obesity is a clear example of a preventable disease that frequently requires further medical treatment. There is a question of whether we should, or even can, require people to change their bad habits and prevent these diseases. While the need for change is evident, there is no ethical way to require people to change. However, campaigns and programs promoting healthier lifestyles could be beneficial in the long term, resulting in a decreased frequency of pharmaceutical interventions and preventable diseases.

There are many diseases that are likely a product of disease-mongering, such as compulsive buying disorder and oppositional defiant disorder. Compulsive buying disorder (CBD) is characterized by excessive shopping despite significant consequences. Oppositional defiant disorder is resistant, vindictive, and argumentative behavior in children.[8, 9] It is debatable if diseases such as these qualify as legitimate medical conditions or if they are common human behaviors and emotions. Conditions such as CBD are profitable for pharmaceutical companies, as the treatment may warrant pharmaceutical intervention. This brings into question whether disease-mongering should be considered a method of social control. However, this does not seem to be the case, as many of these diseases affect consenting adults, who have the right to decline treatment at will.

An interesting proposal is whether resources should be diverted from social illnesses, such as obesity and ADHD, to prevalent conditions for which we do not have efficacious treatments. While resources should be reallocated from disorders such as CBD, they should not be redirected from all social illnesses. Conditions such as obesity are significant and can result in adverse effects that require additional medical treatment. Depending on the severity of the case, many of these illnesses warrant treatment. Prevention is exceedingly important and resources should be directed here to minimize the frequency of the condition.

In the US, there is a prevalence of commonly performed, yet unnecessary, medical procedures conducted to appease patients. Some examples of this are the use of IV fluids in the treatment of intoxicated patients in the Emergency Room and cleansing wounds with saline as opposed to tap water. Data show that IV fluids are inefficacious in reducing how long intoxicated patients remain in the ER, and that tap water is as efficacious, if not more, than saline in cleansing acute injuries.[10, 11] It has been reported that approximately 20% of healthcare procedures in the US are unnecessary, this is a significant contributor to high healthcare costs.[9] There should be a larger emphasis placed on investigating whether current treatments are efficacious and eliminating the practices that hold no purpose.

Works Cited

1. WHO. WHO remains firmly committed to the principles set out in the preamble to the Constitution [5/3/2022]. Available from: https://www.who.int/about/governance/constitution.
2. Fact Sheet: FDA at a Glance 2020 [5/2/2022]. Available from: https://www.fda.gov/about-fda/fda-basics/fact-sheet-fda-glance.
3. Hurt RT, Frazier TH, McClave SA, et al. Obesity epidemic: overview, pathophysiology, and the intensive care unit conundrum. JPEN J Parenter Enteral Nutr. 2011;35(5 Suppl):4S-13S.
4. Wing RR, Phelan S. Long-term weight loss maintenance. Am J Clin Nutr. 2005;82(1 Suppl):222S-5S.
5. NIDDK. Prescription Medications to Treat Overweight & Obesity [5/2/2022]. Available from: https://www.niddk.nih.gov/health-information/weight-management/prescription-medications-treat-overweight-obesity.
6. Panuganti KK, Nguyen M, Kshirsagar RK. Obesity. StatPearls. Treasure Island (FL)2022.
7. Prescription Drugs [5/2/2022]. Available from: https://hpi.georgetown.edu/rxdrugs/.
8. Ghosh A, Ray A, Basu A. Oppositional defiant disorder: current insight. Psychol Res Behav Manag. 2017;10:353-67. Epub 20171129.
9. Carroll AE. The High Costs of Unnecessary Care. JAMA. 2017;318(18):1748-9.

10. Fernandez R, Griffiths R. Water for wound cleansing. Cochrane Database Syst Rev. 2012(2):CD003861. Epub 20120215.
11. Perez SR, Keijzers G, Steele M, et al. Intravenous 0.9% sodium chloride therapy does not reduce length of stay of alcohol-intoxicated patients in the emergency department: a randomised controlled trial. Emerg Med Australas. 2013;25(6):527-34. Epub 20131108.

Essay: The Risks of Overprescribing and Self-Medication

Baden Cruickshank

In the face of discomfort, perceived illness, or any number of other ailments many turn to their healthcare provider for prescription drugs or their nearest drug store for over-the-counter (OTC) drugs. There has been an increase in prescription drug use in the past few decades, from under 40% of US adults taking at least one prescription drug per month in the 1990s, to nearly 50% in 2018, with an even greater proportional increase in the number of US adults taking greater than one prescription drug per month in the same period.[1] The prevalence of OTC drug use is even higher in the US, with nearly 80% of adults consuming them regularly, a value even higher in younger adults and students.[2] The pharmaceutical industry stands to benefit from such large numbers of US adults regularly consuming medications, and thus uses the fears of patients for financial gain.

The pharmaceutical industry is well known to care more about making a profit than helping patients with their legitimate health problems and often uses disease-mongering to increase profits while taking advantage of consumers. Disease mongering is a marketing strategy used by the pharmaceutical industry to manipulate perfectly healthy patients into believing that they are sick and require medication to improve their condition.[3,4] By manipulating the accepted definition of a disease and advertising that manipulated definition, pharmaceutical companies can increase sales of their drugs at the expense of the consumer.[5] This often results in the over-prescription of drugs such as statins, antidepressants, and stimulants due to encouragement by pharmaceutical companies for physicians to diagnose patients and prescribe a drug, and for patients to believe that they have a disease that requires treatment.

These patients that have been tricked by pharmaceutical companies may pressure their prescriber for a prescription that they do not need and may receive a drug that will not benefit them at all. Statin use has been promoted through this method, with lower and lower guidelines being set for "normal" blood cholesterol, which in turn increases the population of patients who may "require" treatment to lower their blood cholesterol to "normal" levels.[6] This manipulation of consumers and prescribers by pharmaceutical companies through disease mongering cannot continue, their only goal should be to produce and advertise drugs to patients who truly need and benefit from them; instead, these companies care solely about profit. These companies should not be able to define and advertise diseases and treatments to fit their goals and should rely on science to make decisions rather than economics.

The pharmaceutical industry's tendency to favor profit over the health of consumers has led to a focus more on drugs that will make a profit and have proven efficacy and less on discovering new drugs to treat diseases that lack effective treatments, such as Alzheimer's or genetic diseases. If there was less focus on profit and more focus on new drug discovery and research, the industry would make a more meaningful impact on the lives of all patients, including those who are currently overlooked. New drug development is incredibly expensive, and pharmaceutical companies rarely focus on discovering new drugs to treat rare diseases because they do not stand to make a profit. Orphan drug approval laws have attempted to motivate these companies to focus research on drug discovery for rare diseases by providing incentives such as tax and other fee exemptions.[7] Rare diseases are defined by the FDA as any disease that affects fewer than 200,000 people in the US, an estimated 25 million are affected by these diseases in the US alone. These laws have encouraged drug research that may not have been done otherwise; however, there needs to be more assistance given to pharmaceutical companies to encourage a shift away from continued research on profitable drugs, to new research on drugs critical to the health of much of the population.

Overprescription of antibiotics has become a major concern worldwide as it has caused increasing antimicrobial resistance. Physicians and other healthcare providers are constantly overprescribing antibiotics due to diagnostic uncertainty and patient pressure in cases where antibiotics are unnecessary.[8] Overprescribing antibiotics can be incredibly dangerous due to the potential to increase antimicrobial resistance, but it can also increase the risk of adverse effects as well as the length and severity of diseases in cases where antibiotics are improperly prescribed.[9] Antibiotic prescribing has become so common that patients have begun to expect them for every surgery, injury, or ailment no matter the severity and regardless of whether or not antibiotics are the proper treatment. The negligence of healthcare providers coupled with patient demands can pose a major problem to global health and must be addressed. Proper patient education is necessary to address misconceptions associated with antibiotic prescribing to ensure that they understand the implications of antibiotic use. Additionally, providers must be properly trained and educated to only prescribe antibiotics in instances where they are completely necessary to improve patient health.

Additionally, the overprescription of opioids plays a significant role in the US opioid epidemic. From 1999–2008 the sale of prescription opioids increased by four times and likely remains severely elevated today.[10] The vast majority of surgical patients receive opioid prescriptions regardless of the surgery type or patient characteristics, likely resulting in unnecessary opioid prescriptions for many patients.[11] Dentists in the US tend to severely overprescribe opioids for third molar removals and other surgeries, ignoring recommendations from the American Dental Association to prescribe nonopioid analgesics instead.[12] This overprescription of opioids is due to a combination of factors, but perhaps a major factor is pressure from patients. Patients expect to receive opioids when they undergo surgery and some likely would push back against any efforts from prescribers to deny them the medication that they expect. Efforts must be made to educate both patients and prescribers to reduce the rates of opioid prescription which would address a contributing factor of the US opioid epidemic.

The pharmaceutical industry is incredibly important for human health, and it is impossible to ignore the accomplishments that have been made in drug research and development by major pharmaceutical companies. However, it is also impossible to ignore the shortcomings of these companies and at times it feels like new drug discovery is grinding to a stop, replaced by the optimization of old drugs for profit. Changes must be made to the system to ensure that the pharmaceutical industry will focus more of its resources on drug development for new diseases and rare diseases, which may require additional incentives or other changes. The pharmaceutical industry must not be allowed to use disease-mongering to increase profits, patients, and prescribers should be educated in the intended uses of drugs and when they are necessary to avoid overprescription.

Works Cited

1. CDC. Prescription drug use in the past 30 days, by sex, race and Hispanic origin, and age: United States, selected years 1988-1994 through 2015-2018 2019. Available from: https://www.cdc.gov/nchs/data/hus/2019/039-508.pdf.
2. Sanchez-Sanchez E, Fernandez-Cerezo FL, Diaz-Jimenez J, et al. Consumption of over-the-Counter Drugs: Prevalence and Type of Drugs. Int J Environ Res Public Health. 2021;18(11). Epub 20210521.
3. Shankar PR, Subish P. Disease mongering. Singapore Med J. 2007;48(4):275-80.
4. Moynihan R, Heath I, Henry D. Selling sickness: the pharmaceutical industry and disease mongering. BMJ. 2002;324(7342):886-91.
5. Dear JW, Webb DJ. Disease mongering -- a challenge for everyone involved in healthcare. Br J Clin Pharmacol. 2007;64(2):122-4.
6. Gonzalez-Moreno M, Saborido C, Teira D. Disease-mongering through clinical trials. Stud Hist Philos Biol Biomed Sci. 2015;51:11-8.
7. Office of Inspector General. The Orphan Drug Act Implementation and Impact 2001. Available from: https://oig.hhs.gov/oei/reports/oei-09-00-00380.pdf.
8. Fiore DC, Fettic LP, Wright SD, et al. Antibiotic overprescribing: Still a major concern. J Fam Pract. 2017;66(12):730-6.
9. Llor C, Bjerrum L. Antimicrobial resistance: risk associated with antibiotic overuse and initiatives to reduce the problem. Ther Adv Drug Saf. 2014;5(6):229-41.
10. Theisen K, Jacobs B, Macleod L, et al. The United States opioid epidemic: a review of the surgeon's contribution to it and health policy initiatives. BJU Int. 2018;122(5):754-9. Epub 20180726.
11. Thiels CA, Anderson SS, Ubl DS, et al. Wide Variation and Overprescription of Opioids After Elective Surgery. Ann Surg. 2017;266(4):564-73.
12. Suda KJ, Zhou J, Rowan SA, et al. Overprescribing of Opioids to Adults by Dentists in the U.S., 2011-2015. Am J Prev Med. 2020;58(4):473-86. Epub 20200204.

Topic: Opioids and The Opioid Epidemic—How Did We Get Here?

Opioids are powerful pain-relieving medications derived from the poppy plant that include morphine, heroin, codeine, hydrocodone, and oxycodone. These drugs have been a component of the US medical arsenal since before the Civil War for reducing pain and increasing human comfort. They are also capable of producing euphoria and a sensation of well-being that can be compelling to the point of addiction. That these drugs, whether prescription or obtained on the street, can be abused is not news to anyone with a modicum of scientific literacy. However, there appears to be a controversy surrounding the most recent surge in addictions and deaths due to opioid abuse.

To avoid addiction problems, stronger opioids and opiates such as hydrocodone and oxycodone have traditionally been restricted to the worst of human pains, such as those associated with severe burns, amputations, and cancer. So, better, longer-lasting, and safer analgesics are a continual focus of drug discovery. To improve the analgesic arsenal, in 1995 a sustained-release formulation of oxycodone (OxyContin) was approved by the FDA.[1] The purpose of this novel compound, according to the advertising accompanying this new dosage form, was to reduce patient dosing.

This could be done, they explained, by significantly increasing the duration of pain relief to up to 12 hours a day, a feature of this novel and expensive new product. This reduced typical patterns of dosing opioids from 4–6 times a day to twice-daily dosing, increasing convenience.[2] Also, such a dosing regimen and the purported slow release of analgesia-inducing medication was anticipated to significantly decrease the drug's abuse liability. Subjects were told that they would not experience the intense withdrawal that was associated with older formulations that cause drug cravings and dependence. However, the pharmacokinetics of OxyContin, or how the drug behaved in the body, was vastly different than advertised. Instead of all-day relief from pain, patients reported needing another drug dose as early as 4–6 hours after the first dose.

This would not be terribly remarkable, that the actual pharmacokinetics of a drug were different than reported in trial data, but what the drug company did to cover up these conflicting reports was controversial. Documents show that drug representatives from Purdue, the manufacturer of OxyContin, falsely claimed a 12-hour half-life for the drug and pressured physicians who prescribed it to dose it according to those false claims. Physicians who wrote prescriptions allowing more frequent dosing were "counseled" to adhere to the pharmaceutical company's suggested dosing regimen and to increase patient doses excessively, perhaps recklessly to make up for the lack of analgesia. This type of coercion, coupled with a wide-spread miscommunication about a poorly worded letter in the *New England Journal of Medicine* was the initiating event that would culminate in a US opioid abuse epidemic.[3]

There created a pattern that is currently evident among today's addicts. First, they present to a clinic with minor or resolvable pain and are given large doses of OxyContin that are inappropriate for their needs. Then, as their tolerance to these large doses increased, even more drug was needed to reduce their pain. Requests for more pain medication began to concern physicians who then began to deny additional prescriptions or extensions of pain therapy. Then, if patients could not "doctor shop" and find other willing providers and their habit had become severe, they could turn to illicit sources of the same drug or a much cheaper alternative, heroin.[4-6] Heroin has no medical use, so the only source for this would be the street corner. Not all heroin is well made, and obtaining and selling it is illegal. So, now addicts have a medical problem as well as a potential legal issue. Thus, the healthcare system created addicts by supplying them with careless amounts of potent drugs and then strung them along until they were hooked. Then they cut off the supply. Pharma is culpable for lying about the drug's pharmacokinetics. Physicians are liable because they did not do the requisite research to verify the pharmaceutical company's false claims and they allowed unschooled reps to "educate" them about OxyContin. When patients became addicted, the physicians simply turned their backs.

Even pharmacies are getting ensnared in litigation over opioid abuse because they are considered product distributors. Pharmacists are responsible for medical management counseling and suggesting safe practices for opioid use, but they cannot control individuals once they leave the pharmacy. Pharmacies have been discussed in the context of having pain-management agreement plans for consumers, but depending on one's viewpoint, they replicate or make redundant patient opioid contracts with physicians or they reinforce the message that addiction is a serious potential consequence of drug over-use.[7] Either way, a piece of paper is not likely to stop an addict, and it at best may only moderately raise awareness of such potential for addiction for a society that is barely scientifically literate.

Much like the lawsuits over tobacco, in which cigarette manufacturers were required to pay public health costs of smoking and fund cessation programs in exchange for immunity from legal action in the future, interest is increasing over suing the pharmaceutical companies who misrepresented OxyContin's abuse potential.[2] Perhaps this will be the best source for financing addiction treatment, deployment of opioid reversal antidotes, and creating educational materials to prevent additional patients from getting hooked on these very powerful medications. Purdue may be getting the message: the company is reported to be slashing its drug representative sales force and requiring remaining representatives to discuss other, non-opioid drugs with physicians instead, but this may be too little intervention, delivered entirely too late.

Writing Prompts

- How do we define a disease and what evidence do we collect that someone has that disease?

- Is it ethical, in the face of a disease, to do nothing?
  - Why or why not?
- The law states that certain opioids cannot be prescribed to "treat" an opioid addiction.
  - What do you think about this logic?
- Should addicts be jailed or treated?
- Are physicians to blame for the opioid addiction crisis?
- Are drug companies to blame for this mess? Are they both complicit?
- MDs argue that long-term opioid use is of no benefit; patients argue that there is no harm.
  - We lack data for both claims….how do we compromise?
- What might happen if physicians changed pain management entirely and used opioids as a backup, last resort measure?
  - Patients could be taught or encouraged to use other non-drug measures.
  - Patients could be told that life cannot be lived pain-free.
  - Patients could be told that no drug can remove all pain; some pain is inevitable and not life-threatening.
- Has the opioid crisis created policies of under-treatment of chronic pain?
- Should all pain be treated or should some of us just "get over it"?
- Is treating pain a medical or moral issue?
- Why should patients expect healthcare professionals to treat their pain?
- Why should MDs expect patients to stop asking for pain relief?
- Should we reframe pain as a fact of life and do a 180° on the current perspective that all pain should be treated and is treatable?
  - How much pain should we endure?
    - All of it; some of it; a little or none of it?
    - For how long?
    - Who should endure the most pain and why?

Works Cited

1. Cicero TJ, Inciardi JA, Munoz A. Trends in abuse of Oxycontin and other opioid analgesics in the United States: 2002-2004. J Pain. 2005;6(10):662-72.
2. Semuels A. Are Pharmaceutical Companies to Blame for the Opioid Epidemic? The Atlantic. 2017.
3. Porter J, Jick H. Addiction rare in patients treated with narcotics. N Engl J Med. 1980;302(2):123.
4. Ponte C, Lepelley M, Boucherie Q, et al. Doctor shopping of opioid analgesics relative to benzodiazepines: A pharmacoepidemiological study among 11.7 million inhabitants in the French countries. Drug Alcohol Depend. 2018;187:88-94.
5. McDonald DC, Carlson KE. Estimating the prevalence of opioid diversion by "doctor shoppers" in the United States. PLoS One. 2013;8(7):e69241.
6. Nordmann S, Pradel V, Lapeyre-Mestre M, et al. Doctor shopping reveals geographical variations in opioid abuse. Pain Physician. 2013;16(1):89-100.
7. Cobaugh DJ, Gainor C, Gaston CL, et al. The opioid abuse and misuse epidemic: implications for pharmacists in hospitals and health systems. Am J Health Syst Pharm. 2014;71(18):1539-54.

Essay: The US Opioid Problem: Overprescription and Overdose

Baden Cruickshank

The US opioid problem has increased dramatically in the past decades, with reported opioid-related deaths reaching over 60,000 in 2020, a dramatic increase from less than 10,000 in 1999.[1] While only making up around 5% of the world population, the US consumes 80% of the world opioid supply.[2] These statistics are concerning and reflect the failures of many, including the pharmaceutical companies, prescribers, and pharmacists dispensing the medication.

A significant example of the role of pharmaceutical companies in the US opioid problem is Purdue Pharmaceutical's handling of advertising for OxyContin, an extended-release version of oxycodone. While advertising their new drug, the company falsely claimed that it had a lower abuse potential and an increased duration of efficacy while also deceiving patients in prescription labeling and advertisement.[3] Through omission and manipulation of critical data, Purdue Pharmaceuticals pressured prescribers with aggressive marketing tactics to prescribe OxyContin to their patients, assuring them that it was safer and more effective than other opioids on the market.[4] This example of strategies used by a pharmaceutical company to unethically promote their product is concerning and is likely not a stand-alone event. The pressure put on prescribers by Purdue Pharmaceuticals lead to the overprescription of OxyContin and contributed to it now being considered a drug that contributes to the US opioid problem due to the masking of its abuse potential from prescribers and patients.[3] Although there are policies in place to regulate the marketing and advertisement of prescription drugs, they were obviously insufficient or inadequately enforced in this case. No pharmaceutical company should be able to lie to prescribers and consumers about the safety and efficacy of their products, and it is shameful that companies are willing to threaten the lives and livelihoods of consumers for financial gain.

Another major contributing factor to the US opioid problem is overprescription, both for medical and nonmedical reasons. Even in cases where it would be considered reasonable for healthcare providers to prescribe opioids for pain management, significant overprescription can still be seen. Physicians, dentists, and other providers can be seen to prescribe opioids at excessively high rates, even in cases where opioids were likely not necessary.[5-7] This overprescription of opioids leads to many patients having a portion left over; in fact, data suggest that greater than 60% of prescribed opioids remain unused after surgeries, which provides a significant quantity available for diversion (movement into the illegal drug market).[8] This "just in case" point of view taken by many healthcare providers is dangerous and likely contributes significantly to the US opioid problem.

This outlook by prescribers is influenced by several factors, including pressure from pharmaceutical companies and patients. There must be significant consideration put into updating policies, re-educating prescribers, and educating patients on proper opioid use and disposal, if there is to be any hope of improving the opioid problem in the US. An additional point of concern is the intentionally fraudulent prescription of opioids by physicians and other healthcare providers for personal gain. The term *pill mill* is often used to describe instances of inappropriate prescription or dispensing of prescription opioids, often used as a gateway for opioid abusers to illegally acquire these prescription medications.[9] These pill mills can significantly contribute to opioid diversion and can involve cooperation between prescribers, pharmacists, and even patients to illegally distribute these drugs.[10] Although efforts have been made at the state and federal level to combat pill mills, they still likely contribute greatly to the US opioid problem.

Patient expectation or demand for opioids following many common surgical procedures contributes to excessive leftover opioids which can lead to diversion and abuse. Opioid prescription has become so common in the past decades that many patients expect them for common surgical procedures such as wisdom teeth removal and other cases that non-opioid analgesics would be a more reasonable treatment with no abuse potential.[11, 12] To decrease the risk of opioid abuse caused by unnecessary prescription, efforts should be made to educate patients both on the proper uses of opioids, and when they are not necessary. If patients had a better understanding of pain and when it is ok to be in pain, there would likely be a decrease in demand for opioid prescriptions by patients, and therefore less pressure on prescribers to provide them.

Community pharmacists also play a major role in the regulation of the US opioid problem, as they evaluate both prescription and patient integrity to determine whether to dispense prescription opioids or not. Pharmacists play this key role by determining prescription validity, providing patient education, and communicating with prescribers to ensure proper medication use.[13] However, many pharmacists find that it is difficult to carry out this role, citing limited continued education, lack of patient interaction opportunities, limited time, and a high burden of responsibilities.[14] Community pharmacists are generally incredibly overworked and overburdened and are forced to fulfill this important role to limit opioid abuse originating from their pharmacy. Pharmacists should not be expected to both regulate opioid abuse and complete the innumerable other tasks present in their pharmacies; they are bound to make mistakes if they are forced to continually split their focus on such an important issue. Pharmacists and retail pharmacy chains have been held legally responsible for their contributions to the US opioid problem in the past, a problem that could be avoided if better policies were in place within both governments and the pharmacy chains.[15, 16] Pharmacists should not be the sole line of defense for the prevention of opioid abuse, and changes must be made to policies to ensure that pharmacist error does not continue to contribute to the US opioid problem.

The US opioid problem is an important issue in this country and has built upon foundations of illegitimate prescribing practices, illegitimate marketing by pharmaceutical companies, overprescription, and errors along the supply chain. This issue can only be addressed by interdisciplinary efforts among governments, prescribers, pharmaceutical companies, pharmacists, and patients through education, re-education, and implementation of new policies.

Through these combined efforts, we can address the US opioid problem by limiting diversion and preventing new opioid abusers from arising.

Works Cited

1. NIH. Overdose Death Rates 2022. Available from: https://nida.nih.gov/research-topics/trends-statistics/overdose-death-rates.
2. Manchikanti L, Singh A. Therapeutic opioids: a ten-year perspective on the complexities and complications of the escalating use, abuse, and nonmedical use of opioids. Pain Physician. 2008;11(2 Suppl):S63-88.
3. Whelan E, Asbridge M. The OxyContin crisis: problematisation and responsibilisation strategies in addiction, pain, and general medicine journals. Int J Drug Policy. 2013;24(5):402-11.
4. Egilman DS, Collins G, Falender J, et al. The marketing of OxyContin(R): A cautionary tale. Indian J Med Ethics. 2019;4(3):183-93.
5. Lozada MJ, Raji MA, Goodwin JS, et al. Opioid Prescribing by Primary Care Providers: a Cross-Sectional Analysis of Nurse Practitioner, Physician Assistant, and Physician Prescribing Patterns. J Gen Intern Med. 2020;35(9):2584-92. Epub 20200424.
6. Suda KJ, Evans CT, Gibson G, et al. Opioid Prescribing by Dentists in the Veterans Health Administration. Am J Prev Med. 2022;63(3):371-83. Epub 20220324.
7. Theisen K, Jacobs B, Macleod L, et al. The United States opioid epidemic: a review of the surgeon's contribution to it and health policy initiatives. BJU Int. 2018;122(5):754-9. Epub 20180726.
8. Schirle L, Stone AL, Morris MC, et al. Leftover opioids following adult surgical procedures: a systematic review and meta-analysis. Syst Rev. 2020;9(1):139. Epub 20200611.
9. Ramirez R. Pill Mills: An Overview of Law Enforcement's Painful Challenge 2020. Available from: file:///Users/badencruickshank/Downloads/Ramirez,-Rick-paper.pdf.
10. Rigg KK, March SJ, Inciardi JA. Prescription Drug Abuse & Diversion: Role of the Pain Clinic. J Drug Issues. 2010;40(3):681-702.
11. Fricova J. [Non-opioid analgesics]. Cas Lek Cesk.157(2):74-8.
12. Clark DJ, Schumacher MA. America's Opioid Epidemic: Supply and Demand Considerations. Anesth Analg. 2017;125(5):1667-74.
13. Gregory T, Gregory L. The Role of Pharmacists in Safe Opioid Dispensing. J Pharm Pract. 2020;33(6):856-62. Epub 20190630.
14. Vadiei N, Eldridge LA, Meyerson BE, et al. "The gatekeepers in prevention": Community pharmacist perceptions of their role in the opioid epidemic. Subst Abus. 2022;43(1):319-27. Epub 20210702.
15. Ault A. Pharmacists May Be Legally Liable for Opioid Overdoses 2017. Available from: https://www.medscape.com/viewarticle/882358.
16. Landi H. Federal jury holds pharmacy chains CVS, Walgreens and Walmart responsible for role in opioid crisis 2021. Available from: https://www.fiercehealthcare.com/finance/federal-jury-holds-cvs-walgreens-and-walmart-responsible-for-role-opioid-crisis.

Essay: The US Opioid Problem—Expect the Expected

Lauren Thompson

Opioids have gotten an immense amount of attention in the media in recent years, yet their use in medicine is far from novel. At first, opium gum, derived from the poppy plant, was used to manage pain and treat diarrhea by physicians caring for soldiers of the Civil War.[1] As time has passed, we have continued to explore opiates and their synthetic counterparts in terms of pain management. So, if this is such an established area of medicine, how come things are suddenly getting so bad?

One of the most pivotal moments regarding opioid use trends can be credited to the approval and marketing of OxyContin, an extended-release oxycodone. The rationale behind making an extended-release version was simple: if patients were able to take a tablet every 12 hours, the common side effects associated with opioid withdrawal would be minimized.[2] Patients would be able to benefit from steadier pain relief, avoiding the highs and lows characteristic of the immediate-release versions. As soon as the drug was approved Purdue Pharmaceuticals, the manufacturer of OxyContin, highlighted all of these features and began to market– and they did so aggressively.

The campaign for OxyContin included substantial financial incentives for the sales representatives and all expenses paid for conferences for healthcare professionals.[3] Purdue representatives and speakers at these conferences stuck to their scripts, using promotional materials and witty slogans in combination with prescriber profiles to advocate for the new drug. Sales representatives emphasized the importance of increasing the dose of OxyContin, not the frequency, and physicians complied. They assured physicians that this was a low-risk and tremendously beneficial drug for a variety of patients.[4]

These marketing tactics were highly effective, and by 2006 extended-release oxycodone made up 28% of all opioid prescriptions.[5] Physicians were prescribing OxyContin as first-line treatment under the impression it did not pose the same risk for abuse or addiction compared to other opioids.[6] The subjectivity of pain along with misleading claims provided by Purdue enabled OxyContin's colossal success. The vision Purdue Pharmaceuticals had was coming to life; however, these utopian ideas about OxyContin were often unsupported scientifically.

The pharmacological properties of OxyContin were dismissed for years and inevitably, as the number of opioid prescriptions began to skyrocket, as did the trends of diversion and abuse of those same prescriptions.[7] The number of prescription opioid-related deaths was rapidly increasing, along with deaths related to heroin and other synthetic opioids.[8] However, it is important to note these statistics increased in direct proportion to the sheer mass of opioid prescriptions being filled. The ease of access and relatively low cost of heroin made the transition from prescription opioids seem logical to some users. Though, this group makes up a minority, for it is estimated only about 4% of prescription opioid abusers make this change to heroin.[9] That is not to insinuate heroin is not a problem, but rather the percentage of people who replace opioid abuse with heroin abuse does not deviate from what would be anticipated.

Despite this being such a small division of heroin users, this is the story we are sold day in and day out in the media. Rather than considering environmental contributions such as socioeconomic barriers or racial inequities, physicians and big pharma became the sole scapegoats.[10] The typical story follows the life of a successful young adult who was prescribed opioids and eventually loses everything. This narrative is popular among the public because it diverts responsibility from the user and assigns it to the provider who wrote the prescription. Details about previous drug use are frequently left out, furthering this idea that there are morally good drug users that were simply dealt an unfair hand.[11] When these circumstances are laid out in such a relatable fashion, it is hard not to sympathize with the user. After all, it could have been any of us, right?

What this attitude fails to take into consideration is the inevitable creation of a conflicting view: all other drug users are bad, immoral, and did it to themselves. Negative bias in healthcare towards drug users already impacts patient care and patient trust in physicians, and this is only exacerbated by this black-or-white type of thinking.[12] If the same understanding was present for all drug users regardless of the way they got there, the stigma surrounding addiction may begin to reduce. Decreased stigma in the general population, as well as healthcare settings, may enable more patients to seek treatment and receive equal care.[13]

When struggling patients receive no or subpar care, they tend to continue the same lifestyle, often filled with damaged interpersonal relationships, financial burdens, and legal troubles.[14] It is proven that punitive measures are significantly less effective at treating opioid use disorders than medical care.[15] For example, medication treatments for opioid use disorder, such as methadone or buprenorphine, can be highly successful.[16] However, even these proven methods of treatment are obstructed by bias surrounding the therapy.[17] People who are misinformed about the mechanism by which these drugs work may claim maintenance therapy does not equal recovery, once again discouraging users from seeking treatment.

In conclusion, countless people and entities contributed to the complex opioid problem we see today. Whether you blame the ill-advised physicians or financially motivated pharmaceutical giants, the issue remains the same. The over-prescribing of OxyContin and other opioids forced the United States to see the repercussions of drug abuse on a large scale. It is crucial to use this as an opportunity for providers to better understand pain management and the properties of the drugs involved. And for the general population, this is a chance to recognize the reality of opioid abuse and all the contributing external factors to drug abuse as a whole. Drugs cannot be inherently good or bad, but the way we approach their misuse can be.

Works Cited

1. Klys M, Maciow-Glab M, Rojek S. On the history of opium. Arch Med Sadowej Kryminol. 2013;63(3):226-35.
2. Kalso E. Oxycodone. J Pain Symptom Manage. 2005;29(5 Suppl):S47-56.
3. Van Zee A. The promotion and marketing of oxycontin: commercial triumph, public health tragedy. Am J Public Health. 2009;99(2):221-7.
4. Egilman DS, Collins G, Falender J, et al. The marketing of OxyContin(R): A cautionary tale. Indian J Med Ethics. 2019;4(3):183-93.
5. Dhalla IA, Mamdani MM, Sivilotti ML, et al. Prescribing of opioid analgesics and related mortality before and after the introduction of long-acting oxycodone. CMAJ. 2009;181(12):891-6. Epub 20091207.
6. Physicians' Desk Reference. OxyContin® Package Insert1997.
7. OxyContin Availability, Diversion, and Abuse. Intelligence Bulletin 2004.
8. Opioid Data Analysis and Resources. Center for Disease Control and Prevention 2022.
9. NIDA. A subset of people who abuse prescription opioids may progress to heroin use. NIH 2022.
10. Mennis J, Stahler GJ, Mason MJ. Risky Substance Use Environments and Addiction: A New Frontier for Environmental Justice Research. Int J Environ Res Public Health. 2016;13(6). Epub 20160618.
11. Szalavitz M. What the media gets wrong about opioids. Columbia Journalism Review. 2018.
12. Dahl RAMV, J. Priyanka PhD; Harland, Karisa K. MPH, PhD; Radke, Joshua MD. Investigating Healthcare Provider Bias Toward Patients Who Use Drugs Using a Survey-based Implicit Association Test: Pilot Study. Journal of Addiction Medicine. 2022.
13. Volkow DN. Addressing the Stigma that Surrounds Addiction. NIDA. 2020.
14. Hagemeier NE. Introduction to the opioid epidemic: the economic burden on the healthcare system and impact on quality of life. Am J Manag Care. 2018;24(10 Suppl):S200-S6.
15. Brinkley-Rubinstein L, Zaller N, Martino S, et al. Criminal justice continuum for opioid users at risk of overdose. Addict Behav. 2018;86:104-10. Epub 20180224.
16. Bell J, Strang J. Medication Treatment of Opioid Use Disorder. Biol Psychiatry. 2020;87(1):82-8. Epub 20190702.
17. Rozner L, Peles E. [Stigma and Misinformation About Methadone Maintenance Therapy]. Harefuah. 2021;160(1):19-23.

Essay: The Opioid Epidemic— What We Aren't Doing

Erica Day

While much of opioid abuse may come from non-prescription sources, health practitioners are not free of blame.[1] Medical use of opioids has increased, along with it the increase of opioid misuse.[2] Proper opioid prescription and attention during care should reduce the amount of misuse and abuse from prescribed sources. While resources are available for patient drug observation, they are not used consistently in many different professions, even in situations involving the high potential for abuse patients.[3-5] With the availability of these resources, and the knowledge of their existence, the blame for prescribed opioid misuse can only fall on the health practitioner. Health practitioners can change their techniques and practices to reduce opioid misuse and subsequent future abuse, to impact the spheres that they have an effect in to reduce the opioid epidemic.

The initial step of reducing opioid misuse is to reduce opioid use. Opioids should be reserved for situations where non-opioid pain management plans have proven ineffective or statistically do not provide enough pain relief. Disappointingly, there is a gap of knowledge in the effectiveness of opioids vs. other analgesics in post-operative acute pain care.[6] In most situations, when proper care is provided, the primary option for pain management should be non-opioid. The impact of opioid misuse is more dangerous than feeling temporary acute pain. In situations where the split between opioid and non-opioid treatment is blurry, the more conservative approach of non-opioid analgesics should be taken. Finding a treatment that does not involve opioids reduces the risks of opioid-related harm, as well as the chance for de facto therapy. Opioids will always be more potent than their other analgesic counterparts, but with their effectiveness comes increased risk.

Not every analgesic will be perfect for each patient. Non-opioids may not be effective in treating the patient's pain, or the health risks of NSAIDs and gastrointestinal or kidney disease.[7] In this case, if a patient has not disclosed prior issues of substance abuse, opioids may be the most effective pain management plan. Treatment does not stop there. Continuous monitoring of the patient is necessary to ensure that the medications are used properly, and pain has been treated satisfactorily. Low doses of opioids should be used as they provide the same level of pain relief, minimizing costs for both patient and producer and ensuring general dose safety.[8] Treatment plans meant to be temporary should include programs that decrease withdrawal symptoms through patient preparation. For longer opioid treatments, a patient analysis should occur to see if opioid therapy is still necessary for pain, especially in non-cancer pain.[9] Techniques like these quickly bring awareness to patients who may have chronic pain or are misusing opioids and in determining the future.

For patients in opioid treatment subject to improper or previous prescribing practices with high-dose opioids, more medical assistance is necessary to reduce opioid use. Dose tapering is successful in these situations, especially when prolonged over large amounts of time.[10] Careful watch of these patients is necessary to reduce potential harm and should only occur if the opioid is no longer necessary for pain management. For situations where craving reduction is necessary, buprenorphine/naloxone and methadone are effective drugs in treating these afflictions.[11] And in situations where those with a history of substance abuse need analgesic different techniques are necessary, including multimodal analgesia and abuse screening tools.[12] Overall, for proper opioid prescription and care medical observation is necessary to mitigate harm from a healthcare standpoint, including proper screening.

Another solution that will reduce harmful opioid prescribing and treatment is proper education. Proper education provides an increase in understanding of opioids [13, 14] which will allow safe prescription and care for those taking opioids. A certification or a mandatory class would be perfect for providing education on the risks and rewards of opioids, and when to prescribe them, as well as a proper understanding of the weight of prescribing an opioid. These are serious drugs that should be saved for the most serious of cases, especially when weaker analgesics are better suited for the situation.

Where health professionals can make an impact on the opioid epidemic, and reduce the inherent harm of prescribing opioids, is through proper treatment of those affected, educated prescription practices, and careful watch of those under care. Increased education on opioid prescribing and care for patients on opioids should be necessary for every doctor prescribing these drugs, requiring a special certification that verifies a full understanding of the risks, as well as when they should be used. Opioids are potent drugs and it's time we treated them so, consciously and ethically.

Works Cited

1. Carise D, Dugosh KL, McLellan AT, et al. Prescription OxyContin abuse among patients entering addiction treatment. Am J Psychiatry. 2007;164(11):1750-6.
2. Atluri S, Sudarshan G, Manchikanti L. Assessment of the trends in medical use and misuse of opioid analgesics from 2004 to 2011. Pain Physician. 2014;17(2):E119-28.
3. Chaudhary S, Compton P. Use of risk mitigation practices by family nurse practitioners prescribing opioids for the management of chronic nonmalignant pain. Subst Abus. 2017;38(1):95-104.
4. Piper BJ, Desrosiers CE, Lipovsky JW, et al. Use and Misuse of Opioids in Maine: Results From Pharmacists, the Prescription Monitoring, and the Diversion Alert Programs. J Stud Alcohol Drugs. 2016;77(4):556-65.
5. Starrels JL, Becker WC, Weiner MG, et al. Low use of opioid risk reduction strategies in primary care even for high risk patients with chronic pain. J Gen Intern Med. 2011;26(9):958-64. Epub 20110224.

6. Mitra S, Carlyle D, Kodumudi G, et al. New Advances in Acute Postoperative Pain Management. Curr Pain Headache Rep. 2018;22(5):35.
7. Ejaz P, Bhojani K, Joshi VR. NSAIDs and kidney. J Assoc Physicians India. 2004;52:632-40.
8. Mohanty S, Shin M, Casper D, et al. Postoperative Prescription of Low-dose Narcotics Yields Equivalent Pain Outcomes Compared to High-dose Narcotics in Opioid-naive Patients Undergoing Spine Surgery. Spine (Phila Pa 1976). 2021;46(24):1748-57.
9. Von Korff M, Saunders K, Thomas Ray G, et al. De facto long-term opioid therapy for noncancer pain. Clin J Pain. 2008;24(6):521-7.
10. Barrett AK, Sandbrink F, Mardian A, et al. Medication Use Evaluation of High-Dose Long-Term Opioid De-prescribing in Multiple Veterans Affairs Medical Centers. J Gen Intern Med. 2022. Epub 20221011.
11. McAnulty C, Bastien G, Eugenia Socias M, et al. Buprenorphine/naloxone and methadone effectiveness for reducing craving in individuals with prescription opioid use disorder: Exploratory results from an open-label, pragmatic randomized controlled trial. Drug Alcohol Depend. 2022;239:109604. Epub 20220817.
12. Vadivelu N, Lumermann L, Zhu R, et al. Pain Control in the Presence of Drug Addiction. Curr Pain Headache Rep. 2016;20(5):35.
13. Marshall KF, Carney PA, Bonuck KJ, et al. Preparing fourth year medical students to care for patients with opioid use disorder: how this training affects their intention to seek addiction care opportunities during residency. Med Educ Online. 2023;28(1):2141602.
14. Barcelona V, Wischik DL, Marshall A, et al. Integration of medication for opioid use disorder training into graduate nursing education. Nurs Forum. 2022;57(5):869-73. Epub 20220526.

Topic: Black and Gray Market Drug Purchasing

The internet has forever changed the way consumers use information and services, especially how individuals learn about and purchase drugs and supplements for personal use. These may be approved drugs that are made in the US and reimported or they may be drugs that are not approved, approved but discontinued, or simply not available on the US market. In this latter case, for drugs unavailable in the US that are shipped from other countries, the drugs are considered to be imported. If the drugs originated in the US, left the country, and were then shipped back to consumers here, they are considered to be re-imported. Imported and re-imported drugs have different rules associated with each type of purchase.

Such online drug purchases have never been easier thanks to cryptomarket digital platforms with anonymizing software such as Tor and the Invisible Internet 2 network layer/browser. Add to this technology encrypted email clients such as proton mail which allows virtually complete user privacy, and we now have almost untraceable methods for inquiring about drugs online.[1, 2] Then, cryptocurrencies such as Bitcoin and other peer-to-peer trade platforms such as Google Wallet and Skrill cloak individual purchases of these substances.[3] These technologies have coalesced to offer consumers access to an unprecedented number of potentially risky compounds and treatments, but data show that only a few deaths have been attributed to such purchases.[4] This fact, however, does not discourage the US government from using hyperbolic scare tactics to reign in drug importation and re-importation and to frighten the small-time user of drugs for therapeutic purposes.

> "Silk Road was founded on libertarian principles and continues to be operated on them. It is a great idea and a great practical system...It is not a utopia. It is regulated by market forces, not a central power (even I am subject to market forces by my competition. No one is forced to be here)."
>
> Ross Ulbricht, Founder, Silk Road website

Happily, such transparent campaigns to control the behaviors of private citizens do not appear to sway those determined to make an online drug purchase, if the proliferating black and gray market is an indicator. Black markets, sources of illegal drug traffic or trade of officially scarce or controlled substances, caught the public's attention with the exposure of Silk Road, an online darknet marketplace initiated in 2011 (shut down in 2013) for selling everything from illegal drugs to stolen money and credit cards and weapons. The ease with which consumers could find and acquire drugs via Silk Road has been likened to 'kids in a candy store'.[5] However, for all of the frightening propaganda launched by the government in the wake of Silk Road's demise, an unlikely but perhaps beneficial outcome of the Silk Road "experiment" was that habitual drug users were less inclined to source their illicit drugs from street drug dealers or to hoard illegal drugs. Silk Road allowed them to feel assured of a reliable supply of drugs and anonymity as a purchaser.[5, 6]

After the shutdown of Silk Road, numerous other sites emerged and then closed in succession as law enforcement was alerted to the sites' presence or because the sites were scams to steal customer bitcoins. This left independent drug sellers who were bold enough to market their wares on the Clearnet (non-Tor/non-dark internet). Most of these vendors transact with gift cards and cash, avoiding cryptocurrency altogether, which is substantially easier for the consumer. Thus, individuals of any age who are sufficiently savvy to use the internet and an online payment scheme can purchase illegal drugs, prescription drugs without a prescription, and research chemicals that are not intended for human consumption at all.[7]

Gray markets, for which there is no federally accepted definition, sell legal substances, but they do so beyond the manufacturer's traditional trade channels. These markets have also been referred to as parallel markets, and they serve a niche in the market when there are drug shortages.[8] For instance, some retail pharmacies exist entirely to purchase scarce drugs from authorized dealers and then sell these at exorbitant markup to wholesalers and others in the drug supply chain.[9, 10] Under this paradigm, a drug can be sold and re-sold as many as five times before it reaches a pharmacy that dispenses it to a patient, with price markups all along the way. Thus, a drug typically selling for $10 can cost $200 when it reaches the end user.[9] Typically, vendors in this space purchase drugs in short supply that are needed by critically ill patients. These gray suppliers "dangle" the exorbitantly marked-up drug to those in the most need, raising questions about product authenticity and safety. After all, if the original manufacturer declares a shortage of a particular drug, how did this gray market supplier acquire so much of it?[8]

"Around the time of the takedown of this site, there were more than 250,000 listings for illegal drugs and toxic chemicals on AlphaBay...As of earlier this year, 122 vendors advertised fentanyl; 238 advertised heroin."

Jeff Sessions, Past US Attorney General

People in desperate need may never stop to ask these types of questions. In fact, studies show that everyone from illicit drug wholesalers to adolescents has been able to use black and gray markets to source and acquire dangerous drugs such as opioids. This appears treacherous, but data show that the internet is actually not the most common source for purchasing drugs.[11] The reasons given by 100 drug addicts who were interviewed for their purchasing histories and habits were that internet purchases were more expensive, more prone to oversight by the authorities, and more likely to be scams; thus, only 11 of the 100 interviewed confirmed internet sourcing for their addictive substances.[11]

Studies also show that consumers are driven to online drug purchasing to save money. People with multiple expensive prescriptions often find unlimited supplies of medicines of interest at vastly lower prices, even with international shipping factored into the price. Also, privacy is maintained with online purchasing. No prescription is required for many black and gray markets, so the onus is entirely on the purchaser to identify the correct drug, the strength, and the dosing regimen. Many savvy patients can do this (and are doing this now), so this appears to contradict FDA claims that US citizens cannot make competent treatment decisions for and by themselves.

Writing Prompts

- Should we allow any adult consumer to purchase any US-approved drug from any source and accept the risk?
    - How about irrespective of approval status?
    - Could we allow re-importation and simply tax it as a revenue source?
- Is the FDA protecting pharma's interests by dissuading consumers from other drug supplies?
- Is the FDA out of bounds by keeping consumers from individual decisions about medications?
- Should "backroom" clinics that use imported drugs that harm be sanctioned more strongly than consumers who purchase online drugs?
- Should the US be a leader in an effort to standardize global drug safety laws?
- Would it be feasible that we'd all agree on what was an acceptable risk/what was dangerous?
- Is it racist or elitist to suggest that a drug from Canada is safer than one from India or Mexico?
- Is it hypocritical for Northern states to bus people to Canada for drug purchases?
- Should all US states have this service?
- Who'd pay for it?
- If a consumer is harmed by a drug from, say, Pfizer, but it was purchased online, with no prescription, is Pfizer liable?
- Should all foreign-made drugs have English patient information?
- Is online drug purchasing a good thing?
    - It stops a co-pay, an insurance claim, a pharmacy bill, and follow-up expenses
    - Are we just so risk-averse we cannot imagine that this is true?
- Should we enact a patient drug strike to get pharma's attention about the predatory pricing that fuels online purchasing?
- What would you be willing to give up for 30 days to stop them from profiting from you?
- Can you imagine that some people would risk online drug purchases to treat problems that are highly stigmatized?
    - What about patients who suffer from conscience clauses and are denied legal treatment?
    - Are they of special consideration for online drug buying?
    - Did the medical profession create this problem?
    - If so, should they be the solution (free samples, no more OC hostage-taking)?
- Should MDs waive multiple appointments for renewing Rx for otherwise stable patients?
- Are women disproportionately affected by drug import restrictions?
- Are the mentally ill disproportionately affected by drug import restrictions?

Works Cited

1. Barratt MJ, Lenton S, Maddox A, et al. 'What if you live on top of a bakery and you like cakes?'- Drug use and harm trajectories before, during and after the emergence of Silk Road. Int J Drug Policy. 2016;35:50-7.
2. Dolliver DS. Evaluating drug trafficking on the Tor Network: Silk Road 2, the sequel. Int J Drug Policy. 2015;26(11):1113-23.
3. Aldridge J, Askew R. Delivery dilemmas: How drug cryptomarket users identify and seek to reduce their risk of detection by law enforcement. Int J Drug Policy. 2017;41:101-9.
4. Ishikawa T, Yuasa I, Endoh M. Non specific drug distribution in an autopsy case report of fatal caffeine intoxication. Leg Med (Tokyo). 2015;17(6):535-8.
5. Van Hout MC, Bingham T. 'Silk Road', the virtual drug marketplace: a single case study of user experiences. Int J Drug Policy. 2013;24(5):385-91.
6. Van Hout MC, Bingham T. 'Surfing the Silk Road': a study of users' experiences. Int J Drug Policy. 2013;24(6):524-9.
7. Festinger DS, Dugosh KL, Clements N, et al. Use of the Internet to Obtain Drugs without a Prescription Among Treatment-involved Adolescents and Young Adults. J Child Adolesc Subst Abuse. 2016;25(5):480-6.
8. Rosenthal ET. The "gray market" raises concerns about cost, safety, and ethics. J Natl Cancer Inst. 2012;104(3):168-70.
9. Barlas S. 'Gray market' not such a gray area anymore: why hospitals are paying exorbitant drug prices. P T. 2012;37(10):544.
10. May D. Plenty of green in gray market. There's more at issue than just inflated prices for drugs in short supply. Mod Healthc. 2011;41(42):25.
11. Inciardi JA, Surratt HL, Cicero TJ, et al. Prescription drugs purchased through the internet: who are the end users? Drug Alcohol Depend. 2010;110(1-2):21-9.

Essay: Black and Gray Drug Purchasing

Ines Studer

The United States (US) is notorious for having high healthcare costs, but the prices have not always been so high. In the 1980s the US, France, Australia, Canada, and the United Kingdom had similar pharmaceutical spending *per capita*. A significant change was evident in the late 1990s and early 2000s when spending in the US grew at a significantly higher pace than the other countries.[1] As a result of these high costs, among residents of high-income countries, US adults are the most likely to omit healthcare because of financial stresses.[2] This has led to many patients opting to obtain drugs from nontraditional sources i.e., Mexico, Canada, and foreign sources through the internet.[3-5] A significant source of online drug purchasing is the Silk Road, which is readily accessible to anyone using Tor software.[6]

The FDA regulation of drugs purchased outside of the United States requires that the imported drugs be for personal use, in no more than a 3-month supply, and not for resale.[7] While, online drug purchasing from foreign sources is illegal in the United States, these packages are not often intercepted, and it is highly unlikely that consumers purchasing their prescription drugs will be prosecuted.[8] The FDA maintains that these drugs may not be safe or efficacious and that they hold no liability.[9] Interestingly, a safe importation plan has been

> "It's crucial to keep in mind that the hundreds of millions of dollars now spent on prescription drug advertisements are ultimately paid for by consumers in the form a higher drug prices."
>
> — Michael K. Simpson, American politician, and dentist

proposed to reduce the cost of drugs. To accomplish this, the plan entails two highly regulated pathways, the first of which involves the importation of drugs from Canada, while the second pathway allows manufacturers of FDA-approved drugs that are sold in foreign countries to be imported at a significantly lower cost.[10, 11]

Many patients in the US cannot afford their drug regimen as evidenced by some diabetic patients rationing their insulin.[12, 13] In the US, patients are permitted to assume risk to their health by testing experimental drugs through clinical trials, expanded access, and Right-to-Try legislation, but are not permitted to purchase drugs online, where the prices are often significantly cheaper than in US pharmacies.[14] It is contradictory that terminally and seriously ill patients are allowed to assess the risk of taking experimental drugs, but other patients are not allowed to decide between the risk of purchasing the drug from foreign sources online or rationing their vitally important medications. This clear contradiction indicates that patients should be permitted to purchase their prescription medications from foreign sources, except highly addictive drugs that are available for purchase on these sites.[15]

Elderly US adults have been taking bus trips to Canada to purchase prescription drugs at a reduced cost. This is a clear sign of discontent with current drug pricing and signifies the need for change.[16,17] While this does not reflect well on drug pricing in the US, this is a very understandable practice and could be a viable option for many elderly people who cannot afford the prices in the US. Unless drugs become commonly affordable, these trips could become more commonplace throughout the US and are currently functioning as a temporary fix for the long-term problem.

To bring attention to the issue of high drug prices charged by pharmaceutical companies and potentially force their hand in making reforms, a patient drug strike has been suggested. While I agree that more attention should be called to the issue, a patient drug strike would likely be more harmful to the patients themselves than to the companies. Many pharmaceutical companies are worth billions of dollars and likely have reserves to withstand long-term shortages of income compared to the short-term need of the patients on daily drug regimens.[18] Changes in drug pricing are especially difficult to bring about because they are not a typical business, human lives are in the balance.

Works Cited

1. Sarnak DO, Squires D, Kuzmak G, et al. Paying for Prescription Drugs Around the World: Why Is the U.S. an Outlier? Issue Brief (Commonw Fund). 2017;2017:1-14. Epub 20171001.
2. Osborn R, Squires D, Doty MM, et al. In New Survey Of Eleven Countries, US Adults Still Struggle With Access To And Affordability Of Health Care. Health Aff (Millwood). 2016;35(12):2327-36. Epub 20161116.
3. de Guzman GC, Khaleghi M, Riffenberg RH, et al. A survey of the use of foreign-purchased medications in a border community emergency department patient population. J Emerg Med. 2007;33(2):213-21. Epub 20070618.
4. Shepherd M. Drug importation and safety of drugs obtained from Canada. Ann Pharmacother. 2007;41(7):1288-91. Epub 20070619.
5. Brown J, Li C. Characteristics of online pharmacy users in a nationally representative sample. J Am Pharm Assoc (2003). 2014;54(3):289-94.
6. Barratt MJ. Silk Road: eBay for drugs. Addiction. 2012;107(3):683.
7. Is it legal for me to personally import drugs? 2021.
8. Wolfson BJ. Shopping Abroad For Cheaper Medication? Here's What You Need To Know 2019. Available from: https://californiahealthline.org/news/shopping-abroad-for-cheaper-medication-heres-what-you-need-to-know/.
9. Buying Medicine from Outside the United States 2013. Available from: https://www.fda.gov/drugs/buying-using-medicine-safely/buying-medicine-outside-united-states.
10. SAFE IMPORTATION ACTION PLAN. Available from: https://www.hhs.gov/sites/default/files/safe-importation-action-plan.pdf.

11. Issue Brief: Safe Importation Action Plan. Available from: https://www.ashp.org/advocacy-and-issues/key-issues/drug-pricing/issue-brief-safe-importation-action-plan?loginreturnUrl=SSOCheckOnly.
12. Herkert D, Vijayakumar P, Luo J, et al. Cost-Related Insulin Underuse Among Patients With Diabetes. JAMA Intern Med. 2019;179(1):112-4.
13. Fralick M, Kesselheim AS. The U.S. Insulin Crisis - Rationing a Lifesaving Medication Discovered in the 1920s. N Engl J Med. 2019;381(19):1793-5.
14. Nagar S. A Silent Killer: The Rise of the Online Prescription Drugs Illicit Market. Available from: https://hir.harvard.edu/the-rise-of-the-online-prescription-drugs-illicit-market/.
15. Dasgupta N, Freifeld C, Brownstein JS, et al. Crowdsourcing black market prices for prescription opioids. J Med Internet Res. 2013;15(8):e178.
16. U.S. Seniors Travel to Canada for Affordable Rx Drugs 2005. Available from: https://www.consumerwatchdog.org/newsrelease/us-seniors-travel-canada-affordable-rx-drugs.
17. Davie E. Quiet resurgence: Americans coming north to fill prescriptions on the rise again 2019. Available from: https://www.cbc.ca/news/canada/nova-scotia/u-s-canada-prescriptions-border-1.5137350.
18. Ledley FD, McCoy SS, Vaughan G, et al. Profitability of Large Pharmaceutical Companies Compared With Other Large Public Companies. JAMA. 2020;323(9):834-43.

Topic: Placebo and Nocebo Effects

When patients are given medications, two therapeutic aspects exist: a drug- or device-induced effect and a non-drug effect that is perceived by the patient due to his/her interaction with a healthcare provider and the drug or device. Such non-drug effects can be broadly classified as placebo or nocebo effects and these subjective perceptions are based on a commonly used tool in clinical drug trials, the placebo. The placebo (from the Latin: "I will please") is a substance that is pharmacologically inert (not a drug) and offers no true medical effects but the individual believes it does. The sense of benefit that it provides to that individual is considered to arise from his/her belief that the substance is effective. Scientists speculate that almost all positive effects of over-the-counter cough "remedies" are due to a placebo effect as a cough is under voluntary control and may be adjusted with the perception that a drug is reducing cough symptoms.[1] If true, researchers should scrutinize and relabel all medications that produce these effects because many individuals may be subjecting themselves to unnecessary drug exposures and expenses for no tangible benefit other than imagined effects.

In contrast, a nocebo (from the Latin: "I will harm") is a substance without medical effects but which is perceived by an individual to worsen their health status, again due to negative perceptions of the individual, not because of actual harm.[2] In fact, the nocebo effect is used to explain patient complaints when they are switched from a more expensive brand name pharmaceutical to a generic and often less expensive drug.[3] This type of nocebo effect can compromise any therapeutic benefit even though generics are required to be bioequivalent to their branded counterparts (within 85–115%) with regard to efficacy and potential side effects.[4]

> "Nocebos often cause a physical effect, but it's not a physically produced effect. What is the cause? In many cases, it's an unanswered question."
>
> Irving Kirsch, Associate Director, Program in Placebo Studies, Lecturer, Harvard Medical School and Beth Israel Deaconess Medical Center

Initially, placebos were used in clinical drug trials as treatments comparable to the drug being investigated. In the trial, a group of subjects is given the drug under study and a separate but similar group of subjects is given an inert placebo. Then, subject groups are compared against one another to determine what effects the experimental drug had compared to the control or placebo and whether it should be tested in larger groups and eventually in patients who have the condition that the experimental drug is anticipated to treat. To have a drug approved, the drug's effects must be statistically different from those effects perceived to be conveyed by the placebo. Often, a drug "fails a trial" or is not approved because its effects are not distinctively different from those of an inert placebo or it is more harmful than the placebo.[1, 5] So, the placebo-controlled approach is not a trivial matter. Therefore understanding why placebo effects are interpreted as real benefits by some people, as well as how to identify these particular individuals, is valuable information for clinical trial specialists.

What we do know about placebo effects includes a bit of humor. For instance, scientists have documented that capsule placebos offer a greater "benefit" than tablets. Also, an injection is more "beneficial" than a capsule or tablet.[6] Likewise, a drug dispensed from a shiny, well-designed box confers a greater placebo effect than one given from a plain or unadorned box.[7, 8] Expensive placebos were thought to be better than less expensive ones and red tablets tended to produce perceived stimulant effects whereas blue tablets appeared to induce sedative or calming effects.[7, 9, 10] Finally, placebo treatments administered with positive verbal cues were more effective than actual drugs given with no positive messaging.[11] For these reasons, scientists attempt to tightly control potential placebo effects by having the experimental medication match the color, weight, consistency, taste, shape, and smell of the placebo.[12] Even with these precautions in place, placebo or nocebo responses are considered to be "real" and as such require a study in the context of human drug use. So far, emerging studies have offered compelling data to suggest why such diverse experiences occur and who is most likely to be susceptible to these types of outcomes.

"A placebo is a phony cure that works. This is very hard for the medical profession to get their teeth around because they hate placebos, but scientifically, placebos work in about 30% of cases that are psychogenic diseases."

Charles Alexander Jencks, postmodern theorist, architectural historian, and author

For instance, inter-individual differences in 5 genes that modify dopamine, 4 that modify serotonin, and one that influences the opioid receptor gene are reported to contribute to the placebo response. Scientists suggest that as many as 34 unique genes have some contribution to placebo perceptions.[13, 14] Dopamine is responsible for a sensation of reward and is important in drug-seeking behavior in addicts. Serotonin is associated with aversive stimuli and this neurotransmitter helps people avoid unpleasant events. Opioid receptor compounds such as endorphins, enkephalins, and opioid drugs reduce pain and can offer a sense of euphoria and well-being.[15] Variations in encephalin degradation cause increased placebo responses with regard to reduced pain. This is thought to be mediated by a faulty endocannabinoid degradation enzyme, leading to more circulating endocannabinoids and greater antinociception or blockade of noxious or painful stimuli.[15] It is therefore very reasonable that differences in neurotransmitters or receptors that modulate "good" and "bad" sensations might play a role in perceived placebo and nocebo effects.

Genes that call for dopamine degradation can cause increased or decreased break down of this hormone. People with greater dopamine degradation and consequently less circulating dopamine are less susceptible to placebo effects.[16, 17] However, people with high activity for dopamine degradation were more susceptible to nocebo effects. Their brains behaved as if they had a reduced capacity for pleasure or good feelings.[18, 19] Understanding underlying causes of placebo and nocebo effects may help clinical trial professionals to screen people with known genetic predispositions to either effect and omit them from clinical trials. The controversy this brings is that then, would the drug trial be relevant for more general populations who would have similar heritable traits toward placebo or nocebo effects caused by non-active substances?

In summary, the placebo has a rightful place in medical research as a non-therapeutic comparator and a replacement for the placebo-controlled trial is not on the immediate horizon. The only other option for clinical trials is comparing a new experimental drug to an existing approved drug with similar indications and efficacy. These types of active comparator or active control trials produce different data: they suggest whether a new, experimental drug is not inferior to the current standard of care, which typically was approved by outperforming a placebo. These trials do not compare experimental therapy to no therapy at all. Therefore, we must decide if omitting genetically predisposed placebo and nocebo responders is ethical and ultimately representative of the patients who will eventually receive the new drug. Or, do we want to radically change the way drugs are approved, eliminating placebo controls entirely and going with active comparator data?

Writing Prompts

- How do we explain unconscious responses to placebo?
    - Do you have any ideas?
- Do you think the placebo effect meets a therapeutic need?
    - Can we exploit it for better public health? How?
- Does knowingly dispensing a placebo for "those types of patients" violate the idea of "do no harm"?
- Should placebos be available without an Rx to remove provider influence/patient harm?
    - Or does the act of receiving an official Rx create this enhanced effect?
- If you accept self-reports that a patient benefitted from a placebo, are you misleading the patient?
    - Does this violate his/her informed consent?
    - Does this undermine patient autonomy?
- How do we identify whether certain drug classes produce the most placebo effects?
- What drug classes would you imagine have the most placebo or nocebo responses?
- Is a placebo legally a drug if it produces an effect?
    - How can something be a drug for one population but not another?
- If the suggestion is enough to make a patient well/ill, should we never again give a life estimate for terminal illnesses?
- Is telling a patient about their imminent death a medical hex?
- Is there any such thing as a terminal illness, given the placebo effect?
- Can spontaneous remission be explained through the lens of the placebo effect?
- Can you see a way to exploit the placebo effect to taper patients off of medications?
    - Should they know that you are decreasing their active dose and substituting a placebo?
- Have we created a rationale for using homeopathy and unproven compounds?

- After all, if "nothing" works, should we endorse quackery as treatment?
- Does the placebo/nocebo effect undermine the authority of medical professionals?
- Should we come clean to the public about how expectation, belief, trust, hope, and suggestibility are determinants of therapeutic outcomes?

Works Cited

1. Eccles R. Importance of placebo effect in cough clinical trials. Lung. 2010;188 Suppl 1:S53-61.
2. Pozgain I, Pozgain Z, Degmecic D. Placebo and nocebo effect: a mini-review. Psychiatr Danub. 2014;26(2):100-7.
3. Bingel U, Placebo Competence T. Avoiding nocebo effects to optimize treatment outcome. JAMA. 2014;312(7):693-4.
4. Kam-Hansen S, Jakubowski M, Kelley JM, et al. Altered placebo and drug labeling changes the outcome of episodic migraine attacks. Sci Transl Med. 2014;6(218):218ra5.
5. Mahmud N, Kamm MA, Dupas JL, et al. Olsalazine is not superior to placebo in maintaining remission of inactive Crohn's colitis and ileocolitis: a double blind, parallel, randomised, multicentre study. Gut. 2001;49(4):552-6.
6. Bannuru RR, McAlindon TE, Sullivan MC, et al. Effectiveness and Implications of Alternative Placebo Treatments: A Systematic Review and Network Meta-analysis of Osteoarthritis Trials. Ann Intern Med. 2015;163(5):365-72.
7. Khan A, Bomminayuni EP, Bhat A, et al. Are the colors and shapes of current psychotropics designed to maximize the placebo response? Psychopharmacology (Berl). 2010;211(1):113-22.
8. Loden M, Buraczewska I, Halvarsson K. Facial anti-wrinkle cream: influence of product presentation on effectiveness: a randomized and controlled study. Skin Res Technol. 2007;13(2):189-94.
9. Espay AJ, Norris MM, Eliassen JC, et al. Placebo effect of medication cost in Parkinson disease: a randomized double-blind study. Neurology. 2015;84(8):794-802.
10. Jacobs KW, Nordan FM. Classification of placebo drugs: effect of color. Percept Mot Skills. 1979;49(2):367-72.
11. Kong J, Spaeth R, Cook A, et al. Are All Placebo Effects Equal? Placebo Pills, Sham Acupuncture, Cue Conditioning and Their Association. Plos One. 2013;8(7).
12. Fai CK, Qi GD, Wei DA, et al. Placebo preparation for the proper clinical trial of herbal medicine--requirements, verification and quality control. Recent Pat Inflamm Allergy Drug Discov. 2011;5(2):169-74.
13. Vance E. People susceptible to the placebo effect may be keeping us from getting new drugs. The Washington Post. 2016.
14. Tiwari AK, Zai CC, Sajeev G, et al. Analysis of 34 candidate genes in bupropion and placebo remission. Int J Neuropsychopharmacol. 2013;16(4):771-81.
15. Pecina M, Martinez-Jauand M, Hodgkinson C, et al. FAAH selectively influences placebo effects. Mol Psychiatry. 2014;19(3):385-91.
16. Hall KT, Nelson CP, Davis RB, et al. Polymorphisms in catechol-O-methyltransferase modify treatment effects of aspirin on risk of cardiovascular disease. Arterioscler Thromb Vasc Biol. 2014;34(9):2160-7.
17. Hall KT, Lembo AJ, Kirsch I, et al. Catechol-O-methyltransferase val158met polymorphism predicts placebo effect in irritable bowel syndrome. PLoS One. 2012;7(10):e48135.
18. Wendt L, Albring A, Benson S, et al. Catechol-O-methyltransferase Val158Met polymorphism is associated with somatosensory amplification and nocebo responses. PLoS One. 2014;9(9):e107665.

19. Hall KT, Tolkin BR, Chinn GM, et al. Conscientiousness is modified by genetic variation in catechol-O-methyltransferase to reduce symptom complaints in IBS patients. Brain Behav. 2015;5(1).

Essay: The Placebo Effect and Placebo Responders in Clinical Trials

Alena LaBree

Placebos are recognized as an irreplaceable tool in the development of medicine because of their use as controls in randomized clinical trials.[1] Placebos are not a new idea; in fact, they have been around for centuries dating back to Ancient Egypt.[2] Today, placebos are still used as controls in clinical trials and continue to be useful in distinguishing a true pharmacological effect of an active compound.[1] However, because of the placebo effect phenomenon, it has been argued whether placebo responders should be excluded from clinical trials. It is believed that the placebo effect is powerful enough to keep certain drugs from being approved, as these drugs may be unable to produce an effect that is statistically significant compared to the effects of a placebo.

Emerging neuroscience data suggest a strong connection between a psychological response and a physiological outcome which can be heightened by genetic variation in some neurological pathways, thus, making certain individuals more likely to respond to a placebo.[1, 3-5] Genetic screening may provide a more accurate way of identifying the individuals who will respond to a placebo so they can potentially be eliminated from clinical trials. However, while there may be potential benefits of excluding placebo responders, such as a cost reduction of a clinical trial due to reduced sample size,[1] excluding placebo responders may not improve a clinical trial's efficacy and could compromise its integrity.

> *"Randomized double blind placebo control studies are considered the "gold standard" of epidemiologic studies. If well designed, (they) provide the strongest possible evidence of causation."*
>
> Hulley, Cummings, Browner, Grady, & Newman, Clinical Research Experts

Attempts to improve the clinical trial design by excluding placebo responders have already occurred via placebo run-in periods; however, these were typically unsuccessful at increasing a clinical trial's efficacy in determining a drug's true pharmacological effect.[1] Because of the recent discovery of genetic variability in certain neurological pathways contributing to the placebo effect, genetic screening may result in a more accurate way to exclude these placebo responders and improve clinical trial efficacy compared to placebo run-in periods. However, the connection between genetic variation in neurological pathways and a placebo response is underdeveloped as there is limited research on this connection.[1] Additionally, using genetic screening to eliminate placebo responders also follows the assumption that only these individuals with certain genetic variations are capable of exhibiting a placebo response, which may not be the case. There are likely multiple psychological mechanisms and responses contributing to a placebo effect;[6] thus, even if placebo responders were to be eliminated, it may not be possible to fully eliminate them from clinical trials as our screening processes may not be effective enough to fully capture and eliminate every individual who is likely to respond.

In clinical trials, placebos are used as controls to represent a group receiving no treatment so it can be determined if a drug in a treatment group is efficacious. However, since the administration of a placebo can elicit effects, it is thought that comparing a treatment group to a placebo group in a clinical trial may not actually be comparing a drug to the absence of treatment.[6] The effects that a placebo can elicit are usually minimal and are rarely powerful enough to treat or cure an illness.[4] Because placebo effects commonly are so minimal, subjects in the placebo control group could become aware they are receiving the placebo and withdraw because they are not experiencing a substantial benefit. This can compromise the blindness that is a hallmark of a clinical trial. The exclusion of placebo responders could make it more evident who is and who is not receiving the placebo, having the effect of a higher percentage of subjects withdrawing due to their lack of results.

Another hallmark of clinical trial design is randomization. Randomization is to ensure that a smaller sample size is an accurate representation of a larger population to avoid selection bias.[7] Eliminating placebo responders from a clinical trial would fail to accurately represent the population that will be using the drug after its approval, as it is likely that placebo responders will be taking the drug. Additionally, preventing placebo responders from enrolling in clinical trials could make recruitment for clinical trials more difficult than it already is because it further limits who can be enrolled, which may also contribute to selection bias.

Researchers have been looking for ways to minimize placebo responses in clinical trials as placebo responses do have the potential to keep certain drugs from getting approved, as the placebo effects may be masking the drug's effects. But even with the issues of placebo responders, placebo-controlled clinical studies are still recognized as the best way to determine a causation effect of a drug under study.[7] While eliminating these responders may seem good in theory, it may be too complicated to eliminate them fully and will likely affect the blindness and randomization aspects that are the hallmark of a clinical trial design.

Works Cited

1. Hall KT, Loscalzo J, Kaptchuk TJ. Genetics and the placebo effect: the placebome. Trends Mol Med. 2015;21(5):285-94.
2. Macedo A, Farre M, Banos JE. Placebo effect and placebos: what are we talking about? Some conceptual and historical considerations. Eur J Clin Pharmacol. 2003;59(4):337-42. Epub 20030627.
3. Wager TD, Atlas LY. The neuroscience of placebo effects: connecting context, learning and health. Nat Rev Neurosci. 2015;16(7):403-18.

4. Cai L, He L. Placebo effects and the molecular biological components involved. Gen Psychiatr. 2019;32(5):e100089. Epub 20190906.
5. Lee HF, Hsieh JC, Lu CL, et al. Enhanced affect/cognition-related brain responses during visceral placebo analgesia in irritable bowel syndrome patients. Pain. 2012;153(6):1301-10. Epub 20120427.
6. Gupta U, Verma M. Placebo in clinical trials. Perspect Clin Res. 2013;4(1):49-52.
7. Misra S. Randomized double blind placebo control studies, the "Gold Standard" in intervention based studies. Indian J Sex Transm Dis AIDS. 2012;33(2):131-4.

Topic: Drug Advertising, Sales, and Prescribing

The US is in the unenviable position of outspending 10 countries that are very similar with respect to healthcare expenditures and quality. Such dubious leadership is due to US healthcare provider salaries, which are high; the most expensive prescription drugs in the world; and burdensome administrative costs to run ever-enlarging hospitals and medical clinics that are continually cannibalized by corporations with profit-making motives. Thus, total US drug spending represents approximately 17% of our healthcare expenditures, and payers such as Medicare spend approximately 2% more because they cover more specialty drugs and medications for the most ill and elderly segment of our population.[1,2]

The newest prescription drugs contribute the most to patient out-of-pocket costs because they are the most expensive drugs on the market, even though they are often not better than a similar drug that costs less and has been on the market for a longer period of time.[3,4] Pharmaceutical companies suggest that these increased costs for new drugs are directly tied to the price of research and development. However, data suggest otherwise—that almost all drug makers spend more on advertising and drug representative activity than scientific research and innovation.[5] More intriguing is that the revenue generated from drug sales is billions more than what is needed to engage in new drug discovery.

> *"Every night I watch the nightly news. It's funded by the pharmaceutical companies. Virtually every ad is a drug ad. They get their say every night on the nightly news through advertising."*
>
> — Michael Moore, American documentary filmmaker, activist, and author

Indeed, direct-to-consumer advertising, which is legal in the US and New Zealand only, drives up drug prices by suggesting drugs for consumers that they may not need, offering more pricey options for patients who may be better served with a cheaper generic, and creating new diseases that appear to require treatment when, in the past, these conditions were mere annoyances. Today, they represent real health threats that must be mitigated, if the ads are to be believed. Additional advertising is more covert in the form of drug representatives who are chiefly schooled in communications, journalism, or another non-scientific field. Hired for their looks and confidence, these non-specialists attempt to "educate" physicians about the latest product by showing up between patient appointments, bribing clinics with free lunches, or more egregiously, asking to follow the physician when he/she sees patients.[6-10] The public perception of these disingenuous representatives is being increasingly soured as emerging data confirm that not only do these "drug pushers" know zero pharmacology but also that they financially reward physicians with "grants" or speaker fees if the physicians promote their products exclusively.[11] Because of these nefarious practices, organizations such as ProPublica and others have created databases for researching physician kickbacks from drug companies.[12] This is important information because physicians routinely claim that they are not swayed by representative visits or information. However, studies confirm the contrary: physicians who engage with drug representatives as purported "thought leaders" about their drugs have increased prescribing of those products.[13, 14] This cannot be good for patients who may not need the drug or cannot afford it. Likewise, giving free samples of new and expensive medications is a form of advertising.[15, 16] Studies show that when patients are given these samples, they request those more expensive medications at follow-up visits.[17, 18] Again, they may not need that particular drug and insurance may not cover it.

Next, the US essentially shoulders the burden and costs of all pharmaceutical innovation but we have the most onerous drug pricing scheme for our customers due to a closed market system unique to pharmaceutics.[19] In fact, this industry is the only one that enjoys product exclusivity, lengthy patent protection, and price controls within an otherwise free capitalistic market.[20] This causes US consumers to subsidize drug costs for the rest of the globe, something that is a great concern because the US hosts the most children living in poverty as well as has the greatest incidence of obesity, lung disease, heart disease, and diabetes for people across all spectra of socioeconomic circumstances. It would seem that in a pharmaceutically resource-rich environment, we'd have better health outcomes.[21]

Also, Pharma takes advantage of our broken drug regulatory system when possible. After President Ronald Reagan signed into law the Orphan Drug Act of 1983 to encourage drug makers to create drugs to treat small populations of patients with few therapeutic options, Pharma was granted tax breaks and patent exclusivity for an additional seven

"There seems to be no logic—or warning—to these price spikes...Sunlight is needed to help respond to price shifts, because if the pricing trends continue, patients and communities will not be able to afford life-saving drugs."

Barbara L. McAneny, MD, AMA President-elect

years for any orphan drug approved. The spirit of the Act was to incentivize Pharma to develop drugs that essentially had no hope of paying for the research invested in them because they would not be in widespread use. This is not what happened, however. Instead, drug companies "re-invented" old drugs that were already available and very inexpensive in other countries as "new" drugs for the US market. Then, they exorbitantly raised the prices of these specialty medications under the guise of having too few patients to recoup research costs that were never incurred in the first place.

Finally, again due to mismanaged governance over the pharmaceutical and healthcare industry, pharmacy benefit managers have insinuated themselves into healthcare by insisting that we need third-party administration of all of our health plans, something that appeared to function fine before the introduction of these dubious partners.[22] Pharmacy benefit managers report that they exist to bargain with pharm to drive down drug costs and increase consumer confidence in our drug supply, but studies confirm something else.[23] For instance, pharmacy benefit managers often keep drug company rebates that should rightfully go to the pharmacy and be passed on to the customer.[24] They also charge pharmacies, insurers, and employers special fees for drugs that they claim to price-negotiate for patient discounts. Because these managers are entirely for-profit, they are motivated to keep any differences in discounts and to ask for even more from drug companies. This produces a sinister relationship between managers and drug companies who keep drug cost formulas away from consumers, enabling them to collude to increase drug prices. Then, public pharmacy benefit managers blame drug companies for high prices that they drove upwards by asking for discounts. Meanwhile, Pharma points the finger back at benefit managers as being the ones to blame for soaring medication prices.

Writing Prompts

- Should we ban direct-to-consumer ads for drugs?
- Should patients be "re-educated" as to who the health expert is (their MD)?
- Should MDs turn away patients who request specific drugs?
  - Is the US correct in clawing back time and space for reps?
- Should MDs list on their office door who they take money from?
- Should MDs have to disclose that they get money from a drug maker every time they Rx that drug to a patient?
  - All scientific papers have such mandatory disclosure agreements.
- Should Pharma have to underwrite a certain percent of US prescription costs considering that they cause the high prices and force-feed the public propaganda?
  - Should this be levied as an annual tax?
- Should all drug companies post all R&D expenditure data next to sales and advertising costs in an effort of transparency?
- Is healthcare a service for which we should pay or is it a human right?
  - At what price point is profiting from a drug unethical?
- Health insurance companies and health maintenance organizations (HMOs) can negotiate lower prices for consumers but Medicare cannot; is this fair?
- When US Pharma companies merge with those outside the US, they can benefit from an inversion transaction, allowing relinquishing of US corporate citizenship in exchange for paying no taxes here...is this fair?
  - What could we have done with that money in the US?
  - Fund drugs for the poor and elderly?
  - Spend it on university-based scientific research as grants?
  - Set up free clinics in poor areas of the country?
- Should Pharma mergers be allowed only to a point to prevent monopolies and anti-competitive outcomes?
  - What is that point?

Works Cited

1. Evaluation OotASfPa. Observations on Trends in Prescription Drug Pricing. 2016.
2. MedPAC. Overview: Medicare drug spending 2016.
3. Gastala NM, Wingrove P, Gaglioti A, et al. Medicare Part D: Patients Bear The Cost Of 'Me Too' Brand-Name Drugs. Health Aff (Millwood). 2016;35(7):1237-40.

4. Regnier S. What is the value of 'me-too' drugs? Health Care Manag Sci. 2013;16(4):300-13.
5. Hansen RA, Schommer JC, Cline RR, et al. The association of consumer cost-sharing and direct-to-consumer advertising with prescription drug use. Res Social Adm Pharm. 2005;1(2):139-57.
6. Spurling GK, Mansfield PR, Montgomery BD, et al. Information from pharmaceutical companies and the quality, quantity, and cost of physicians' prescribing: a systematic review. PLoS Med. 2010;7(10):e1000352.
7. Restricted contact with drug company representatives influences future physicians. Am J Health Syst Pharm. 2001;58(24):2366.
8. Davis GF. Physicians and drug company sales representatives. Am J Med. 2000;108(5):432-3.
9. Rosner F. Physicians and drug company representatives. Am J Med. 2000;108(3):263.
10. Chren MM. Interactions between physicians and drug company representatives. Am J Med. 1999;107(2):182-3.
11. Blake RL, Jr., Early EK. Patients' attitudes about gifts to physicians from pharmaceutical companies. J Am Board Fam Pract. 1995;8(6):457-64.
12. Norris SL, Holmer HK, Ogden LA, et al. Characteristics of physicians receiving large payments from pharmaceutical companies and the accuracy of their disclosures in publications: an observational study. BMC Med Ethics. 2012;13:24.
13. Freemantle N, Johnson R, Dennis J, et al. Sleeping with the enemy? A randomized controlled trial of a collaborative health authority/industry intervention to influence prescribing practice. Br J Clin Pharmacol. 2000;49(2):174-9.
14. Towards better patient care: drugs to avoid. Prescrire Int. 2013;22(137):108-11.
15. Allou KRS, Iraqi H, Cherrah Y, et al. [Which place occupies the free drug sample in the prescription of the physicians in Morocco?]. Therapie. 2018.
16. Hurley MP, Stafford RS, Lane AT. Characterizing the relationship between free drug samples and prescription patterns for acne vulgaris and rosacea. JAMA Dermatol. 2014;150(5):487-93.
17. Morgan MA, Dana J, Loewenstein G, et al. Interactions of doctors with the pharmaceutical industry. J Med Ethics. 2006;32(10):559-63.
18. Hall KB, Tett SE, Nissen LM. Perceptions of the influence of prescription medicine samples on prescribing by family physicians. Med Care. 2006;44(4):383-7.
19. Huskamp HA, Epstein AM, Blumenthal D. The impact of a national prescription drug formulary on prices, market share, and spending: lessons for Medicare? Health Aff (Millwood). 2003;22(3):149-58.
20. Levy MS. Bib Pharma Monopoly: Why Consumers Keep Landing on "Park Place" and How the Game is Rigged. Am Univ Law Rev. 2016;66(1):247-303.
21. Berndt ER, Mortimer R, Bhattacharjya A, et al. Authorized generic drugs, price competition, and consumers' welfare. Health Aff (Millwood). 2007;26(3):790-9.
22. Sumida WK, Taniguchi R, Juarez DT. The Daniel K. Inouye College of Pharmacy Scripts: Prescription Drug Pricing. Hawaii J Med Public Health. 2016;75(1):25-30.
23. Cohen JP, Khoury CE, Milne CP, et al. Rising Drug Costs Drives the Growth of Pharmacy Benefit Managers Exclusion Lists: Are Exclusion Decisions Value-Based? Health Serv Res. 2017.
24. Gabay M. Direct and Indirect Remuneration Fees: The Controversy Continues. Hosp Pharm. 2017;52(11):740-1.

Essay: Deceptive Drug Marketing

Why is DTCA potentially harmful to a patient's health?

Jason Canizales

The development of new drugs and bringing them to market is a lengthy process that requires on average 10–15 years of careful research to assess safety and efficacy.[1, 2] Due to an extensive pharmacological background required to understand the nuances of drug approval, medical professionals have been majorly in charge of safeguarding the public from potential dangers they may not fully understand. For this reason, pharmaceutical companies had exclusively directed promotional material of new drugs (products) to physicians who have direct control over their prescription/sales. However, over the past decade, with an increasing number of people having more agency over their own healthcare decisions, the marketing of drugs to patients/consumers have brought pharmaceutical companies better avenues to promote their remedies to a rather informatically-vulnerable audience.[3] In the world, only the US and New Zealand allow direct-to-consumer advertising (DTCA) of drugs. In doing so pharmaceutical companies have been financially impacted by an increase in sales revenue with limited legislative involvement over its ethical practice. In wake of the positive reinforcement of DTCA, overly disproportionate expenditure of DTCA vs research and development (R&D) suggests a continually profitable practice that may promote the dissemination of deceptive information in favor of a profitable business model.[4, 5]

Regulation of DTCA

In 1985 the FDA rescinded the moratorium of DTCA, albeit concerns of its potential repercussions were still a cause for concern.[6] To mitigate future problems, advertisements were to meet the same legal requirements directed to physicians. Thus, product-claim advertisements—regardless of the medium used—have been required to provide the brand and generic name of a drug, at least 1 FDA-approved use and presentation of a balanced ratio of potential risks and benefits.[7] By 1997 the pressure on the FDA to loosen restrictions in DTCA came as a result of greater consumer involvement in healthcare and other interested parties. At the time, policy reduction advocates promoted the idea of providing a summary of the general risks in ads to involve both consumers and physicians in the decision-making process of whether to buy or prescribe a drug respectively. To comply with the surging demands, the FDA allowed broadcasts to refer consumers to a toll-free telephone number, print ads, a website, and/or their pharmacist or physician instead of providing a full debrief of a drug's labeling.[6, 8] Because of this, dilution of the FDA's direct policing of DTCAs progressively diminished allowing pharmaceutical companies to ease their way into the media.

What Ads Are Not Required to Tell You
Rx advertisement is regulated by the FDA while over-the-counter medication is monitored by the FTC.[9] Amidst efforts placed to require drug manufacturers to report factual, transparent, and accurate information in DTCAs, sometimes loopholes in policy may be exploited. Although the FDA oversees advertisement for prescription drugs, the manufacturing company is not required to provide pre-release authorization for FDA compliance before its advertisement to the public.[10] However, if the FDA deems an ad unacceptable for public display, a letter can be sent to the drug company to request its immediate removal. In addition, even if serious adverse effects, addiction, or withdrawal effects are known, federal law is unable to ban a company from advertising its drug.[9] The only exception is drugs with black box warnings.

As a result of the further branching of policy, several other forms and regulations for advertising arose. Reminder advertisements were originally designed for medical journals to prompt physicians to recall a medication about a specific condition. Nowadays, this form of advertisement works to bring to mind medications the public already recognizes. This means that only the name of the drug is provided and no form of allusion to its use or risks is included. In contrast, help-seeking ads operate by describing a condition without directly mentioning a drug's name. These usually recommend patients to seek medical counseling, but in doing so, a patient may associate a drug company with a potential treatment for their condition.[7, 11]

Among other concerns, drug companies are not obligated to disclose a drug's price or whether a generic version exists. This is a particular disadvantage to patients who may not be able to afford their medication and are ultimately forced to purchase the "only" alternative for their condition. Prevalence of a condition treated by the drug, its mechanism of action, and how quickly a drug works (although what is meant by "quickly" has to be stated) are also some other features that can be omitted in DTCAs.[7]

Concerns of Exponential Increase in DTCA Investment
Ever since FDA regulation over DTCA became more flexible in 1997, pharmaceutical companies have continued to increase investment in all 3 categories of advertising. Between 1996 and 2003, there was a 400% increase in pharmaceutical DTCA ranging from $791 million to $3.2 billion.[11, 12] For comparison, in 2000 marketing efforts of retailing companies were about $160 million (Dell), $146 million (Budweiser), $125 million (Pepsi), and $78 million (Nike).[13] In the same year, advertisement dollars towards Rofecoxib (Vioxx)—a selective COX-2 inhibitor—were $161 million yet it was withdrawn from the market in 2004 after a study that showed its long-term use associated with twice the risk of having a heart attack compared to placebo.[14] For this reason, calls for the FDA to delay DTCA of new drugs to better assess post-marketing safety surveillance were stated. Despite the endorsement of the idea by multiple sources including the Institute of Medicine, no government regulation has been established on the issue.[15]

DTCA is a fraction of the total money spent on advertising. Between 1997–2016, advertising increased from $17.7–$29.9 billion of which close to $10 billion was directed towards DTCA in 2016 alone.[16] While DTCA supporters may claim that advertising efforts are continually being directed toward medical professionals, the 460% increase in DTCA (in the same time period) seems to suggest a greater preference/priority to consumers rather than prescribers. The global pharmaceutical industry was valued at $816 billion in 2016. However, top pharmaceutical companies only spend 20.5% of their revenue on R&D.[5] Because pharmaceutical companies spend large sums of money in bringing new drugs to market ($314 million to $2.8 billion), they are compelled to gain a return on investment greater than what is originally spent.[17] Given a lack of government financial support (orphan drugs being an exception) has driven these companies to resort to strategies that will produce them the most money. Therefore, if a deficit in drug promotion exists, this will translate into overall lesser profits. Unfortunately, this practice inevitably affects the quality and transparency of R&D.[5]

Patents exist to allow pharmaceutical companies to financially recover from the high-cost process of bringing a new drug into the market. While primary patents allow for the 20-year protection of an active ingredient of a drug, companies have been trying to seek additional secondary patents to protect other aspects of a drug to prolong their exclusivity in the market.[18] This means that even if the primary exclusivity of a drug ends, secondary patents which may cover formulation or manufacturing processes can delay the generic variations of that drug from coming to market. This is particularly a dangerous practice because it monopolizes the circulation of a single drug for a long time allowing the company to have a considerable influence over its pricing.[19]

Clinical Significance

Effective pharmaceutical advertising can work as an effective psychological tool that can impact the judgment of both a patient and a physician. While DTCAs may help inform and empower patients in taking charge of their health, omission of quintessential information may lead a patient to reach inaccurate conclusions.[20] Overemphasis on a drug's benefits can negatively condition a patient to disproportionately recall more of the desirable aspects rather than its risks. Physicians also corroborate this appeal whenever a patient suggests the advertised medication.[21]

A study found that 82% of the claims in televised DTCAs were mostly factual and provided a credible rationale, but only 26% disclosed potential risk factors that could potentially influence a patient's opinion on the drugs advertised.[22] In addition, DTCAs suggest that a solution to a particular problem is linked to their product; however, information related to simple lifestyle changes or behaviors as an alternate solution to a condition may not be mentioned. If the media were to be devoid of inaccurate and predatory information, perhaps arguments in favor of DTCAs would be more agreeable in defense of healthcare.

Some studies have shown that DTCA-lead conversations are likely to result in a prescription of the drug advertised despite a physician's awareness of alternative options.[23,24] Data suggests that patients who request a particular brand or generic drug are more likely to have their request accepted in comparison to those who do not.[20] In some instances, physicians may not be fully knowledgeable of a new drug's physiological action and safety profile. This can be particularly problematic when a patient purposely withholds important "unappealing" information from a DTCA drug in pursuit of acquiring a prescription believed to be suitable for them.[25] Although physician reports surrounding inappropriate prescriptions tend to vary, repercussions of patient compliance with suggested medications can be harmful to public health.

If a physician was to decline a patient's suggestion, this may also negatively impact the relationship between them. From a clinician's point of view, studies show a particular distaste whenever patients begin to talk about DTCA drugs. A physician may also grow frustrated if an argument about a drug's effectiveness leads a patient to question their authority over "evidence" heard or found from the media.[26] Conversely, if a clinician were to deny their request, a patient could proceed to dismiss any warnings and acquire the prescription from another source or switch physicians.[27] Due to the unreliability of DTCAs, patients unaware of the potential dangers should be more understanding of their physician's comments and concerns to avoid unnecessary complications.

Concluding Remarks

The growing financial interests of pharmaceutical companies have had a direct impact on the safety profile of the drug development process. This poses a risk to the public if misleading or omitted information is present in DTCA. Due to a lack of government scrutiny and restricted FDA oversight, the accuracy of the information presented in DTCAs cannot be guaranteed. For this reason, concerns of a receptive audience to a misleading façade of DTCAs may indirectly harm a population that is not aware of the underlying dangers of a particular drug.

Works Cited

1. How long a new drug takes to go through clinical trials: Cancer Research UK; 2022 [cited 2022]. Available from: https://www.cancerresearchuk.org/about-cancer/find-a-clinical-trial/how-clinical-trials-are-planned-and-organised/how-long-it-takes-for-a-new-drug-to-go-through-clinical-trials.
2. Development & Approval Process 2022. Available from: https://www.fda.gov/drugs/development-approval-process-drugs.
3. The Impact of Direct-to-Consumer Advertising: US Food & Drug Administration; 2015 [cited 2022]. Available from: fda.gov/drugs/information-consumers-and-patients-drugs/impact-direct-consumer-advertising.
4. Spurling GK, Mansfield PR, Montgomery BD, et al. Information from pharmaceutical companies and the quality, quantity, and cost of physicians' prescribing: a systematic review. PLoS Med. 2010;7(10):e1000352.
5. Jacob NT. Drug promotion practices: A review. Br J Clin Pharmacol. 2018;84(8):1659-67. Epub 20180220.
6. Donohue J. A history of drug advertising: the evolving roles of consumers and consumer protection. Milbank Q. 2006;84(4):659-99.
7. Basics of Drug Ads: US Food & Drug Administration; 2015 [cited 2022]. Available from: https://www.fda.gov/drugs/prescription-drug-advertising/basics-drug-ads.
8. Feather KR. Oral History Interview with Ken Feather. Rockville, Md: US Food and Drug Administration. 1997.
9. Prescription Drug Advertising: US Food & Drug Administration; 2015 [cited 2022]. Available from: https://www.fda.gov/drugs/prescription-drug-advertising/prescription-drug-advertising-questions-and-answers#:~:text=The%20Federal%20Trade%20Commission%20(FTC,LASIK%20procedures%2C%20and%20contact%20lenses.
10. Sullivan HW, Aikin KJ, David KT, et al. Consumer understanding of the scope of FDA's prescription drug regulatory oversight: A nationally representative survey. Pharmacoepidemiol Drug Saf. 2020;29(2):134-40. Epub 20191212.

11. Gellad ZF, Lyles KW. Direct-to-consumer advertising of pharmaceuticals. Am J Med. 2007;120(6):475-80.
12. Querna B. The big pill pitch. US News World Rep. 2005;138(21):52-3.
13. Rosenthal MB, Berndt ER, Donohue JM, et al. Promotion of prescription drugs to consumers. N Engl J Med. 2002;346(7):498-505.
14. Sibbald B. Rofecoxib (Vioxx) voluntarily withdrawn from market. CMAJ. 2004;171(9):1027-8.
15. Shuchman M. Drug risks and free speech--can Congress ban consumer drug ads? N Engl J Med. 2007;356(22):2236-9. Epub 20070502.
16. Franquiz MJ, McGuire AL. Direct-to-Consumer Drug Advertisement and Prescribing Practices: Evidence Review and Practical Guidance for Clinicians. J Gen Intern Med. 2021;36(5):1390-4. Epub 20200915.
17. Wouters OJ, McKee M, Luyten J. Estimated Research and Development Investment Needed to Bring a New Medicine to Market, 2009-2018. JAMA. 2020;323(9):844-53.
18. Gurgula O. Strategic Patenting by Pharmaceutical Companies - Should Competition Law Intervene? IIC Int Rev Ind Prop Copyr Law. 2020;51(9):1062-85. Epub 20201028.
19. Atkinson JD, Moodie RS. Legitimate patent extension or patent system abuse? Pharm Pat Anal. 2013;2(3):317-24.
20. Almasi EA, Stafford RS, Kravitz RL, et al. What are the public health effects of direct-to-consumer drug advertising? PLoS Med. 2006;3(3):e145. Epub 20060328.
21. Davis J. The effect of qualifying language on perceptions of drug appeal, drug experience, and estimates of side-effect incidence in DTC advertising. J Health Commun. 2007;12(7):607-22.
22. Frosch DL, Krueger PM, Hornik RC, et al. Creating demand for prescription drugs: a content analysis of television direct-to-consumer advertising. Ann Fam Med. 2007;5(1):6-13.
23. Mintzes B, Barer ML, Kravitz RL, et al. How does direct-to-consumer advertising (DTCA) affect prescribing? A survey in primary care environments with and without legal DTCA. CMAJ. 2003;169(5):405-12.
24. DeFrank JT, Berkman ND, Kahwati L, et al. Direct-to-Consumer Advertising of Prescription Drugs and the Patient-Prescriber Encounter: A Systematic Review. Health Commun. 2020;35(6):739-46. Epub 20190411.
25. Connors AL. Big bad pharma: an ethical analysis of physician-directed and consumer-directed marketing tactics. Albany Law Rev. 2009;73(1):243-82.
26. Delbaere M, Smith MC. Health care knowledge and consumer learning: the case of direct-to-consumer drug advertising. Health Mark Q. 2006;23(3):9-29.
27. Frosch DL, Grande D, Tarn DM, et al. A decade of controversy: balancing policy with evidence in the regulation of prescription drug advertising. Am J Public Health. 2010;100(1):24-32.

Topic: Supplements and Homeopathy

Supplements, as defined by the US FDA, are adjuncts to the daily human diet, and as such are not regulated in the same manner as drugs. This distinction was formalized by President Clinton in 1994 with the promulgation of the Dietary Supplement Health and Education Act (DSHEA).[1] With this act, the government attempted to accomplish two goals: to ensure continued consumer access to dietary supplements and to provide consumers with more information about their intended use. This new legislation, however, did not modify the regulatory status of supplements as a subcategory of foods, which are governed by unique laws and have particular safety issues.[1] Therefore, supplements did not need to meet new standards of efficacy, safety, or purity but they could be subjected to oversight by the FDA and withdrawn from the market if they were found to cause harm.[2] Such after-the-fact problem-solving put the burden on the consumer to report adverse events, and it did nothing to protect anyone from new and untested supplements or dubious or dangerous ingredients. Still, this legislation is in place today, and supplements must be determined to be dangerous before any action can be taken by the US government, and by that time, it may be too late.

"It's (homeopathy) exactly equivalent to taking one 325 milligram aspirin tablet, throwing it into the middle of Lake Tahoe, and then stirring it up... Then, when you get a headache, you take a sip of this water, and—voila!—it is gone...(t)hat is what homeopathy is all about."

James Randi, Canadian-American retired stage magician and a scientific skeptic

Supplements, due to their non-drug status, cannot make label claims that the compounds can be used to treat or mitigate disease; however, supplement labels can offer structure and function claims. With these types of claims, the manufacturer of the supplement can describe the role of a nutrient or dietary ingredient (iron is required for blood cell formation), mention how that nutrient contributes to a function (fiber supports digestive regularity), and suggest a benefit of that nutrient for addressing a deficit (folate prevents neural tube defects). Unfortunately, structure and function claims are often indistinguishable from drug-like claims to the general consumer. Finally, such label claims do not suggest the product at hand contains the labeled nutrient at all, or that the product contains sufficient quantities of any nutrient to prevent a deficiency or support any function.[3] On the rare occasion when a supplement makes prohibited drug-like claims that are noticed and documented to be false, or when a supplement is found to be harmful and removed from the market, other supplement manufacturers will fill this new void in the market space. Such a rush to put products in front of consumers virtually guarantees that most of what is sold is hastily planned, poorly studied, not well-understood, and lacking efficacy and safety data.[4]

These liabilities are especially true for a category of supplements loosely referred to as traditional Chinese medicines (TCM) that appeal to consumers who erroneously assume that these products are time-tested remedies. That these products are neither traditional nor particularly Chinese does not appear to discourage consumers from beliefs in their ability to "heal" or produce meaningful changes in the body. Because TCM products are often derived from plants or plant combinations that vastly differ by growing season, latitude and longitude of plant origin, plant maturity, harvesting technique, plant component (root versus leaf versus stem), and plant blending ratios, there is no standardized and acceptable method for comparing TCM products to one another.

For this reason, scientists who submit papers about these products to prestigious Western journals frequently have their manuscripts returned unread because they have not produced meaningful science that can be peer-reviewed. Without this peer-review, nothing can be said with certainty about the function and structure claims for such supplements.[5] Perhaps more telling is that no TCM product has—to date—survived the rigor of a US FDA approval process and been approved as a new chemical entity (new drug product). This is true despite the strong desire of and multiple attempts by TCM manufacturers to have their supplements achieve drug status here and abroad.[6,7]

Such confusion about TCM's lack of efficacy and acceptance in Western science may stem from the lack of rigor and reproducibility across Asia with respect to drug innovation and testing. For instance, in 2010, China had no method for recalling dangerous or tainted drugs or foods in its very own supply chain. Because China is one of the top exporters of consumer products across the globe, it almost always falls to countries that import these products to do the policing that China will not or cannot do. And the problem is not insignificant. For instance, in 2007, a top Chinese food and drug regulator, Mr. Zheng Xiaoyu, was executed after he admitted to taking bribes in exchange for approving untested drugs in the China Food and Drug Administration (CFDA) system.[8] Then, in larger and formal clinical trials of Chinese drugs, data integrity is known to be problematic or entirely lacking. Chinese clinical trial subjects themselves are often the cause of misconduct by faking or tampering with their urine samples to mask smoking and drinking habits, which are common practices even in the face of indisputable evidence of adverse health effects associated with these activities.[9] Because trial subjects are well compensated for faking data, this fraudulent trend is unlikely to cease soon.

In an attempt to raise the integrity of China's science and drug discovery process, the Chinese government in 2018 issued a warning to all Chinese drug development scientists—if their applications for drug approval within the CFDA were found to be inauthentic or to have fraudulent data, they could be punished by time in prison or by death.[10] In response to this edict, more than 80% (1,193) of 1,622 submitted CFDA applications were immediately withdrawn. This suggests that little science underlies many applications for Chinese drug products and that the laboratories that submit these applications are complicit in this fraud. Because this criminal activity reflects actual drug approval applications in the CFDA pipeline, there is ample reason to assume that TCM supplement manufacturers have little interest in honesty, authenticity, and safety.

Fortunately, scientists with expertise in nutrition and supplementation are often unanimous and vocal on the topic of supplements, irrespective of their purported source. These experts suggest that vitamins and mineral supplements are largely a waste of money and do not offer additional health benefits that cannot be obtained in a regularly consumed, relatively nutritionally complete diet.[11-17] Thus, scientists suggest that most of the hype surrounding supplements is mythical and at best, these additives do little more than generate expensive urine. More frightening perhaps than unnecessarily spending money on supplements is the adverse effects that these products may have on specific populations. For instance, for people who are receiving treatment for cancer, antioxidant supplements, which are largely misunderstood by most of the lay public, may block the chemotherapeutic effects of very expensive cancer drugs and prevent tumor cells from being removed by protecting them from selective drug toxicity. Thus, some vitamins and antioxidants may actually promote certain types of tumors[16, 18, 19] Therefore, following the lead of top scientists, consumers may completely avoid the risk associated with unnecessary supplement use by simply abstaining from using them at all.

Similar to the supplement racket, another medical treatment augmentation is homeopathy which was founded more 200 years ago by Dr. Samuel Hahnemann.[20] Homeopathy was and continues to be based on the

"I also turn to homeopathic remedies for the treatment of indigestion, travel sickness, insomnia and hay fever just to name a few. Homeopathy offers a safe, natural alternative that causes no side effects or drug interactions."

Cindy Crawford, model and non-scientist

ancient, but now thoroughly disproven theory that "like treats like". Thus, treating someone with influenza should, according to homeopathy, cure the flu. Furthermore, homeopathy suggests that the more dilute a substance is, the more (paradoxically) potent it is for curing illness.[21] For instance, a homeopathic product such as *Oscillococcinum* is, as the label indicates, a 30C liquid preparation of duck liver (regarded to be a natural avian flu reservoir). Homeopathic protocols and peer-reviewed science confirms that a 30C homeopathic product is diluted at approximately $1:100^{30}$ (for this particular supplement: one part duck liver to 10^{60} parts water).[22, 23] This represents a greater dilution than what would be represented by a one-milliliter drop of India ink in an Olympic swimming pool.

Ridiculous dilutions aside, another problem for the consumer who purchases such products is that the original solution from which all subsequent homeopathic dilutions were made is never disclosed to the buyer. Thus, the original solution may contain no active molecules at all before the dilution steps are initiated. Avogadro's number, which underpins all chemistry, suggests that one mole of any element or compound is 6.022×10^{23}. So, any dilution of a substance that exceeds this value contains only the possibility of that molecule remaining. Put another way, the most dilute an element or compound can be and still contain any possible residue of that element or compound is approximately 12C. That the only positive studies in the literature regarding *Oscillococcinum* are from the product manufacturer, Boiron, suggests significant study bias or outright fraud.[24] Also, only 11 studies in the scientific literature mention the product at all, and most are short commentaries about the deceptiveness of homeopathy. Thus, this is likely sufficient evidence that the public should put no faith or money into this product or similar compounds.[24]

Therefore, the chemical and pharmacological underpinnings of homeopathy are not scientific or founded on known scientific explanations, so homeopathy is not considered medicine in any form. Rather, it is an exercise in fraud and dishonest or ignorant self-reporting. Even with these truths in evidence, homeopathy is enjoying a resurgence among non-scientifically trained people who seek "natural" remedies to their illnesses and annoyances. This creates a conflict and a controversy for scientists, especially pharmacologists, who are less inclined to align their scientific viewpoints with quackery and who are more predisposed to call homeopathic "responses" what they truly are: placebo outcomes or manifestations of self-limiting conditions that improve over time irrespective of the treatment given. When pressed, a few pharmacologists are probably comfortable with assigning homeopathic self-reports of a cure as a third category of non-drug somatic response. However, the disdain of the expert for sham medicine has done little to dispel fake practitioners, and currently we "honor" unorthodox and unschooled approaches to healthcare as "complementary and alternative medicine".

This nomenclature arose and was modified over time as quack practitioners, often people with zero medical training but a sole desire to make money from a gullible public, demanded labels of legitimacy.[25] First, those who plied the trade of homeopathy and other dubious practices were dubbed alternative medical practitioners. This did not mollify the quacks for too long because, to them, it suggested that what they did was not actual medicine, or that it could be omitted from a healthy lifestyle. Thus, complementary medicine was applied to their machinations, but this also failed to satisfy those who saw their education and approach as being equal to or better than conventional (Western) medicine. The idea that it was complementary again suggested that it was not required. Giving in to pandering by the homeopathic community and the increasing distrust by the public that evidenced-based medicine was a failure because it did not produce a cure for every person every time, the homeopathic process was finally dubbed "integrative" medicine.

What homeopathic specialists and their victims cannot appear to understand is that if the "medicine" offered by homeopathy was efficacious and offered reproducible effects, it would cease to be "alternative", "complementary", or "integrative" and instead would just be classified as "medicine" in the manner of all scientifically derived treatments so named.[26] Supporters of quack medicine are often quick to ascribe cynicism to scientists who will not bend to their discipline's false claims. Again, this is a point of ignorance. Cynicism is the closing of the mind to all possibilities. In contrast, scientific skepticism calls for approaching claims with an open mind but accepting only those claims that can survive the scrutiny of rigorous scientific tests.[27]

Then, most "evidence" for efficacious homeopathy appears in self-titled alternative and complementary medical journals, which is additional support for selection bias in reporting homeopathy outcomes.[28] In agreement with this harsh assessment of homeopathy, the British Medical Association refers to homeopathy as "witchcraft".[29] Also, in the US, there is a $1 million award for any person or organization who can prove that homeopathy is efficacious—and no one has taken up the challenge to date—which may suggest that homeopathy is not a legitimate path to health and wellness.[30] Finally, the New Zealand Medical Council requested that all medical practitioners cease recommending homeopaths to their patients unless the patients were informed that homeopathy could offer no more than a placebo-mediated effect.[29, 31] Thus, it seems clear that the controversial practice of selling patients false hope in the form of watered-down substances of homeopathy is biologically implausible and inconsistent with how experts understand medicine, biology, pharmacology, and pathology.[31]

Writing Prompts

- Is homeopathy and supplement "prescribing" unethical?
- Does advocating either of these practices run counter to the oath to "do no harm"?
- Is seeking homeopathic remedies akin to a failure to seek effective healthcare?
- Should parents be jailed for using homeopathic "remedies" for minor children?
- Is homeopathy a waste of resources?
  - What are the most wasted ones?
- Is advocating homeopathy promoting false beliefs?
- How do you explain the homeopathic benefits people claim to receive?
- Should naturopaths and homeopaths be banned from patient care?
- Should we strive to omit courses on this topic from research-intensive medical colleges?
  - Why or why not?
- If homeopathy causes death, is it as grave as a medical error-induced death?
  - Why or why not?
- Should we request legislation to shut down homeopathic and naturopathic "training centers"?
- Should we forbid any licensing of these graduates?
- Should all practitioners of this field have to post disclaimers in plain sight of "patients"?
- Should practitioners be banned from dispensing any supplement from their office or having ties to any dispensary?
  - If not, how do we keep the focus on patient well-being and not financial gain?
- Is it unethical for pharmaceutical laboratories to support supplement labels for "purity" when they know there is no test for efficacy?
- Chiropractic "medicine" is viewed by many as quackery, too. Because the nation's first chiropractic school was allowed at the U of Florida (Tallahassee), should we let all universities have chiropractic colleges?
  - Then, by extension, would we have to train naturopaths? Herbalists? Crystal healers? Astrologists?
  - Where do we draw the line and re-establish the boundary of science to magic?

Works Cited

1. Dickinson A. History and overview of DSHEA. Fitoterapia. 2011;82(1):5-10.
2. McNamara SH, Siegner AW, Jr., Phelps EP. DSHEA provisions confine FDA's authority to issue regulations that concern allegedly adulterated dietary supplements. Food Drug Law J. 1999;54(4):595-8.
3. Chirumbolo S. Bias and adverse effects of homeopathy: is scientific criticism in homeopathy a "mission impossible"? Int J Clin Pract. 2013;67(9):924-6.

4. Seamon MJ, Clauson KA. Ephedra: yesterday, DSHEA, and tomorrow--a ten year perspective on the Dietary Supplement Health and Education Act of 1994. J Herb Pharmacother. 2005;5(3):67-86.
5. Chang J. Scientific evaluation of traditional Chinese medicine under DSHEA: a conundrum. Dietary Supplement Health and Education Act. J Altern Complement Med. 1999;5(2):181-9.
6. Jarvis WT. Quackery: a national scandal. Clin Chem. 1992;38(8B Pt 2):1574-86.
7. Pigliucci M. Scientism and Pseudoscience: A Philosophical Commentary. J Bioeth Inq. 2015;12(4):569-75.
8. Kahn J. China Quick to Execute Drug Official. The New York Times. 2007.
9. Liu A. Dishonest participants, another chapter of China's fake data story. FierceBiotech. 2017.
10. Fellows M. China threatens prison time and death penalty to fight fraudulent trial data. PharmaFile. 2017.
11. El Hadi H, Vettor R, Rossato M. Vitamin E as a Treatment for Nonalcoholic Fatty Liver Disease: Reality or Myth? Antioxidants (Basel). 2018;7(1).
12. Palermo A, Tuccinardi D, D'Onofrio L, et al. Vitamin K and osteoporosis: Myth or reality? Metabolism. 2017;70:57-71.
13. Duque G, Daly RM, Sanders K, et al. Vitamin D, bones and muscle: myth versus reality. Australas J Ageing. 2017;36 Suppl 1:8-13.
14. Moyer MW. The myth of antioxidants. Sci Am. 2013;308(2):62-7.
15. Talaulikar V, Manyonda I. The myth of vitamins C and E for the prevention of preeclampsia: just when will the penny drop? Am J Obstet Gynecol. 2010;203(6):e7-8; author reply e.
16. Herbert V. The antioxidant supplement myth. Am J Clin Nutr. 1994;60(2):157-8.
17. Randolph PM. Exploring the vitamin myth. RDH. 1986;6(2):30, 5, 7-8.
18. Talaulikar VS, Manyonda IT. Vitamin C as an antioxidant supplement in women's health: a myth in need of urgent burial. Eur J Obstet Gynecol Reprod Biol. 2011;157(1):10-3.
19. Busby JE, Kamat AM. Chemoprevention for bladder cancer. J Urol. 2006;176(5):1914-20.
20. Jobst KA. Homeopathy, Hahnemann, and The Lancet 250 years on: a case of the emperor's new clothes? J Altern Complement Med. 2005;11(5):751-4.
21. Haustein KO. [Homeopathy from the viewpoint of the clinical pharmacologist]. Z Arztl Fortbild (Jena). 1996;90(2):97-101.
22. Weissmann G. Homeopathy: Holmes, Hogwarts, and the Prince of Wales. FASEB J. 2006;20(11):1755-8.
23. Vickers AJ, Smith C. Homoeopathic Oscillococcinum for preventing and treating influenza and influenza-like syndromes. Cochrane Database Syst Rev. 2006(3):CD001957.
24. Chirumbolo S. Oscillococcinum(R): Misunderstanding or biased interest? Eur J Intern Med. 2014;25(3):e35-6.
25. Loudon I. A brief history of homeopathy. J R Soc Med. 2006;99(12):607-10.
26. Atwood KC. "Neurocranial restructuring" and homeopathy, neither complementary nor alternative. Arch Otolaryngol Head Neck Surg. 2003;129(12):1356-7.
27. Schmaltz R, Lilienfeld SO. Corrigendum: Hauntings, homeopathy, and the Hopkinsville Goblins: using pseudoscience to teach scientific thinking. Front Psychol. 2017;8:1982.
28. Fisher PA. What about the evidence base for homeopathy? BMJ. 2011;343:d6689; author reply d93.
29. Holt S, Gilbey A, Colquhoun D, et al. Call for doctors not to practice homeopathy or refer to homeopaths. N Z Med J. 2011;124(1332):87-8.
30. Poynton L, Dowell A, Dew K, et al. General practitioners' attitudes toward (and use of) complementary and alternative medicine: a New Zealand nationwide survey. N Z Med J. 2006;119(1247):U2361.

31. Ernst E. A systematic review of systematic reviews of homeopathy. Br J Clin Pharmacol. 2002;54(6):577-82.

Essay: Traditional Chinese Herbal Medicine as Dietary Supplements in the US

Can they replace conventional medical therapies and what are the potential risks?

Nanase Toda

Introduction

Herbal products have substantially grown in popularity, and are currently used by nearly 1 in 5 US adults.[1] In the US, these products are classified as dietary supplements and contain various parts of one or more plants including leaves, flowers, roots, and stems.[1-3] Interestingly, there has been a perception that regards those products as "natural" and thus safe, leading to their administration as an alternative to conventional medical treatments to prevent, treat, and cure diseases.[4]

What is Traditional Chinese Medicine?

The most historic and well-known herbal remedies include traditional Chinese medicine (TCM), which originated in ancient China more than 2,000 years ago as a medical system based on empirical knowledge and ideas derived from Chinese philosophical theories such as Yin-Yang and its foundational concepts, namely, Qi.[5] A conceptual skeleton of TCM is the Yin-Yang theory, which states that opposing forces, Yin and Yang, compose the universe. The interaction between these contradictory forces generates Qi, the vital substances flowing in the body.[6] These ideas are currently unmapped or not elucidated in scientific terms.[5]

As opposed to Western medicine, which usually targets a specific disease by establishing standard medical care, TCM customizes treatment for each individual based on "Syndrome differentiation."[5] Syndrome differentiation refers to the analysis of clinical data obtained by TCM diagnostic procedures including observation of tongue appearances and pulse analysis.[7,8] Usually, the same disease diagnosed by Western medicine varies in TCM syndromes. For instance, according to TCM, rheumatoid arthritis can be classified into either cold or heat patterns. Contingent upon these patterns, different TCM herbal formulations might be prescribed for the same disease.[7]

Currently, in the US, TCM herbal products are consumed as dietary supplements whereas in China, they are regarded as drugs.[9] A few TCM herbal formulations have been assessed in FDA clinical trials for their efficacy in treating medical conditions such as cardiovascular disease, cancer, and hyperlipidemia.[5] Also, studies have been conducted to evaluate the efficacy of TCM in treating other medical conditions including mental illnesses and respiratory disorders such as bronchitis.[10]

According to the definition of dietary supplements under the Dietary Supplement Health and Education Act and the FDA's definition of drugs, dietary supplements cannot affect body structure or function, nor can they be used to diagnose, cure, mitigate, treat, or prevent diseases because they are not drugs.[11, 12] Hence, because of the classification of TCM herbal products under current US laws, they are unable to replace conventional medical treatments. Furthermore, even people who plan to use dietary supplements to benefit from placebo effects should not use TCM herbal supplements in particular, due to the potential toxic contaminants.[10]

Lack of Robust Evidence for the Safety, Efficacy, and Quality

Due to the globally expanding consumption of herbal products for promoting health, assuring their safety, efficacy, and quality is crucial, and a rising number of published studies and systematic reviews suggests that efforts have been undertaken to verify them.[4, 13] In addition, several studies have been conducted to identify the constituents in TCM herbal formulations, isolate active components, and evaluate their biological activities for potential drug discovery.[5] Despite these efforts, the outcomes of these studies were inconclusive because of the poor quality and quantity of the trials.[13] Most systematic reviews for TCM discuss the insufficiency of high-quality trials using an appropriate methodology, which prevents any definitive conclusions from being made about the efficacy of TCM herbal products. These reviews also mention specific limitations of the studies including a lack of the quantity of testing for the same herbal formulations, potential bias, and an insufficient number of subjects to be able to stratify them into subgroups for analysis.[5] This lack of robust evidence for the safety, efficacy, and quality of TCM herbal products is hampering the acceptance of TCM by mainstream medicine. For TCM to be integrated into the US healthcare system, the safety, efficacy, and quality of TCM must be demonstrated with robust evidence.[5]

Lack of Regulations for Dietary Supplements in the US

The complex chemical compounds in TCM and a lack of standardized characterization protocols cause difficulty for regulatory agencies to inspect ingredients, active compounds, and adulterants in TCM herbal supplements.[14, 15] Because TCM herbal products are currently classified as dietary supplements, they are not required to be approved by the FDA; thus, they do not undergo preclinical studies using animal models or clinical trials involving humans. The lack of FDA surveillance possibly leads to variations in the efficacy, purity, quality, and storage of the products.[16] Therefore, under current regulations, these products may not meet safety, quality, and efficacy expectations.[4]

Moreover, the lack of regulations for dietary supplements potentially leads to the addition of contaminants to the products.[16] Indeed, some TCM herbal products have been contaminated with drugs such as warfarin and diclofenac that are undeclared in the ingredient list, and toxic nonessential metals including arsenic, cadmium, lead, and pesticides.[10] These contaminants are problematic because they potentially cause toxicity in humans.

Conclusion

The lack of surveillance for TCM herbal products in the US and robust evidence for their safety, efficacy, and quality is evident. In addition, there is a potential risk of contaminants, which may cause toxicity in humans. Given this information, it is extremely unlikely that TCM herbal products are qualified to replace conventional medical therapies in the US. Also, their consumption should be avoided to prevent possible toxicity.

Works Cited

1. Bent S. Herbal medicine in the United States: review of efficacy, safety, and regulation: grand rounds at University of California, San Francisco Medical Center. J Gen Intern Med. 2008;23(6):854-9. Epub 20080416.
2. Hawks MK, Crawford PF, 3rd, Moss DA, et al. Integrative Medicine: Herbal Supplements. FP Essent. 2021;505:23-7.
3. National Center for Complementary and Integrative Health. Dietary and Herbal Supplements Bethesda, MD2022 [cited 2022 October 26]. Available from: https://www.nccih.nih.gov/health/dietary-and-herbal-supplements.
4. Liu SH, Chuang WC, Lam W, et al. Safety surveillance of traditional Chinese medicine: current and future. Drug Saf. 2015;38(2):117-28.
5. Fung FY, Linn YC. Developing traditional chinese medicine in the era of evidence-based medicine: current evidences and challenges. Evid Based Complement Alternat Med. 2015;2015:425037. Epub 20150408.
6. Leong PK, Wong HS, Chen J, et al. Yang/Qi invigoration: an herbal therapy for chronic fatigue syndrome with yang deficiency? Evid Based Complement Alternat Med. 2015;2015:945901. Epub 20150211.
7. Wu G, Zhao J, Zhao J, et al. Exploring biological basis of Syndrome differentiation in coronary heart disease patients with two distinct Syndromes by integrated multi-omics and network pharmacology strategy. Chin Med. 2021;16(1):109. Epub 20211026.
8. Jiang M, Lu C, Zhang C, et al. Syndrome differentiation in modern research of traditional Chinese medicine. J Ethnopharmacol. 2012;140(3):634-42. Epub 20120201.
9. Lu WI, Lu DP. Impact of chinese herbal medicine on american society and health care system: perspective and concern. Evid Based Complement Alternat Med. 2014;2014:251891. Epub 20140227.
10. National Center for Complementary and Integrative Health. Traditional Chinese Medicine: What You Need To Know Bethesda, MD2019 [cited 2022 October 26]. Available from: https://www.nccih.nih.gov/health/traditional-chinese-medicine-what-you-need-to-know.
11. Administration USFaD. FDA 101: Dietary Supplements: U.S. Food and Drug Administration; 2022 [cited 2022 November 5]. Available from: https://www.fda.gov/consumers/consumer-updates/fda-101-dietary-supplements.
12. Lopez MJ, Tadi P. Drug Labeling. StatPearls. Treasure Island (FL)2022.
13. Xue CC, Zhang AL, Greenwood KM, et al. Traditional chinese medicine: an update on clinical evidence. J Altern Complement Med. 2010;16(3):301-12.
14. Coghlan ML, Maker G, Crighton E, et al. Combined DNA, toxicological and heavy metal analyses provides an auditing toolkit to improve pharmacovigilance of traditional Chinese medicine (TCM). Sci Rep. 2015;5:17475. Epub 20151210.
15. Zhong XK, Li DC, Jiang JG. Identification and quality control of Chinese medicine based on the fingerprint techniques. Curr Med Chem. 2009;16(23):3064-75.
16. Donoghue TJ. Herbal Medications and Anesthesia Case Management. AANA J. 2018;86(3):242-8.

Topic: Personal Choices that Enforce Medical Care

For most US adults, healthcare needs arise from lifestyle and personal choices. From smoking to obesity, or from alcoholism to drug abuse, we are creating most of our maladies. The question then arises as to whether these deliberate or ignorant missteps deserve the same intensity of healthcare resources as "unearned" illnesses and disabilities. The medical literature features many inquiries similar to this, but few policies shaped by these questions are available. For instance, the literature offers plenty of ethical queries into withholding rehabilitating treatments from patients who, in the eyes of providers, are "unmotivated", "denying", or "inappropriate".[1] Such medically important categories of patients who fall under this perception of "noncompliant" and "resource intensive" include alcoholics, smokers, the obese, and those with type II diabetes.[2]

First, the consensus among medical professionals is that smoking is the worst habit for human health and it is entirely avoidable. Indeed, socially, smoking has rapidly disappeared from vogue as restaurants and other public gathering spaces have banned the practice. The immediate consequence of these public bans was that smokers took their habit outdoors. Subsequent enforcement of outdoor bans for many open-air spaces has helped reduce smoking, too.[3-6] Even so, current tobacco use estimates for the US suggest that about 13% of adults are still smokers.[7] Traits of current smokers are these: they are mostly male, uneducated, and poor.[7] This is unfortunate because smoking is unequivocally confirmed to cause lung cancer and various head and neck cancers,

"You cannot control everything in your life but, you can control what you put in your body."

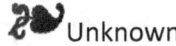Unknown

especially if chronically co-consumed with alcohol and tobacco is considered to be a known human carcinogen.[8]

E-cigarettes or vaping of aerosolized nicotine is more popular with those 18–24 years-of-age who often have no prior history of smoking. This is ironic because vaping was designed and promoted to help current smokers to stop using cigarettes, cigars, and other tobacco products.[9] Vaping nicotine or inhaling it from a special device allows enjoyment of positively reinforcing and addictive nicotine but does not provide the carcinogenic aspect of tobacco which is due to the incomplete combustion of the plant material to yield polycyclic aromatic hydrocarbons, volatile N-nitrosamines, and specific N-nitrosamines and along with concomitant inhalation of carbon monoxide, and benzene.[10, 11] Hence, the switch to e-cigarettes being preferred by healthcare experts and many past tobacco users who wish to avoid cancers. Because tobacco smoking can be avoided entirely and because the warnings have been clearly communicated for decades, lung transplants are withheld from smokers until they can demonstrate a lengthy period of abstinence. This often breeds dishonesty as many (almost 80%) smokers falsely declare that they are not smoking but nicotine metabolite, or cotinine tests, conducted before transplants confirmed that smoking was recent.[12] Preventing smokers from having lung transplants is prudent, as smokers who receive the transplants are likely to resume smoking and even if they do not, they have worse outcomes than nonsmokers or never smokers. Specifically, they have longer hospital stays after transplant surgery and most often need more ventilation.[13]

Likewise, liver transplants have been denied to alcoholics because the liver is the chief detoxification site of all forms of ethanol.[14-17]

"Our bodies are our gardens—our wills are our gardeners."

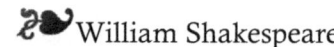William Shakespeare

Because of the scarcity of healthy human transplant organs, especially livers due to the high prevalence of obesity and associated fatty liver disease, these considerations are common.[18-20] Similar to lung transplant programs for past smokers, liver transplant requirements include at least a 6-month abstinence from drinking for potential transplant recipients to qualify for care.[21] The argument for this is that alcoholics will very likely relapse and resume drinking, damaging the healthy transplanted liver.[22] In fact, data from some studies revealed that 100% of alcoholics resumed drinking post-transplantation.[23] Thus, current practices suggest that offering a healthy liver to anyone with cirrhosis, which is almost exclusively caused by alcohol abuse, is highly controversial.[23]

For the obese, science is steadfast: over-fueling past one's needs is the sole source of excess weight gain and sedentary lifestyles promote this. Genetic issues related to weight gain are clear as well: genes can alter signals of satiety which can promote more food consumption but entirely, over-fueling is behavioral and a choice. While the psychology of overeating is complex, the fact remains that one human activity contributes to unhealthy body weights. Thus, the first law of thermodynamics is not under siege. This is deeply troubling because the obese cost the healthcare system dearly. Even attempts to analyze the cost of obesity and its common comorbidities are extraordinary—thought to account for 10% of all US healthcare dollars spent.[24] In many studies, obese patients required resource-intensive mobility assistance to obtain anthropometric measurements, and staff time was increased for patient interactions.[25] Then, obesity causes strain on the US workforce in the form of absenteeism, disabilities, and higher insurance premiums.[26-29]

The obese are particularly challenged in a healthcare setting when requesting surgery. Similar to alcoholics, liver transplants have been denied to the [30]obese who needed liver replacement due to non-alcoholic fatty liver disease. Some obese patients have agreed to gastric sleeve weight loss surgery in tandem with liver transplantation, effectively increasing their odds of reaching a healthy weight with a new liver.[31] Similar to pre-surgical health approaches for smokers and alcoholics—to abstain and prove the ability to resist the drug of choice—obese individuals are often asked to reduce their weight to specific thresholds to qualify for surgery. This protects the patient because obesity is an avoidable risk factor for surgical problems that can be fatal.[32-34]

Next, diabetes type II which is a state of acquired carbohydrate intolerance, glucose elevations, and insulin insensitivity, is also behaviorally derived and can be reversed by non-carbohydrate fuel choices as proteins and fats are not insulinogenic and do not promote diabetes type II. That the medical community is not trained in nutrition and instead reaches for pharmacological interventions (metformin, insulin) which do not solve the problem but extend it, is not a valid excuse for the continuation of this type of response. Thus, perhaps obese and diabetic patients, if also ignorant of nutrition and human biochemistry, are essentially complicit with their healthcare providers for not truly addressing the root cause of the issue. Seemingly, the medical community only seeks to get these problematic patients out the door quickly but with no real solutions for their highly reversible condition.

Nonetheless, not challenging type II diabetics about their lifestyle and perhaps believing that they are not redeemable is effectively stigmatizing this problem which is often referred to as the "blame and shame disease."[35] The result of this type of discrimination and denial of lasting solutions causes obese and type II diabetics to have greater stress and to avoid future healthcare interactions and follow-up consultations. This allows comorbidities associated with diabetes such as kidney failure, blindness, and non-healing wounds to progress, something that, eventually, costs more to address than if it had been prevented.[36]

Writing Prompts

- Would healthcare cost much less if we partitioned lifestyle/behavioral indulgences that lead to illness in a non-insurable category
- Should people who paid to drink, smoke, and overeat be asked to pay more for insurance
  - We already surcharge smokers $20/month at UA
- Should they pay more for the more complex care they need?
  - Are some conditions true disabilities and denying patients care is running afoul of the Americans with Disabilities Act?
- If all MDs must offer evidence-based care to all patients, why do they repeatedly tell obese/diabetics to do the WRONG thing; tell drug addicts and alcoholics they are helpless; and tell smokers that they cannot receive care until they stop altogether?
  - Is this malpractice or discrimination?
- Can providers delay care until a patient "shapes up" behavior-wise?
- When all MDs are cautioned to tell any patient they do not want to see, "go to the ER" are we perpetuating the problem?
- Is denying care to the most expensive patients a form of discrimination or is it prudent?
- Can we deny ER admissions OR
  - Observational admissions OR
  - A hospital bed OR
  - Homecare OR
  - Hospice?
- Who can do this?
  - Politicians?
  - MDs?
  - Specialists only?

- ANPs?
- Hospital administrators (not MDs most of the time)
- What are some consequences to patients who are denied care?
- Should these categories of patients be umbrellaed under Medicaid/care like the elderly and poor?
  - All insurance costs would plummet
  - Premiums will drop
  - Coverage would be more for health maintenance than disease fix-its
- What return on investment do we get from medical services that end up being wasted in the end?
  - How do we evaluate "wasted" resources?
- If resources are tight for HEALTHY people, should care be rationed in SOME manner?
  - How?

Works Cited

1. Caplan B, Shechter J. Reflections on the "depressed," "unrealistic," "inappropriate," "manipulative," "unmotivated," "noncompliant," "denying," "maladjusted," "regressed," etc patient. Arch Phys Med Rehabil. 1993;74(10):1123-4.
2. Scarborough P, Bhatnagar P, Wickramasinghe KK, et al. The economic burden of ill health due to diet, physical inactivity, smoking, alcohol and obesity in the UK: an update to 2006-07 NHS costs. J Public Health (Oxf). 2011;33(4):527-35. Epub 20110511.
3. Laugesen M. Tobacco advertising bans cut smoking. Br J Addict. 1992;87(7):965-6.
4. Borland R, Owen N, Hill D, et al. Changes in acceptance of workplace smoking bans following their implementation: a prospective study. Prev Med. 1990;19(3):314-22.
5. Rosner R, Magee WE, Bard JW. Successful smoking bans. N Engl J Med. 1988;318(24):1622.
6. Strasser AL. Smoking bans protect non-smokers; more reports identify fumes' dangers. Occup Health Saf. 1987;56(4):20.
7. Cornelius ME, Wang TW, Jamal A, et al. Tobacco Product Use Among Adults - United States, 2019. MMWR Morb Mortal Wkly Rep. 2020;69(46):1736-42. Epub 20201120.
8. Dal Maso L, Torelli N, Biancotto E, et al. Combined effect of tobacco smoking and alcohol drinking in the risk of head and neck cancers: a re-analysis of case-control studies using bi-dimensional spline models. Eur J Epidemiol. 2016;31(4):385-93. Epub 20150409.
9. Wang TW, Gentzke AS, Neff LJ, et al. Characteristics of e-Cigarette Use Behaviors Among US Youth, 2020. JAMA Netw Open. 2021;4(6):e2111336. Epub 20210601.
10. Starek A, Podolak I. [Carcinogenic effect of tobacco smoke]. Rocz Panstw Zakl Hig. 2009;60(4):299-310.
11. Rehan HS, Maini J, Hungin APS. Vaping versus Smoking: A Quest for Efficacy and Safety of E-cigarette. Curr Drug Saf. 2018;13(2):92-101.
12. Veit T, Munker D, Leuschner G, et al. High prevalence of falsely declaring nicotine abstinence in lung transplant candidates. PLoS One. 2020;15(6):e0234808. Epub 20200618.
13. Corbett C, Armstrong MJ, Neuberger J. Tobacco smoking and solid organ transplantation. Transplantation. 2012;94(10):979-87.
14. Bromberg JS, Baliga PR. Renal transplantation in a noncompliant patient. N Engl J Med. 1994;330(5):371-2.
15. Edwards SS. The "noncompliant" transplant patient: a persistent ethical dilemma. J Transpl Coord. 1999;9(4):202-8.

16. Seiden DJ, Frader J, Gatter R, et al. Retransplantation and the "noncompliant" patient. Camb Q Healthc Ethics. 1999;8(3):375-81.
17. Weinrieb RM, Lucey MR. Treatment of addictive behaviors in liver transplant patients. Liver Transpl. 2007;13(11 Suppl 2):S79-82.
18. Obed A, Stern S, Jarrad A, et al. Six month abstinence rule for liver transplantation in severe alcoholic liver disease patients. World J Gastroenterol. 2015;21(14):4423-6.
19. Fleming A. When Alcoholism Ruins Someone's Liver, Should They Qualify for a Transplant? The Chicago Tribune. 2017.
20. Al-Saeedi M, Barout MH, Probst P, et al. Meta-analysis of patient survival and rate of alcohol relapse in liver-transplanted patients for acute alcoholic hepatitis. Langenbecks Arch Surg. 2018;403(7):825-36. Epub 20181022.
21. Bramstedt KA, Jabbour N. When alcohol abstinence criteria create ethical dilemmas for the liver transplant team. J Med Ethics. 2006;32(5):263-5.
22. Van Thiel DH. Liver Transplantation for Alcoholics with Terminal Liver Disease. Alcohol Health Res World. 1996;20(4):261-5.
23. Gish RG, Lee AH, Keeffe EB, et al. Liver transplantation for patients with alcoholism and end-stage liver disease. Am J Gastroenterol. 1993;88(9):1337-42.
24. TH Chan School of Public Health. Obesity Prevention Source. Harvard: 2022.
25. Tan WSY, Young AM, Di Bella AL, et al. Exploring the Impact of Obesity on Health Care Resources and Coding in the Acute Hospital Setting: A Feasibility Study. Healthcare (Basel). 2020;8(4). Epub 20201104.
26. Withrow D, Alter DA. The economic burden of obesity worldwide: a systematic review of the direct costs of obesity. Obes Rev. 2011;12(2):131-41.
27. Durden ED, Huse D, Ben-Joseph R, et al. Economic costs of obesity to self-insured employers. J Occup Environ Med. 2008;50(9):991-7.
28. Colditz GA. Economic costs of obesity and inactivity. Med Sci Sports Exerc. 1999;31(11 Suppl):S663-7.
29. Thompson D, Edelsberg J, Kinsey KL, et al. Estimated economic costs of obesity to U.S. business. Am J Health Promot. 1998;13(2):120-7.
30. Moctezuma-Velazquez C, Marquez-Guillen E, Torre A. Obesity in the Liver Transplant Setting. Nutrients. 2019;11(11). Epub 20191023.
31. Nesher E, Mor E, Shlomai A, et al. Simultaneous Liver Transplantation and Sleeve Gastrectomy: Prohibitive Combination or a Necessity? Obes Surg. 2017;27(5):1387-90.
32. Pasulka PS, Bistrian BR, Benotti PN, et al. The risks of surgery in obese patients. Ann Intern Med. 1986;104(4):540-6.
33. Flancbaum L, Choban PS. Surgical implications of obesity. Annu Rev Med. 1998;49:215-34.
34. Ri M, Aikou S, Seto Y. Obesity as a surgical risk factor. Ann Gastroenterol Surg. 2018;2(1):13-21. Epub 20171028.
35. Browne JL, Ventura A, Mosely K, et al. 'I call it the blame and shame disease': a qualitative study about perceptions of social stigma surrounding type 2 diabetes. BMJ Open. 2013;3(11):e003384. Epub 20131118.
36. Puhl RM, Phelan SM, Nadglowski J, et al. Overcoming Weight Bias in the Management of Patients With Diabetes and Obesity. Clin Diabetes. 2016;34(1):44-50.

Essay: Personal Choices and Consequences in Medicine

Teresa Noll

Personal choices take place every day, from choosing what television shows to watch for the evening to deciding whether to move to a different location. Choices require a bit of thought and contemplation before they are acted upon. However, people may not understand the consequences of their actions and may be surprised by the outcome, especially regarding their health. Deciding what to eat, even though it seems like a minor choice, can have complications later in life. The personal choices that one makes over time may also affect another person, and vice versa. In healthcare, these choices may affect how the medical personnel treat you, both socially and medically.

A person's weight, whether it is above or below the average for their BMI, will be considered during visits to the physician's office, especially when they are above the average. This is because having a larger body mass tends to be a prerequisite for many health complications such as hypertension, obesity, and cardiovascular disease.[1] Obesity is mostly caused by the overconsumption of calories and lack of exercise.[2] People can prevent obesity by eating in moderation, as well as engaging in physical activity. Exercise and conscious eating begin with a choice. There is a choice to eat a salad or a milkshake, as well as a choice to take a 30-minute walk or to watch a TV show while sitting. Constantly neglecting one's health will cause negative effects such as weight gain, lethargy, and depressed moods.[3]

How one treats their health and the services they seek may impact other people. People who frequently access emergency rooms for minor concerns may take up space needed for those who need immediate medical attention.[4] Under the Emergency Medical Treatment and Active Labor Act of 1986 (EMTALA), anyone who enters an emergency room must be treated and deemed stable before they are discharged from the hospital. EMTALA is another cause of overcrowded emergency rooms because everyone is seen and treated regardless of the severity, or lack thereof, of their qualm.[5] EMTALA and frequent usage of emergency rooms may cause longer wait times for those who are in true need.

Personal choices may not only impact oneself, but also they may impact the healthcare of others. This has been observed when parents choose not to vaccinate their children.[6] Diseases and illnesses that were rarely heard about begin to reappear, such as measles which was observed to be spreading in Disneyland [7]. Children who are unable to be vaccinated are the most at risk when herd immunity is not observed. Parents are responsible for their children's healthcare, neglecting vaccination may not only put their children at risk but the children of others as well.

Overall, choosing to eat ice cream over going for walk will not immediately cause Type II diabetes, nor will deciding to stay in for the day will cause obesity. However, chronically choosing a poor diet and sedentary lifestyle will increase the risk of developing health complications. Regarding emergency services, abuse of the emergency room is detrimental to those who are in true need since overcrowding in hospitals can extend the wait time for all involved. The healthcare of the public is reliant on everyone, choices regarding not being immunized may be harmful to those who cannot get vaccinated. There is always a choice to develop better habits, prevent debilitating diseases, and live life with fewer complications.

Works Cited

1. Wijayatunga NN, Dhurandhar EJ. Normal weight obesity and unaddressed cardiometabolic health risk-a narrative review. Int J Obes (Lond). 2021;45(10):2141-55. Epub 20210518.
2. Wright SM, Aronne LJ. Causes of obesity. Abdom Imaging. 2012;37(5):730-2.
3. Carek PJ, Laibstain SE, Carek SM. Exercise for the treatment of depression and anxiety. Int J Psychiatry Med. 2011;41(1):15-28.
4. Moe J, Kirkland SW, Rawe E, et al. Effectiveness of Interventions to Decrease Emergency Department Visits by Adult Frequent Users: A Systematic Review. Acad Emerg Med. 2017;24(1):40-52.
5. Brown HL, Brown TB. EMTALA: The Evolution of Emergency Care in the United States. J Emerg Nurs. 2019;45(4):411-4. Epub 20190320.
6. Nelson R. US measles outbreak concentrated among unvaccinated children. Lancet Infect Dis. 2019;19(3):248.
7. Doll MK, Correira JW. Revisiting the 2014-15 Disneyland measles outbreak and its influence on pediatric vaccinations. Hum Vaccin Immunother. 2021;17(11):4210-5. Epub 20210908.

Essay: Misinformation about Vaccination and Ethical Conundrums of Treating Unvaccinated Patients

Jason Canizales

Healthcare providers strive to provide the best treatment to safeguard a patient's health while upholding an equal standard of care for any individual. Despite great efforts to minimize discriminatory treatment in the medical field, the topic of vaccination has led medical professionals to take a stand on whether it is ethical to denote lower-priority hospital admission to unvaccinated patients. The global COVID-19 pandemic made hospital evaluation of patient priority a great concern because larger proportions (up to 94% in a population study of 271 people) of unvaccinated patients began to occupy most intensive care unit (ICU) beds after vaccination became widely available.[1]

Hospitals were progressively forced to deny priority treatment to unvaccinated individuals in favor of vaccinated and other non-COVID-related illness patients. This was a result of underlying frustrations stemming from having a problem that could have been otherwise prevented, an increased chance for COVID-19 mutability and transmission among unvaccinated patients, and resource allocation management towards patients that also required care for other diseases.[2, 3] Although controversial decisions have to be made for the security and well-being of the population, the repercussions of not vaccinating should be communicated to show patients about their critical role in preserving the health of their community.

Vaccination Rationale and Misconceptions
Vaccination against disease at an early age is crucial to preventing life-threatening diseases from emerging later in life. Diseases such as polio, tetanus, chickenpox, smallpox, measles, mumps, and many others have almost if not entirely have been no cause for concern due to vaccination.[4] However, just because the threat of these diseases is not as prevalent as they were before, this may create a false sense of confidence that vaccination may not be needed. Skepticism surrounding vaccines may stem from a variety of different reasons; each questioning the science behind the efficacy of vaccines in acclimating the immune system to potential threats. Reasons that help explain why people may refuse to get themselves or their children vaccinated extend

from religious, personal/philosophical, safety, and inconclusive information backgrounds surrounding vaccination.[5]

People who refuse vaccination due to religious beliefs tend to be a complicated population to convince because the reasoning paradigm at its core may not coincide with the scientific ideology required to understand how a vaccine works. A complete refusal of all vaccines is expected while others may compromise by accepting a few. Although the decision may not come from a point of ignorance, it can be attributed to an individual's decision to uphold the restrictions posed upon their beliefs. For instance, some components utilized for specific vaccine manufacture may not be deemed acceptable to use for some belief systems. Animal-derived gelatin in addition to human fetal tissue used in rubella vaccines can be seen as abhorrent which has driven research toward finding ways to comply with acceptable ingredients to increase vaccination rates in this population.[5, 6]

Regarding personal/philosophical decisions as to why someone may refuse to vaccinate can be linked to a lack of understanding of immunological processes or fear communicated through outdated science. This population tends to believe that vaccines pose a deleterious effect contrary to natural immunity and thus place into question the need to vaccinate against "rare" diseases when natural immunity is more advantageous.[7] Although there is an indication of partial understanding that natural immunity can provide similar effects to vaccines in promoting the creation of memory leukocytes to assist in future infections, this is only useful if a host survives the initial threat which may not be the case for severe diseases. Given that in some instances vaccines may induce an overreactive immune response, this has become a suitable excuse with which to corroborate vaccine side effects as a distinguishable danger that does not outweigh its "suggested" benefit.[8]

Misinformation is potentially the greatest factor that influences a person's decision on whether vaccination is safe. Multiple outlets such as television, social media, everyday conversations, and a plethora of other sources of opinion may dilute the accuracy of vaccine information available.[9] There is still a fearmongering idea of live viruses being used in vaccines. Although this is a half-truth, only some vaccinations (e.g., measles, mumps, rubella, and varicella) utilize a live-attenuated virus, meaning that the virulence factor responsible for causing disease has been deactivated and can only be a serious issue in already immunocompromised individuals.[10, 11] In the case of the Pfizer-BioNTech COVID-19 mRNA vaccine and other new forms of vaccine technology provide the same advantages of immunity without introducing a virus. Rather, only an antigen component is necessary to elicit an immune response.[12] For these reasons, concerns regarding the introduction of live viruses into one's body are inaccurate and should be disregarded given contemporary vaccine technology that is continuously pushing away from using attenuated vaccines.

Another important popularized concern among mainstream media is the extrapolation of very rare cases where serious side effects are present to spotlight a distasteful narrative against vaccination. News about neuronal damage or autism as a result of vaccination prompts parents towards questioning the safety of vaccines while also adopting a protective mindset in the interest of their child's health. Thimerosal, a preservative component of vaccines responsible for evoking the public's concerns has shown no substantial evidence of toxicity when used at intended doses. Moreover, the only toxicity reports found have been in accidental high-dose exposure in humans of about 100–1000 times the amount found in vaccines.[13] Although there is a robust body of peer-reviewed studies that show thimerosal as non-toxic for humans, it has not been used in vaccines in children under 6 years-of-age for over a decade.[14] Ambiguity and fear surrounding the information an individual has at hand may influence their decision in delaying immunization. Conflicting ideas may shroud a person's judgment leading to partial mistrust in physician instruction due to expected bias from a healthcare provider's supportive opinion on vaccines. For this reason, it is important to stay informed about relevant/objective science to prevent unnecessary concerns to arise.

Ethical Implications of Triaging in Unvaccinated Patients
Selection of patient priority for treatment in situations of resource scarcity is a tough position medical professionals are forced to face in times of crisis. The subjective threshold defining priority is oftentimes not clear and malleable depending on the situation. The establishment of a triage plan amidst a public health emergency is important because it allows patients to be treated based on the severity of their condition rather than being subject to a less optimal first-come, first-serve system.[15] Regardless of a patient's medical situation, objective criteria are followed to dictate the urgency of treatment required in comparison to other patients. Sorting, prioritizing, and resource allocation are the 3 main components to consider when clinicians face an emergency that requires a shift in perspective to address the needs of the population rather than the individual.[16] In particular, COVID-19 brought forth the ethical framework of triaging into question through a surge of controversies among medical practitioners in response to "inadequate" distribution of resources to unvaccinated individuals. Given that a large proportion of hospital beds remained to be occupied by severe cases of COVID-19 by unvaccinated individuals, providing treatment to what could otherwise have been an avoidable hospitalization began to question the prioritization status given to these patients.[17,18]

Before the pandemic struck, it was not immediately possible to determine the extent of a patient's responsibility in the outcome of their hospitalization. For instance, there is no direct way to predict whether the result of a broken bone is due to patient negligence or as a result of a deliberate accident. In mid-2021, about 6% of COVID-19 hospitalizations in ICUs were reported to be occupied by vaccinated patients.[1] The disproportionate amount of unvaccinated COVID-19 cases led to the idea of establishing new triage protocols to hold those people accountable for negatively impacting the health of their community. Not only would their choice impact the severity of their condition, but also place neonates under 6 months who are ineligible for vaccination at risk.[19] Furthermore, hypermutability of a virus may ensue when a large number of susceptible—mostly unvaccinated—subjects allow a virus to be transmitted among a population allowing it "learn" and develop into variants that help boost its immune-escape potential; contributing to the loss of herd immunity.[20,21] Thus diluting the effectiveness of newly developed vaccines that target a specific strain of a virus.

When unvaccinated individuals travel from places where vaccine coverage against a disease is relatively controlled to regions of low vaccine coverage, localized outbreaks may spread among a population with a resistant strain of the virus. For this reason, a disease of no critical concern due to widely available vaccine coverage may resurface again in a vaccinated population.[21, 22] In Brazil, a country in which vaccination is mandatory and regulated by legislation, measles (eliminated from the Americas since 2002) began to reemerge between 2013 and 2015 leading to more than 1000 reported cases in young and infant populations as a result of voluntary non-vaccinations.[23] To minimize the incidence of transmission, some triaging practices have shifted focus to reduce the priority of care to unvaccinated patients.

Triaging regulation in unvaccinated patients may seem ethically unfair given that any patient in need of medical attention should have the same access to healthcare as any other patient; however, overemphasis on this issue may also inadvertently result in the dismissal of other important ethical considerations unrelated to communicable diseases.[24] In a survey conducted by the WHO for over 155 countries, it was found that the disruption of non-communicable health services was substantially reduced during the COVID-19 pandemic. For instance, 53% of countries had reduced or halted services crucial for hypertension treatment, 49% for diabetes and related complications, 42% for cancer care, 31% for cardiovascular emergencies, and 53% for rehabilitation services.[25] Repercussions of healthcare service unavailability resulted in the fatality of a great number of non-COVID-19 related fatalities. In Italy, where COVID-19 had a ravaging impact in comparison to others, studies showed an overall 43.2% increase in out-of-hospital mortality. Specifically, most deaths were linked to endocrine, nutritional, and metabolic complications.[26, 27] Although there is limited literature-based evidence that non-COVID-19 fatalities may have inadvertently increased due to triaging procedures during the pandemic, it can be inferred based on the overarching evidence that this may have been the case.[28]

Clinician sentiments over non-vaccinated COVID-19 hospitalizations are relatively similar. The overly exhaustive responsibility of taking care of ICU patients for a job that is already demanding can be overwhelming when surges of unvaccinated patients start to take valuable space otherwise necessary for other critically ill patients.[29-31] Although they are ethically and lawfully obliged to care for these patients, they still have to negate healthcare access to incoming patients regardless of their emergency needs.[32] In some cases, new patients in emergency departments must wait for days before being admitted due to the limited availability of resources or healthcare providers.[33] It must be placed into consideration that clinicians and staff are subject to prolonged times of service with minimal breaks between shifts. Despite being quintessential for the well-being of the community, this can also be detrimental to their health through overwork and stress. Hence, the development of a shared and justifiable moral outrage among clinicians may negatively impact the quality of care provided by reducing overall empathy towards patients which is necessary for the establishment of trust and security.[34] Holding unvaccinated patients accountable for limiting their potential to save most lives is a direct response to the frustrating situations healthcare providers are placed in and forced to comply. Medical accountability for the ethical decisions in priority treatment becomes less one-sided whenever the repercussions of the latter are far more detrimental to the health of the population.

Concluding Remarks

In short, lower priority admission of unvaccinated patients to hospitals is justifiable if careful consideration of the objective rationale is placed at par with its ethical implications. Although healthcare providers generally agree in providing equal opportunity treatment to all patients, appropriate triaging protocols should be followed whenever a public health crisis may arise. Although vaccination is not mandatory, those unwilling to do so should be aware of the potentially fatal consequences of their choice in addition to being able to discern between verifiable and ungrounded science to reduce vaccination hesitancy based on misinformation. This way, the extent of misguided fear towards vaccination may increasingly reduce and prompt more people to simultaneously protect themselves and their communities.

Works Cited

1. Abdelmalek M. Vast majority of ICU patients with COVID-19 are unvaccinated, ABC News survey finds: Hospitals report few fully vaccinated people are sick with COVID-19 in the ICU. ABC News. 2021.
2. Iserson KV. Ethics, Personal Responsibility and the Pandemic: A New Triage Paradigm. J Emerg Med. 2022;62(4):508-12. Epub 20220120.
3. Fully Vaccinated Adults 65 and Older Are 94% Less Likely to Be Hospitalized with COVID-19: Centers for Disease Control and Prevention; 2021 [cited 2022].
4. Diseases You Almost Forgot About (Thanks to Vaccines): Centers for Disease Control and Prevention; 2022. Available from: https://www.cdc.gov/vaccines/parents/diseases/forgot-14-diseases.html.
5. McKee C, Bohannon K. Exploring the Reasons Behind Parental Refusal of Vaccines. J Pediatr Pharmacol Ther. 2016;21(2):104-9.
6. Wombwell E, Fangman MT, Yoder AK, et al. Religious barriers to measles vaccination. J Community Health. 2015;40(3):597-604.
7. Fredrickson DD, Davis TC, Arnould CL, et al. Childhood immunization refusal: provider and parent perceptions. Fam Med. 2004;36(6):431-9.
8. Saada A, Lieu TA, Morain SR, et al. Parents' choices and rationales for alternative vaccination schedules: a qualitative study. Clin Pediatr (Phila). 2015;54(3):236-43. Epub 20140907.
9. Dube E, Gagnon D, Nickels E, et al. Mapping vaccine hesitancy--country-specific characteristics of a global phenomenon. Vaccine. 2014;32(49):6649-54.
10. Justiz Vaillant AA, Grella MJ. Vaccine (Vaccination). StatPearls. Treasure Island (FL)2022.
11. Understanding Six Types of Vaccine Technologies: Pfizer; 2022. Available from: https://www.pfizer.com/news/articles/understanding_six_types_of_vaccine_technologies.
12. Understanding How COVID-19 Vaccines Work: Centers for Disease Control and Prevention; 2022 [cited 2022]. Available from: https://www.cdc.gov/coronavirus/2019-ncov/vaccines/different-vaccines/how-they-work.html?CDC_AA_refVal=https%3A%2F%2Fwww.cdc.gov%2Fcoronavirus%2F2019-ncov%2Fvaccines%2Fdifferent-vaccines%2Fmrna.html.
13. Thimerosal in Vaccines Questions and Answers: US Food & Drug Administration; 2018. Available from: https://www.fda.gov/vaccines-blood-biologics/vaccines/thimerosal-vaccines-questions-and-answers#:~:text=Data%20reviewed%20did%20not%20demonstrate,times%20that%20found%20in%20vaccines.

14. Thimerosal and Vaccines: US Food & Drug Administration; 2018 [cited 2022 November 7]. Available from: https://www.fda.gov/vaccines-blood-biologics/safety-availability-biologics/thimerosal-and-vaccines#bib.
15. Maves RC, Downar J, Dichter JR, et al. Triage of Scarce Critical Care Resources in COVID-19 An Implementation Guide for Regional Allocation: An Expert Panel Report of the Task Force for Mass Critical Care and the American College of Chest Physicians. Chest. 2020;158(1):212-25. Epub 20200411.
16. Christian MD. Triage. Crit Care Clin. 2019;35(4):575-89. Epub 20190727.
17. Bahl A, Johnson S, Maine G, et al. Vaccination reduces need for emergency care in breakthrough COVID-19 infections: A multicenter cohort study. Lancet Reg Health Am. 2021;4:100065. Epub 20210909.
18. Bibler TM, Nelson RH, Schuman O, et al. Caring for Unvaccinated Patients in the ICU: Beyond Frustration, Toward Beneficial Relationships. Crit Care Explor. 2021;3(12):e0581. Epub 20211202.
19. CDC Recommends COVID-19 Vaccines for Young Children: Centers for Disease Control and Prevention; 2022 [cited 2022]. Available from: https://www.cdc.gov/media/releases/2022/s0618-children-vaccine.html.
20. Angius F, Pala G, Manzin A. SARS-CoV-2 and Its Variants: The Pandemic of Unvaccinated. Front Microbiol. 2021;12:749634. Epub 20210924.
21. Aps L, Piantola MAF, Pereira SA, et al. Adverse events of vaccines and the consequences of non-vaccination: a critical review. Rev Saude Publica. 2018;52:40. Epub 20180412.
22. Gangarosa EJ, Galazka AM, Wolfe CR, et al. Impact of anti-vaccine movements on pertussis control: the untold story. Lancet. 1998;351(9099):356-61.
23. Leite RD, Barreto JL, Sousa AQ. Measles Reemergence in Ceara, Northeast Brazil, 15 Years after Elimination. Emerg Infect Dis. 2015;21(9):1681-3.
24. Shaw D. Journal of Medical Ethics: BMJ Blogs. 2020. [cited 2022]. Available from: https://blogs.bmj.com/medical-ethics/2020/06/22/triaging-ethical-issues-during-a-pandemic-a-rough-guide/.
25. COVID-19 significantly impacts health services for noncommunicable diseases: World Health Organization; 2020 [cited 2022]. Available from: https://www.who.int/news/item/01-06-2020-covid-19-significantly-impacts-health-services-for-noncommunicable-diseases.
26. Clerk AM. Beware of Neglect of Non-COVID Patients in COVID Era. Indian J Crit Care Med. 2021;25(8):837-8.
27. Santi L, Golinelli D, Tampieri A, et al. Non-COVID-19 patients in times of pandemic: Emergency department visits, hospitalizations and cause-specific mortality in Northern Italy. PLoS One. 2021;16(3):e0248995. Epub 20210322.
28. Jacobson SH, Jokela JA. Non-COVID-19 excess deaths by age and gender in the United States during the first three months of the COVID-19 pandemic. Public Health. 2020;189:101-3. Epub 20201010.
29. Davidson R. I'm an E.R. Doctor in Michigan, Where Unvaccinated People Are Filling Hospital Beds. New York Times. 2021.
30. Doctors Refusing to Treat the Unvaccinated? YouTube: The View; 2021.
31. Jayakumar KL, Lipoff JB. Declining care to unvaccinated patients: Ethical and legal considerations. J Am Acad Dermatol. 2017;77(6):1188-90.
32. McKoy M. Obligation To Provide Services. Ethics Journal of the American Medical Association. 2006:332-4.
33. Armstrong D. Unvaccinated Covid Patients Push Hospital Systems Past the Brink. Bloomberg. 2021 December, 14.

34. Dudzinski DM. Moral Outrage Toward Willfully Unvaccinated COVID-19 Patients. J Gen Intern Med. 2022;37(8):2070-1. Epub 20220401.

Topic: Physical and Mental Enhancements—When is It Just Therapy?

No one wants to be average, but most people are. This truth has vexed humans since we could draw on cave walls: to be better, faster, smarter, and stronger has always been a goal for most people. But, what is considered fair and just personal improvement versus an enhancement that is out of reach for others, due to timing, pricing, or access? These topics get much more attention in the athletic realm, but with the internet and globalization of information, even regular Joes and Janes are asking how they, too, can improve their lives and lifespans. Where we traditionally used socialization, education, and parental supervision for the betterment of humankind, we are now reaching into pharmacological interventions and even genetic modifications to change our bodies and minds.

First, for athletic performance enhancement, drugs are popular, so popular—and unethical or risky—that the World Anti-Doping Agency has banned a host of many compounds that have been shown to improve strength (anabolic steroids), endurance (erythropoietin), and speed (beta agonists). Some may suggest that the entire professional sports area is tainted with the whiff of chemistry as so many famous sports figures have come forward or been forced into the spotlight due to illegal drug use. These public figures have induced college and high school athletes to similarly indulge and data suggest that most young adults who play sports engage in some type of performance enhancement.[1-4] These attempts to improve appearance or performance are often relegated to the physical: compounds to produce changes in the body that are used with training programs and precise nutrition to achieve personal goals.

"Performance-enhancing drugs are an illusion. I wish I had never gotten involved with steroids. It was wrong. It was stupid."

Mark McGwire, American former professional baseball player

In the workplace and on college campuses, cognitive enhancements are desired.[5-7] even though there are no *bona fide* cognitive enhancers, drugs designed to help people think more clearly, faster, and with greater understanding and retention, people seem very willing to believe the myth that some drugs, or worse some completely ineffective supplements, can offer cognitive improvement. Because of this misapprehension, college students are particularly susceptible to trying "study drugs" or purloined controlled substances/scheduled drugs from friends who have been diagnosed with attention deficit disorder or something similar and prescribed therapy for it. This is unfortunate because, similar to the illegal status of many physical performance enhancers, almost every drug used to treat attention disorders is Schedule II and a felony to buy, sell or possess without a valid and current prescription from a medical provider.

Along the lines of enhancement have emerged some scientific techniques, notably genetic modification via CRISPR technology.[8] While at this time, genetic editing of germ-line cells or heritable cells that form products of conception is illegal and regarded as highly unethical, it has been done with success in China. The scientist who forayed into this fraught area was sanctioned and pilloried by the scientific community but his accomplishment resonated.[9] It can be done. This may be why the public opinion of this technology, when used in this way, is changing. For instance, most adults believe that germline editing is proper for devastating genetic diseases but less acceptable for curing infectious diseases and largely unacceptable for human enhancement.[10] At this time animals have been enhanced for agriculture and laboratory animals (rabbits, monkeys, and mice) have been manipulated

"Lance Armstrong admitted he used performance-enhancing drugs throughout his career. He confessed in front of the most respected judge in the land, Oprah Winfrey."

Craig Ferguson, Scottish-American comedian, actor, writer, and television host of *The Late Show with Craig Ferguson*

genetically to study changes in muscle tissue growth, blood-oxygen capacity, and endurance, but these discoveries are far off for humans who are vastly more complex and live much longer lives, lives that would be lived with these genetic changes.[11-17] Because changing a gene in a human is indescribably complicated, and genetic edits cannot likely be reversed, much more consideration should be made about these scientific possibilities. As Dr. Ian Malcom, the chaos theorist in the first *Jurassic Park* (1993) movie wisely said in a highly memorable scene: "Your scientists were so preoccupied with whether or not they could, they didn't stop to think if they should." Maybe we are at that moment in time now, obligated to consider this very thing.

Writing Prompts

- What is the difference between therapy and enhancement?
  - How safe are these interventions?
- Is the use of nootropics cheating?
- Would entering a high-demand academic program be considered mental stress?
- The effects of doing such mimic the use of stimulants (insomnia, dyspepsia, headache, reduced appetite)
- Would enhancers further divide social inequality?
  - Only the wealthy/educated have access?
- Should all healthy people have unobstructed access to cognitive enhancers?
  - Should they be restricted to only people with high IQ?
  - Would they represent the elite and as such as a special class?
  - Is there a ceiling on IQ that cannot be surpassed?
  - Should they be restricted to those with lower IQ's as they have the most to gain?

- Because the academic playing field is uneven right now, should universal access to drug enhancements be made available or free to all?
    - Should they only be free to people with "neurological handicaps"?
    - What is the threshold for this "disability"?
- If access was ubiquitous, how do we define "normal" intelligence and cognition?
- Should high-risk jobs require cognitive enhancement therapy (soldiers, security guards, surgeons)?
- Should employers REQUIRE employees to supplement with cognitive enhancers to stay productive?
- Should students have to declare enhancer use on all exams?
    - Could this cause peer-pressure to take these drugs?
- Do these drugs represent an unfair advantage for those with money and access to the drugs?
    - Would this create another health (social) disparity of haves and have-nots?
- What is the difference between therapy and enhancement?
- How safe are these interventions?
- Is the use of nootropics cheating?
- Will enhanced people horde enhancements, not sharing with others so they can leverage their enhancement for gain?
- Will/do enhanced people have less empathy for those not similarly situated (by choice or inability to afford this)?
- But what about using this to create people more suited for living in outer space (or for spaceflight), under water, on the moon, in low-oxygen environments?
    - Would this be good?
    - How will this upend democracy?
        - We will cease to be equal, more so than now
- If you are not enhanced, are you subhuman? Less than?
- Is personal enhancement the ultimate form of autonomy and self-determination?
- Who gets to say if/when we "upgrade" our bodies or minds?
- Is this a simple path for reaching personal goals?
    - Is this living an authentic life?
    - Is this expressing morphological freedom?
- Is enhancement an upgrade or a correction?
- What is "better than well"?
- Is it good for an individual, a community, or society?
- If I enhance, must I disclose it to the public?
- Should be allowed to enhance as much as we can afford or expend the effort to?
- Are some forms of enhancement charades, misrepresenting who we are?
    - Why?
- How is physical enhancement different than cognitive enhancement?
- Are people more willing to change their bodies or their minds
    - Why?
- Should the government stop intervening at all in personal decisions about enhancement?
    - Why/why not?

- Is genetic manipulation of embryos ethical if it eradicates lethal disease?
- When might disease eradication NOT be ethical?
- Should some babies just be allowed to die?
- Where does enhancement begin?
- Is transgender transformation a form of enhancement?
  - Is it instead the correction of a defect?
  - Who defines the defect?
- When does editing an unborn child to correct a life-threatening disease morph into creating no children with the potential for depression, acne, short stature, and ugliness?
- What if gene manipulation corrects a fatal disease initially but causes immense suffering over the lifetime
- Say a gene editing that stops Tay Sachs causes hyperalgesia, depression, and suicidality as an adult?
  - Is it ethical?
- At what age should children be permitted physical modifications?
  - Should parents be allowed to intervene?
  - What if reversal is desired?

Work Cited

1. Yesalis CE, Bahrke MS. Doping among adolescent athletes. Baillieres Best Pract Res Clin Endocrinol Metab. 2000;14(1):25-35.
2. Mulcahey MK, Schiller JR, Hulstyn MJ. Anabolic steroid use in adolescents: identification of those at risk and strategies for prevention. Phys Sportsmed. 2010;38(3):105-13.
3. Anawalt BD. Detection of anabolic androgenic steroid use by elite athletes and by members of the general public. Mol Cell Endocrinol. 2018;464:21-7. Epub 20170921.
4. Teetzel S. Philosophical Perspectives on Doping Sanctions and Young Athletes. Front Sports Act Living. 2022;4:841033. Epub 20220318.
5. Garasic MD, Lavazza A. Performance enhancement in the workplace: why and when healthy individuals should disclose their reliance on pharmaceutical cognitive enhancers. Front Syst Neurosci. 2015;9:13.
6. Peterkin AL, Crone CC, Sheridan MJ, et al. Cognitive performance enhancement: misuse or self-treatment? J Atten Disord. 2011;15(4):263-8.
7. Pomportes L, Brisswalter J, Casini L, et al. Cognitive Performance Enhancement Induced by Caffeine, Carbohydrate and Guarana Mouth Rinsing during Submaximal Exercise. Nutrients. 2017;9(6).
8. Ormond KE, Mortlock DP, Scholes DT, et al. Human Germline Genome Editing. Am J Hum Genet. 2017;101(2):167-76.
9. Raposo VL. The First Chinese Edited Babies: A Leap of Faith in Science. JBRA Assist Reprod. 2019;23(3):197-9. Epub 20190822.
10. Houtman D, Vijlbrief B, Polak M, et al. Changes in opinions about human germline gene editing as a result of the Dutch DNA-dialogue project. Eur J Hum Genet. 2022:1-8. Epub 20220512.
11. Lv Q, Yuan L, Deng J, et al. Efficient Generation of Myostatin Gene Mutated Rabbit by CRISPR/Cas9. Sci Rep. 2016;6:25029. Epub 20160426.
12. Guo R, Wan Y, Xu D, et al. Generation and evaluation of Myostatin knock-out rabbits and goats using CRISPR/Cas9 system. Sci Rep. 2016;6:29855. Epub 20160715.

13. Sebestyen MG, Hegge JO, Noble MA, et al. Progress toward a nonviral gene therapy protocol for the treatment of anemia. Hum Gene Ther. 2007;18(3):269-85.
14. Ohde D, Moeller M, Brenmoehl J, et al. Advanced Running Performance by Genetic Predisposition in Male Dummerstorf Marathon Mice (DUhTP) Reveals Higher Sterol Regulatory Element-Binding Protein (SREBP) Related mRNA Expression in the Liver and Higher Serum Levels of Progesterone. PLoS One. 2016;11(1):e0146748. Epub 20160122.
15. Ohde D, Brenmoehl J, Walz C, et al. Comparative analysis of hepatic miRNA levels in male marathon mice reveals a link between obesity and endurance exercise capacities. J Comp Physiol B. 2016;186(8):1067-78. Epub 20160609.
16. Brenmoehl J, Ohde D, Walz C, et al. Analysis of Activity-Dependent Energy Metabolism in Mice Reveals Regulation of Mitochondrial Fission and Fusion mRNA by Voluntary Physical Exercise in Subcutaneous Fat from Male Marathon Mice (DUhTP). Cells. 2020;9(12). Epub 20201216.
17. Kumaravel J, Sowmini K, Avti P, et al. Marathon mice: researcher view on potential roles in preclinical research. Indian J Pharmacol. 2021;53(2):99-102.

Essay: The Ethics of Human Enhancement

Is the further exploration of the genetic frontier going too far?

Jason Canizales

Any individual should have the opportunity to live a normal life, but if biomedical enhancements provide a person with an opportunity to live a better one, this could be considered an unethical and unacceptable practice of science.[1] Efforts to restore motor and other physiological deficiencies (e.g., eyesight, mobility, hearing, among others) have allowed science to explore approximate solutions to provide individuals with a 'normal life' or in some cases benefit them in ways beyond its intended design. Genetic engineering is a form of restorative/enhancing technology that allows for the direct manipulation of genetic material to prevent certain diseases among many other applications.[2] A great number of people are born with genetic anomalies that may strongly impact their quality of life or even their life expectancies. Although its therapeutic capabilities provide an efficient avenue to combat disease, this technology can also be repurposed to enhance standard physiological functions. The ethical, political, and evolutionary debate between *transhumanists* and *bioconservatives* about the implications of human enhancement presents important considerations for regulating its use. While genetic therapy may be a useful biomedical tool, the risk of disrupting the natural limits of human function may be overall detrimental to the population and the environment.[3,4]

Technological Influence on Healthcare

For centuries, medical technology has had a prevalent impact in providing patients with finer solutions to a variety of conditions. In particular, continued innovation of medical tools aims to improve patient quality of life through increasingly better diagnostic and treatment options. For instance, the identification of reliable biomarkers for diseases such as Alzheimer's has been of great importance given its prevalence in the US accounting for approximately 5.3 million people suffering from this condition.[5] Advancements in ophthalmology research have also aimed to restore partial sight to blind patients with the implantation of artificial retinas.[6] Moreover, stem-cell research presents an opportunity for promoting tissue repair in cases where irreparable damage can be fatal. Prospective applications in cancer treatment may also transcend the need for conventional chemotherapy-based treatments.[7,8] Regardless of its application, the future of medicine appears to be inclined towards advancements in technology as the leading influence in patient care.

Enhancement Concerns and Limitations

While the primordial focus of biotechnology has been to safeguard the health of patients, it has also inevitably found its use to "enhance" other aspects of human function. Technological applications in pharmaceutics are vast and subject to controversy if used in unintended ways as prescribed. Nootropics or "smart drugs" are used to augment cognitive function, particularly in cases of impaired functionality such as dementia or Alzheimer's. However, the use of this drug in academia may also provide students with an unfair advantage over others by increasing the processing power of their brains.[9] Other performance-enhancing drugs such as growth hormone, steroids, erythropoietin, and others have their respective clinical applications and although their chronic misuse may result in future medical complications or fatality, they are unrefutably effective in athletic performance.[10-12]

Providing a clear definition of normality as a comparative baseline for enhancement is an ambiguous task in itself. The human population contains variants in most of its genes and there is no such thing as a "normal" human genome sequence.[13] Phenotypically speaking, what is considered to be normal in a species could be interpreted as the frequency of a trait or capability prevalent within a population.[14] Yet this may not prove to be a reliable interpretation. For example, normal eyesight is considered to be 20/20 although only about 35% of American adults have "normal" vision.[14, 15] Also, consumption of certain psychostimulants such as caffeine is socially accepted despite its known pharmacological ability to heighten alertness.[16] This shows that not all forms of enhancement are unacceptable and a standard measure for "normality" is also not well established.

In pursuit of better defining the negative aspects of human enhancement, the absence of a clear objective approach to this controversy has led the scientific community to debate the extent of its permissibility and prohibition.[17] However, this suggests that perhaps a variable limit to an enhancement spectrum is enigmatically present. To define this concept for this discussion, the difference between standard therapeutic use and enhancement can be considered to be an improvement of basic physiologic functions beyond what is necessary to restore or sustain health.[18, 19]

While recent technological advancements in psychopharmaceuticals, steroids, fertility treatments, cosmetic procedures, preventive medicine, obstetrics, ophthalmology, and many more have valid pragmatic counterarguments over their continued practice, perhaps tampering with the scaffold of biology may be a far more sensible topic with risks transcending those of a single individual.[3] Genetic engineering has brought forth a plethora of innovative possibilities to combat disease. Since the dawn of genetic therapy in the 1960s with the use of recombinant DNA technology, the precision of gene manipulation and editing has increasingly improved and continues to do so.[20, 21] Despite its favorable prospective application in medicine, scientists fear that in search of unlocking its full potential, this may also inevitably compromise public health and the authenticity of human nature.[19]

Genetic Engineering

The technological ability to modify the human genome can be both an exciting and terrifying concept to ponder. Genetic engineering offers humans the ability to have direct control over their biological deficits and limitations. This is possible through gene editing technology (e.g., CRISPR-Cas9) that allows for precise insertion, deletion, or replacement of "faulty" DNA fragments.[22] DNA functions as an instruction manual on how to build anything that comprises the complexity of human design (or biological entity). The addition of desirable genetic material would permit humans to acquire permanent enhancing traits such as increased muscle growth, memory retention, eyesight, disease immunity, and cancer treatment, among many others.[23] In turn, this could also lead to a permanent and radical change of the status quo. Unvoiced requirements for select enhancements in certain areas of society would be in high demand while economic disparities would further the exclusivity of a myriad of genetic advantages.[24] In the interest of utilizing genetic engineering to further the repertoire of healthcare treatment, this has raised a conglomerate of concerns concerning risks and ethical implications of its use.[14]

Objective Assessment
Despite variable sentiments towards tampering with genetics, the scientific debate has been prominently divided into 2 groups: transhumanists and bioconservatives.[25] Advocates for genetic enhancement nurture the argument that increased protection against diseases could raise the life expectancy of humans in tandem with contented lives. Given the stress of pathogenic diseases in healthcare, fortified defenses using genetic technology would substantially reduce the prevalence of diseases in the population.[26] As tempting as it may sound, this could also lead to an opposite state of affairs. Theoretically, regardless of how remarkably evolved humans could be, it would be nearly impossible to keep up with the rate of mutations leading to the development of pathogenic resistance. Being already observed in genetically engineered crops, the transfer of resistance genes between viruses or bacteria is a serious concern.[27] Because humanity would have developed potent resistance to a variety of biological threats, this would also entail similar pathogenic resistance exposing humans to far more perilous diseases.[28, 29]

Germline alterations have surfaced as a promising avenue in preventative medicine; however, the difference between its therapeutic and enhancement use is not substantially dissimilar. While the intended purpose of germ-line therapy is to artificially design future generations of humans with select immunities, long-term side effects of the procedure cannot be predicted. In addition, while live patients may be able to consent to or decline a particular treatment, an unborn child does not have the same luxury of choice. For this reason, the US does not fund any type of research involving germ-line therapy in humans.[30] In fact, any form of germline modification has been subject to strict government regulation (or ban altogether) in over 40 jurisdictions/countries such as Australia, Canada, France, and Germany although sanctions in some Asian countries may not be reprehensive enough to avoid its practice.[31]

An example of germline therapy interest concerns CCR5-Δ32, a 32-bp deletion using CRISPR-Cas9 (a low-cost and accurate gene editing technology) of the CCR5 receptor protein targeted by certain strains of HIV to gain access to leukocytes. In the absence of CCR5, it has shown promise in providing heritable resistance against HIV infection.[32, 33] In 2018, this gene editing procedure was performed in China on 2 non-identical twin embryos of which the father was known to be

HIV positive (despite knowing that if sufficient suppression of HIV is achieved, transmission to the offspring can be negligible).[3] However, deletion of CCR5-Δ32 has also been associated with an increased risk of fatal reactions to other serious diseases (e.g., influenza) questioning the reliability of gene editing in the absence of a clear understanding of the knockout function of a particular gene.[34]

Pleiotropy is a concern because researchers have no way to predict if a deleted gene pertains to a singular function.[35] Thorough research surrounding its pathway(s) is advised to prevent serious outcomes, but this is an arduous task and it may not always be possible. Moreover, despite the prospective effectiveness of CRISPR-Cas9, its gene-cutting precision is not perfect. CRISPR-Cas9 technology is fairly new (appearing in the literature in 2012) meaning that studies surrounding its safety/effectiveness are limited. Off-target mutagenesis is an unintended problem resulting from a change of closely matching gene sequences. While some studies suggest large overestimations attributed to off-target mutagenesis, others report largely the opposite leading to a hazy comprehension of the extent of CRISPR-Cas9 precision for gene editing.[36,37]

Subjective Assessment

The differences between health-oriented and enhancement applications of genetic engineering are vague but seem to have a recurrent feature distinguishing their acceptance among the public and the medical field. Restorative medicine seems to have a positive reception whenever its use is restricted to "normalizing" a deficiency in an individual.[14] As previously described, normal vision is considered to be 20/20 which means that interventions correcting eyesight may be deemed more ethical in comparison to enhancing eyesight to 40/20. In the same light, reconstructive surgery performed on a burn victim rather than installing cybernetic enhancements to one's body may also be found to be a more acceptable practice. If the same approach is to be applied to genetic therapy, perhaps interventions for patients with genetic deficiencies such as sickle cell anemia or Tay-Sachs disease are more likely to be used than providing genetic immunity to general diseases. In the argument of normalcy, it could be advocated that being infected by severe diseases such as HIV or COVID-19 is neither normal nor typically occurs in humans.[38,39] While this holds true to an extent, continued justification of surging life-threatening diseases as "not normal" to human health could inadvertently lead to the fortified enhancement of humans. Thus, contributing to the puzzling dilemma of gene editing in preventative medicine.

Concerning the topic of deliberate enhancement in humans, genetic engineering could have a profound impact on societal norms and regulations. The utilization of CRISPR-Cas9 has the potential to improve multiple desirable traits including those of particular interest to legislature such as lessening of violent behavior tendencies, and substance dependence.[40] If a judge were to decide a person to be dangerous to the community or prone to a repeated offense—similar to mandatory actions or rehabilitation programs imposed by the court of law—the utilization of genetic engineering may be required to "fix" these undesirable attributes. While the morality behind this probable rehabilitation method has yet to be discussed and is possibly subject to regulation, the widespread use of gene editing technology may incentivize its use in the political landscape.

Genetic enhancement for military purposes may opt for the optimization of human performance rather than outweighing the potential risks in favor of military power. Although weaponry has been highly sophisticated, the extent of its destructive power (e.g., nuclear and biochemical weapons) has led to a backlash in the ethical and moral implications of its use. Therefore, soldiers continue to be at the forefront of military operations leading countries to compete over the strength of their military forces. In science fiction, a glimpse of the desirable attributes for a soldier such as increased strength, stamina, attention/awareness, obedience, vision, and limited psychosomatic reactions to the brutality of war has been shown. In addition, resistance to biochemical poisons may also be of relevant interest. Despite its great potential for military might, there is also a concern for the safety (given the current limitations/risks of gene editing technology) and consent of military personnel. Due to the highly stratified chain of command, soldiers are expected to obey the decisions of high-ranking officers. If genetic modification were to be required, soldiers would have minimal liberty to deny enhancement(s).[41,42]

From a philosophical point of view, the very nature of humanity can be compromised by the continued development of bioengineering technology. In religion, it can be considered a serious offense because it is a direct distortion of God's creation and will.[43] Depending on an individual's opinion in natural ethics, tampering with the human body can be seen as depravity regardless of the intended good. Some may advocate for the "wisdom of nature" meaning that things that are naturally occurring should continue to run their course because nature "knows" what is best for all beings. While much of the scientific decisions rely on objective evidence, it is also important to address public sentiment despite conflicting views. The future of science can deliver humanity to a new evolutionary phase (even if by artificial means), but in doing so it may also gain the resentment of the population.

Concluding Remarks
Genetic therapy has great potential to deliver highly efficacious treatment to patients suffering from genetic diseases. However, gene editing technology can also serve a variety of different purposes, and not all of them are ethically suitable. Human enhancement is a practical use of gene editing, but despite its attractive qualities, it may unintentionally result in further subdivision of society, compromise the nature of species, and accelerate the mutation of pathogens resulting in a healthcare crisis. The continued refinement of this technology as shown by the discovery of CRISPR-Cas9 seems to be an unavoidable field of scientific and medical interest which means that the potential for misuse is to be expected. For this reason, strict regulations over the use of this technology should continue to be pursued in the interest of safeguarding the public from the uncertain risks of this technology.

Works Cited
1. Fukuyama F. Our posthuman future: Consequences of the biotechnology revolution: Farrar, Straus and Giroux; 2003.

2. Lanigan TM, Kopera HC, Saunders TL. Principles of Genetic Engineering. Genes (Basel). 2020;11(3). Epub 20200310.
3. Almeida M, Diogo R. Human enhancement: Genetic engineering and evolution. Evol Med Public Health. 2019;2019(1):183-9. Epub 20190928.
4. Brans YW. Biomedical technology: to use or not to use? Clin Perinatol. 1991;18(3):389-401.
5. Karlawish J, Jack CR, Jr., Rocca WA, et al. Alzheimer's disease: The next frontier-Special Report 2017. Alzheimers Dement. 2017;13(4):374-80. Epub 20170314.
6. Pham P, Roux S, Matonti F, et al. Post-implantation impedance spectroscopy of subretinal micro-electrode arrays, OCT imaging and numerical simulation: towards a more precise neuroprosthesis monitoring tool. J Neural Eng. 2013;10(4):046002. Epub 20130530.
7. Aly RM. Current state of stem cell-based therapies: an overview. Stem Cell Investig. 2020;7:8. Epub 20200515.
8. Hayat H, Hayat H, Dwan BF, et al. A Concise Review: The Role of Stem Cells in Cancer Progression and Therapy. Onco Targets Ther. 2021;14:2761-72. Epub 20210420.
9. Malik M, Tlustos P. Nootropics as Cognitive Enhancers: Types, Dosage and Side Effects of Smart Drugs. Nutrients. 2022;14(16). Epub 20220817.
10. Zaami S, Minutillo A, Sirignano A, et al. Effects of Appearance- and Performance-Enhancing Drugs on Personality Traits. Front Psychiatry. 2021;12:730167. Epub 20210924.
11. Handelsman DJ. Performance Enhancing Hormone Doping in Sport. In: Feingold KR, Anawalt B, Boyce A, Chrousos G, de Herder WW, Dhatariya K, Dungan K, Hershman JM, Hofland J, Kalra S, Kaltsas G, Koch C, Kopp P, Korbonits M, Kovacs CS, Kuohung W, Laferrere B, Levy M, McGee EA, McLachlan R, Morley JE, New M, Purnell J, Sahay R, Singer F, Sperling MA, Stratakis CA, Trence DL, Wilson DP, editors. Endotext. South Dartmouth (MA)2000.
12. Hunter M. Athletes risk their lives by routine use of performance enhancing drugs, says BMA. BMJ. 2002.
13. Human Genome Editing: Science, Ethics, and Governance. National Library of Medicine: National Academies Press (US); 2017.
14. Mehlman MJ, Berg JW. Human subjects protections in biomedical enhancement research: assessing risk and benefit and obtaining informed consent. J Law Med Ethics. 2008;36(3):546-9.
15. 20/20 Vision: Visual Acuity, Testing, and More myvision.org2022 [cited 2022]. Available from: https://myvision.org/eyesight/20-20-vision/#:~:text=About%2035%20percent%20of%20adult,5%20vision%20have%20better%20eyesight.
16. Rosenfeld LS, Mihalov JJ, Carlson SJ, et al. Regulatory status of caffeine in the United States. Nutr Rev. 2014;72 Suppl 1:23-33.
17. Giubilini A, Sanyal S. The ethics of human enhancement. Philosophy Compass. 2015;10(4):233-43.
18. Parens E. The goodness of fragility: on the prospect of genetic technologies aimed at the enhancement of human capacities. Kennedy Inst Ethics J. 1995;5(2):141-53.
19. Juengst E. Human Enhancement Standford Encyclopedia of Philosophy2019. 2015. Available from: https://plato.stanford.edu/entries/enhancement/.
20. Szybalska EH, Szybalski W. Genetics of human cell line. IV. DNA-mediated heritable transformation of a biochemical trait. Proc Natl Acad Sci U S A. 1962;48(12):2026-34.
21. Tamura R, Toda M. Historic Overview of Genetic Engineering Technologies for Human Gene Therapy. Neurol Med Chir (Tokyo). 2020;60(10):483-91. Epub 20200908.
22. Gaj T, Gersbach CA, Barbas CF, 3rd. ZFN, TALEN, and CRISPR/Cas-based methods for genome engineering. Trends Biotechnol. 2013;31(7):397-405. Epub 20130509.

23. Human Enhancement: The Scientific and Ethical Dimensions of Striving for Perfection Pew Research Center2016 [cited 2022]. Available from: https://www.pewresearch.org/science/2016/07/26/human-enhancement-the-scientific-and-ethical-dimensions-of-striving-for-perfection/.
24. Rothschild J. Ethical considerations of gene editing and genetic selection. J Gen Fam Med. 2020;21(3):37-47. Epub 20200529.
25. Persson I, Savulescu J. The perils of cognitive enhancement and the urgent imperative to enhance the moral character of humanity. Journal of applied philosophy. 2008;25(3):162-77.
26. Harris J. Enhancing evolution. Enhancing Evolution: Princeton University Press; 2010.
27. Genetically Engineered Crops: Experiences and Prospects. NCBI: National Academies of Sciences, Engineering, and Medicine; 2016. Available from: https://www.ncbi.nlm.nih.gov/books/NBK424534/.
28. Rom Z. Genetic Engineering: A Serious Threat to Human Society: University of Maryland Department of English; 2011 [cited 2022]. Available from: https://english.umd.edu/research-innovation/journals/interpolations/interpolations-spring-2011/genetic-engineering-serious#:~:text=Genetically%20engineered%20organisms%20pose%20an,to%20kill%20millions%20of%20people.
29. Dona A, Arvanitoyannis IS. Health risks of genetically modified foods. Crit Rev Food Sci Nutr. 2009;49(2):164-75.
30. What are the ethical issues surrounding gene therapy? MedLine Plus: National Library of Medicine; 2022 [cited 2022]. Available from: https://medlineplus.gov/genetics/understanding/therapy/ethics/.
31. Araki M, Ishii T. International regulatory landscape and integration of corrective genome editing into in vitro fertilization. Reprod Biol Endocrinol. 2014;12:108. Epub 20141124.
32. So D, Kleiderman E, Toure SB, et al. Disease Resistance and the Definition of Genetic Enhancement. Front Genet. 2017;8:40. Epub 20170410.
33. Kang X, He W, Huang Y, et al. Introducing precise genetic modifications into human 3PN embryos by CRISPR/Cas-mediated genome editing. J Assist Reprod Genet. 2016;33(5):581-8. Epub 20160406.
34. Falcon A, Cuevas MT, Rodriguez-Frandsen A, et al. CCR5 deficiency predisposes to fatal outcome in influenza virus infection. J Gen Virol. 2015;96(8):2074-8. Epub 20150427.
35. Galis F, Metz JA. Evolutionary novelties: the making and breaking of pleiotropic constraints. Integr Comp Biol. 2007;47(3):409-19. Epub 20070820.
36. Iyer V, Boroviak K, Thomas M, et al. No unexpected CRISPR-Cas9 off-target activity revealed by trio sequencing of gene-edited mice. PLoS Genet. 2018;14(7):e1007503. Epub 20180709.
37. Fu Y, Foden JA, Khayter C, et al. High-frequency off-target mutagenesis induced by CRISPR-Cas nucleases in human cells. Nat Biotechnol. 2013;31(9):822-6. Epub 20130623.
38. National Academies of Sciences E, Medicine. Human genome editing: science, ethics, and governance: National Academies Press; 2017.
39. Cascella M, Rajnik M, Aleem A, et al. Features, Evaluation, and Treatment of Coronavirus (COVID-19). StatPearls. Treasure Island (FL)2022.
40. Rodriguez E. Ethical issues in genome editing using Crispr/Cas9 system. Journal of Clinical Research and Bioethics. 2016;7(2).
41. Greene M, Master Z. Ethical Issues of Using CRISPR Technologies for Research on Military Enhancement. J Bioeth Inq. 2018;15(3):327-35. Epub 20180702.
42. Greene M. Ethical Issues of Using CRISPR Technologies for Research on Military Enhancement. Journal of Bioethical Inquiry. 2018.

43. Bioethics NCo. (un) natural: Ideas about Naturalness in Public and Political Debates about Science, Technology and Medicine: Nuffield Council on Bioethics; 2015.

Essay: Physical Enhancement in Response to Climate Change

Erica Day

Evolution is a slow process, but the effect humanity has on the planet is not. The global mean temperature is expected to increase by 1.6° C by 2050 and by 3.3° C from 2051–2100.[1] Other, more temperature-narrow species are facing the effects and are forced to evolve in response to human-created climate change.[2,3] The impact of humanity on its surroundings is not negligible, and we are already feeling the effects of climate change. Heat-related mortality has increased in many areas of the world, especially in vulnerable populations.[4-7] Increased temperatures are also associated with food and water-related diseases, causing increased childhood mortality, which we are already seeing now.[8,9] As climate change ravages the world, and with insufficient policy in reversing these issues, humanity may need to artificially evolve. Physical enhancement through gene editing may be our quickest solution in addressing the incompatibility of the human species to the new world.

Genome editing today, seen with much success, is common in industrial agriculture as traits that provide disease resistance and increased production are artificially selected.[10-12] The end goal of these genomic modifications is to increase survival until harvest, editing out common ailments that lead to lost profit and resources. Climate change is now considered one of the problems that gene editing will need to target, and artificial physical adaptions within the agriculture industry are on the rise. In the hopes of decreasing increased rates of heat stress within cattle, coat colors have been genetically modified to select lighter colors over the solar radiation-absorbing black.[13] Staple crops for human and animal consumption are edited to be drought resistant as freshwater sources diminish due to increased temperature.[14-17] As our world changes around us in response to global warming and becomes more hostile, and as permanent changes to our environment become more severe, the need for humanity to adjust themselves to this new world will rise to ensure species survival. Various physical adaptions including increased thermotolerance and disease resistance should reduce mortality and other climate-related stresses.

One main component of climate change and the effects humanity has upon the world is increased temperature. Already temperature-related mortality has increased and will increase unless a change is enacted. Gene editing may be key in this area as genes related to thermotolerance are selected artificially, key to surviving in a hotter environment. Hsp70, a gene family within humans and other animals, is one specific gene to target as it protects against heat and other environmental-related stresses which are sure to be common in the new world.[18,19] Other species that have survived global temperature stresses, and indicate further survival, possess overexpression of these heat shock proteins in response to environmental indicators.[20, 21] These traits are deemed valuable and then passed to their offspring at high rates. Humanity may find it necessary to follow suit and edit genes for increased temperature resistance, by choosing genes that encourage overexpression of heat shock proteins. Heat stress, a common problem within a world heated with global warming should be a primary physical enhancement that enhances survivability.

Increased temperatures invite other problems: water scarcity and disease. Freshwater sources, polluted or not, begin to evaporate, turning life-supporting land into a barren desert. With water sources gone, as well as drought-caused famine, disease is sure to follow. Already a rise in tropical diseases related to climate change has occurred and will only continue to increase with global warming.[22] In industrial livestock, genes that provide disease resistance or prevention, in general, are artificially selected.[23] Already tested within livestock we humans can follow suit by selecting genes that provide general disease resistance as well as diseases that will be common without water security, diarrheal diseases, and tropical diseases caused by heat and humidity. Genes that provide disease resistance will decrease the mortality rates of humans and the impact that water scarcity will have on the population.[24, 25] Selecting genes that provide resistance and avoiding those that increase susceptibility will only be beneficial in situations of water scarcity and impurity.

Of course, these are predictions and suggestions for a future that hopefully will not come to pass. The changes made to the climate today are irreversible but with aggressive sustainability practices the effect humanity has upon the environment should slow or stop.[26] But currently, the changes necessary are not in place, and a devastated planet becomes ever closer to reality. Mankind is adaptive and resilient, and physical enhancement may be the answer to survival in a super-heated world, but the healthiest solution, for both humanity and the planet, is to work to reduce and reverse damages. Physical enhancement is the way of the future, it should not be humanity's only future.

Works Cited

1. Diaz J, Saez M, Carmona R, et al. Mortality attributable to high temperatures over the 2021-2050 and 2051-2100 time horizons in Spain: Adaptation and economic estimate. Environ Res. 2019;172:475-85. Epub 20190227.
2. Bassitta M, Brown RP, Perez-Cembranos A, et al. Genomic signatures of drift and selection driven by predation and human pressure in an insular lizard. Sci Rep. 2021;11(1):6136. Epub 20210317.
3. Vicenzi N, Bacigalupe LD, Laspiur A, et al. Could plasticity mediate highlands lizards' resilience to climate change? A case study of the leopard iguana (Diplolaemus leopardinus) in Central Andes of Argentina. J Exp Biol. 2021;224(14). Epub 20210722.
4. Rahman MM, Garcia E, Lim CC, et al. Temperature variability associations with cardiovascular and respiratory emergency department visits in Dhaka, Bangladesh. Environ Int. 2022;164:107267. Epub 20220502.
5. Jahan S, Cauchi JP, Galdies C, et al. The adverse effect of ambient temperature on respiratory deaths in a high population density area: the case of Malta. Respir Res. 2022;23(1):299. Epub 20221031.

6. Vicedo-Cabrera AM, Scovronick N, Sera F, et al. The burden of heat-related mortality attributable to recent human-induced climate change. Nat Clim Chang. 2021;11(6):492-500. Epub 20210531.
7. Zhan ZY, Tian Q, Chen TT, et al. Temperature Variability and Hospital Admissions for Chronic Obstructive Pulmonary Disease: Analysis of Attributable Disease Burden and Vulnerable Subpopulation. Int J Chron Obstruct Pulmon Dis. 2020;15:2225-35. Epub 20200922.
8. Ebi KL, Hess JJ, Watkiss P. Health Risks and Costs of Climate Variability and Change. In: rd, Mock CN, Nugent R, Kobusingye O, Smith KR, editors. Injury Prevention and Environmental Health. Washington (DC)2017.
9. Caminade C, McIntyre KM, Jones AE. Impact of recent and future climate change on vector-borne diseases. Ann N Y Acad Sci. 2019;1436(1):157-73. Epub 20180818.
10. Van Eenennaam AL. Application of genome editing in farm animals: cattle. Transgenic Res. 2019;28(Suppl 2):93-100.
11. Yang H, Zhang J, Zhang X, et al. CD163 knockout pigs are fully resistant to highly pathogenic porcine reproductive and respiratory syndrome virus. Antiviral Res. 2018;151:63-70. Epub 20180111.
12. Wang S, Qu Z, Huang Q, et al. Application of Gene Editing Technology in Resistance Breeding of Livestock. Life (Basel). 2022;12(7). Epub 20220718.
13. Laible G, Cole SA, Brophy B, et al. Holstein Friesian dairy cattle edited for diluted coat color as a potential adaptation to climate change. BMC Genomics. 2021;22(1):856. Epub 20211126.
14. Chen YN, Lu J. [Application of CRISPR/Cas9 mediated gene editing in trees]. Yi Chuan. 2020;42(7):657-68.
15. Cao HX, Vu GTH, Gailing O. From Genome Sequencing to CRISPR-Based Genome Editing for Climate-Resilient Forest Trees. Int J Mol Sci. 2022;23(2). Epub 20220116.
16. Zenda T, Liu S, Dong A, et al. Advances in Cereal Crop Genomics for Resilience under Climate Change. Life (Basel). 2021;11(6). Epub 20210529.
17. Numan M, Serba DD, Ligaba-Osena A. Alternative Strategies for Multi-Stress Tolerance and Yield Improvement in Millets. Genes (Basel). 2021;12(5). Epub 20210514.
18. Harrison GS, Drabkin HA, Kao FT, et al. Chromosomal location of human genes encoding major heat-shock protein HSP70. Somat Cell Mol Genet. 1987;13(2):119-30.
19. Tavaria M, Gabriele T, Kola I, et al. A hitchhiker's guide to the human Hsp70 family. Cell Stress Chaperones. 1996;1(1):23-8.
20. Falfushynska HI, Phan T, Sokolova IM. Long-Term Acclimation to Different Thermal Regimes Affects Molecular Responses to Heat Stress in a Freshwater Clam Corbicula Fluminea. Sci Rep. 2016;6:39476. Epub 20161220.
21. Lardies MA, Arias MB, Poupin MJ, et al. Heritability of hsp70 expression in the beetle Tenebrio molitor: Ontogenetic and environmental effects. J Insect Physiol. 2014;67:70-5. Epub 20140623.
22. Mahmud AS, Martinez PP, He J, et al. The Impact of Climate Change on Vaccine-Preventable Diseases: Insights From Current Research and New Directions. Curr Environ Health Rep. 2020;7(4):384-91. Epub 20201025.
23. Singh P, Ali SA. Impact of CRISPR-Cas9-Based Genome Engineering in Farm Animals. Vet Sci. 2021;8(7). Epub 20210630.
24. Arama C, Skinner J, Doumtabe D, et al. Genetic Resistance to Malaria Is Associated With Greater Enhancement of Immunoglobulin (Ig)M Than IgG Responses to a Broad Array of Plasmodium falciparum Antigens. Open Forum Infect Dis. 2015;2(3):ofv118. Epub 20150826.
25. Moller M, Kinnear CJ, Orlova M, et al. Genetic Resistance to Mycobacterium tuberculosis Infection and Disease. Front Immunol. 2018;9:2219. Epub 20180927.
26. Solomon S, Plattner GK, Knutti R, et al. Irreversible climate change due to carbon dioxide emissions. Proc Natl Acad Sci U S A. 2009;106(6):1704-9. Epub 20090128.

Essay: Designer Babies—Gene Editing and Enhancement

Baden Cruickshank

Designer babies, or CRISPR babies, have become a trendy topic in the past decades, particularly in the non-scientific community. The idea of being able to genetically assemble a child to look and act exactly how you desire has become an appealing idea for many prospective parents. Interest in being able to change hair color, eye color, physical fitness, strength, and disease resistance before birth may be enticing, but it certainly does not come without risks. The idea is to use CRISPR-Cas9, a gene-editing technology that was originally developed to edit the genomes of animal models in laboratory settings, to produce desired outcomes in the human genome.[1]

CRISPR-Cas9 technology was developed relatively recently, but its precursors have been studied for decades. The system involves the utilization of a specific RNA sequence to guide an endonuclease Cas9 protein that is used to cleave DNA and allow for subsequent modification.[1-3] This technology has allowed for unique research that was impossible before its creation, as it permits researchers to specifically edit the genome of laboratory cells or animal models to meet their needs precisely. One researcher has already attempted to use CRISPR-Cas9 to edit the genome of human babies before birth and was met with backlash and criticism from the scientific community. His goal was to create HIV-resistant children by inactivating the CCR5 gene which encodes proteins that many strains of HIV use to enter the cell in multiple human embryos.[4]

Though he was somewhat successful in editing the genomes of two children, he was met with outrage and denounced by the majority of the scientific community. Most developed countries have laws or other regulations prohibiting human genome editing at this point, citing a lack of knowledge of the risks involved.[5] It is simply irresponsible and unethical to make an outright attempt to edit the genome of human embryos without further research into potential unknown consequences. The action of CRISPR-Cas9 has been thoroughly researched and is relatively understood in other mammals, but it is still unknown whether it will function the same way in the human genome.[6]

Editing the human genome may seem appealing to many at face value, it seems like the key to irradiating disease, both genetic and otherwise, and would allow for a "perfect" society with ideal physical and mental attributes for all. In an ideal world, it would be wonderful to have a simple way to ensure that no child suffers from illness again, to eliminate genetic diseases by simply removing it from an embryo's genome, or to allow parents to design their child to be an ideal human specimen. Reality is harsher than an ideal world, and there is no way to ensure that any editing of the human genome would be safe, effective, or controlled at this time. What if altering the genome of a child to prevent transmission of HIV from a parent would lead to depression, anxiety, or other ailments later in life that would not have occurred otherwise? There is simply no way to know based on current knowledge, and significant research would need to be done to determine the potential effects of editing the genome. Additionally, without clear enforcement and regulation, the idea of physical and mental enhancement and the creation of "designer babies" may begin to border on eugenics. If the idea of designer babies becomes acceptable and practical in the future without regulation it would likely become polarized based on socioeconomic status, with children of the wealthy being designed to be superior physically and mentally to all others.

Perception of the acceptability of gene editing for either personal enhancement or treatment of diseases varies between the public and scientific communities. The public is generally more accepting than scientists, with many supporting gene editing for physical and mental enhancement and a greater portion supporting it for the treatment of diseases.[7] Scientists are much more hesitant to support gene editing for physical and mental enhancements for non-medical uses and tend to be less supportive than the public of its use for the treatment of diseases.[8] The public tends to consider only positive outcomes while not focusing on potential negatives, and that is likely what leads to a greater portion of public support for gene editing in humans. Scientists tend to focus more on potential negatives than positives, considering unintended consequences and negative outcomes instead of positive ones. Public and scientific perception varies greatly on the topic, and discussions and additional research must be conducted to further understand the appeal of human genome editing within both communities.

The idea of gene editing for designer babies is an interesting and appealing topic, but at this time it is underdeveloped and under-researched. There is significant work to be done before serious considerations can be made to apply CRISPR-Cas9 technology to the human genome. Research into the consequences of gene editing must be conducted to determine the potential effects of editing the human genome, and policies and regulations must be put in place to ensure that the technology is not abused or used incorrectly in the future. There is much to consider before designer babies hit the production lines, and until there is comprehensive knowledge and proper governance of the topic, it should not be considered.

Works Cited

1. Redman M, King A, Watson C, et al. What is CRISPR/Cas9? Arch Dis Child Educ Pract Ed. 2016;101(4):213-5. Epub 20160408.
2. Lau V, Davie JR. The discovery and development of the CRISPR system in applications in genome manipulation. Biochem Cell Biol. 2017;95(2):203-10. Epub 20161028.
3. Adli M. The CRISPR tool kit for genome editing and beyond. Nat Commun. 2018;9(1):1911. Epub 20180515.
4. Rose BI, Brown S. Genetically Modified Babies and a First Application of Clustered Regularly Interspaced Short Palindromic Repeats (CRISPR-Cas9). Obstet Gynecol. 2019;134(1):157-62.
5. Araki M, Ishii T. International regulatory landscape and integration of corrective genome editing into in vitro fertilization. Reprod Biol Endocrinol. 2014;12:108. Epub 20141124.
6. Ma Y, Zhang L, Qin C. The first genetically gene-edited babies: It's "irresponsible and too early". Animal Model Exp Med. 2019;2(1):1-4. Epub 20190111.

7. Delhove J, Osenk I, Prichard I, et al. Public Acceptability of Gene Therapy and Gene Editing for Human Use: A Systematic Review. Hum Gene Ther. 2020;31(1-2):20-46.
8. Waltz M, Juengst ET, Edwards T, et al. The View from the Benches: Scientists' Perspectives on the Uses and Governance of Human Gene-Editing Research. CRISPR J. 2021;4(4):609-15.

Essay: Genetic Editing of Humans

Brianna Hunt

For years, the concept of gene editing human embryos and creating "designer babies" seemed like nothing more than a science fiction cautionary tale, or an unachievable goal. However, after researcher He Jiankui genetically edited two human embryos in hopes to confer immunity to HIV infection, it is time that society confronts the reality that the age of gene editing has already arrived.[1] Thanks to the CRISPR-Cas 9 system, scientists can modify genomes simply and efficiently.[2] In addition to being used for research, there is the possibility to use this system for therapeutic applications in the future.[3] This is a new technology that has not yet been thoroughly explored for human use, so scientists must tread especially carefully and avoid unethical experiments if we are to proceed down this path.

Editing the genes of humans indeed holds the potential to greatly benefit society. With this technology, we could potentially eradicate genetic disorders and reduce the likelihood of developing disorders (such as diabetes) later in life.[4] The most reasonable therapeutic use for this technology soon is the elimination of monogenic diseases, such as sickle cell anemia or cystic fibrosis.[5] For example, CRISPR-Cas9 technology has already been used to improve cardiac function in mice with Duchenne muscular dystrophy, another monogenic disease.[6] If this technology were to be used in humans as well, it could potentially save the lives of thousands of patients with this condition.[7] At first, it seems clear that we should use the CRISPR system to its full potential to create a healthier world.

However, this issue is not that simple. With the ability to genetically edit embryos, we could select traits that have nothing to do with future health. We could select certain traits of appearance or personality. Currently, the position taken by many geneticists is that genome editing should only be done with a clear medical rationale.[8] Even so, if there are potential profits to be made from this technology, it is only a matter of time before the wealthy will use it for non-medical purposes. These advancements would likely only be available to the people who can afford them, which would only widen the divide between socioeconomic classes. Before allowing genetic editing of humans, we would have to ensure that legislation is in place to prevent this from happening.

In addition to the socioeconomic considerations that must be made, we must also consider the safety of using this experimental technology. With the CRISPR system, there is always the possibility of introducing off-target mutations, which could cause deleterious effects even worse than the genetic disease that the editing was meant to cure.[9] This is especially worrisome in the case of germline editing. In this case, changes made to the genome are irreversible and can be passed down to further generations.[9] This is also concerning because any human born after germline editing would not have consented to these modifications. We have no way of knowing the potential consequences until it is already too late. Therefore, it may be too dangerous to pursue therapeutic uses of genetic editing in humans.

There is another important consideration to be made. Without proper regulations, genetic editing technology could be easily exploited for eugenics purposes. This technology could be used to eliminate certain genes, which would severely limit human diversity.[10] The goal of eugenics also holds the implication that society would be better without people who have disabilities or illnesses. This is an incredibly dangerous—not to mention entirely false—mindset to have. Disabled and ill people are perfectly capable of contributing to society, so instead of aiming to eradicate these disabilities or conditions, we should be focusing on ways we can improve current society to be more accommodating to these people. Additionally, genetic editing is not the be-all and end-all for creating a healthier society. Several conditions can develop throughout a person's life as a result of environmental factors, rather than being caused by genes. It makes more sense to prioritize improving the lives of these people after birth, rather than performing dangerous experiments on embryos.

We are not ready to take the plunge into a future where genetic editing of humans is an accepted practice. Even if we have the tools at our disposal, we need to be cautious. While using CRISPR has great potential to do good, it could just as easily be used to the detriment of society. Before proceeding, it is essential for there to be regulations in place to ensure any gene editing of humans is done safely and ethically.

Works Cited

1. Greely HT. CRISPR'd babies: human germline genome editing in the 'He Jiankui affair'. J Law Biosci. 2019;6(1):111-83. Epub 20190813.
2. Hryhorowicz M, Lipinski D, Zeyland J, et al. CRISPR/Cas9 Immune System as a Tool for Genome Engineering. Arch Immunol Ther Exp (Warsz). 2017;65(3):233-40. Epub 20161003.
3. Gagnon KT, Corey DR. Stepping toward therapeutic CRISPR. Proc Natl Acad Sci U S A. 2015;112(51):15536-7. Epub 20151207.
4. Dabi YT, Degechisa ST. Genome Editing and Human Pluripotent Stem Cell Technologies for in vitro Monogenic Diabetes Modeling. Diabetes Metab Syndr Obes. 2022;15:1785-97. Epub 20220611.
5. Doudna JA. The promise and challenge of therapeutic genome editing. Nature. 2020;578(7794):229-36. Epub 20200212.
6. El Refaey M, Xu L, Gao Y, et al. In Vivo Genome Editing Restores Dystrophin Expression and Cardiac Function in Dystrophic Mice. Circ Res. 2017;121(8):923-9. Epub 20170808.
7. Choi E, Koo T. CRISPR technologies for the treatment of Duchenne muscular dystrophy. Mol Ther. 2021;29(11):3179-91. Epub 20210403.
8. Ormond KE, Mortlock DP, Scholes DT, et al. Human Germline Genome Editing. Am J Hum Genet. 2017;101(2):167-76.
9. Shinwari ZK, Tanveer F, Khalil AT. Ethical Issues Regarding CRISPR Mediated Genome Editing. Curr Issues Mol Biol. 2018;26:103-10. Epub 20170907.
10. Pollack R. Eugenics lurk in the shadow of CRISPR. Science. 2015;348(6237):871.

Topic: Transgender Controversies

Although transgender as a topic in society is not new, it is apparently a minimally studied topic in medicine. In fact, many medical school curricula do not offer teaching in transgender aspects of medicine at all.[1] Thus, in the US, we are graduating healthcare providers with almost zero sophistication and knowledge in how to care for a rapidly emerging population who require medical interventions, specifically if they wish to physically transition to the gender to which they identify. Indeed, 40% of LGBTQ patients have complained that there are no healthcare providers at all who can meet their needs appropriately. This dearth of caregivers may have many causes: poor or no training of providers, little general awareness by providers of these populations and their needs, and insurance company refusals to cover care for transgendered and LGBTQ people.[2]

"I've never been interested in being invisible and erased."

— Laverne Cox, actress and LGBTQ advocate

This results in discrimination against these populations in the form of denial of fertility treatments, counseling, screening for routine health problems, opioid abuse treatment, and even pediatric care for children.[3-5] This almost certainly means that acquiring care for gender reassignment (surgical or pharmacological) and transition care is either difficult or impossible.[6] Specifically, complaints about providers included that clinicians lacked knowledge about drugs and correct dosing, general endocrinology, how to take an appropriate medical history, gender-affirming surgical options, and social issues.[7] An argument has been made that these deficits in healthcare options are not due to provider intolerance but due to ignorance, something which is easily fixable via targeted medical curricula. How effective these curricular changes may be is uncertain as politicians have weighed in on the issue with a pronounced lack of scientific or medical background, allowing them to push forward laws to prevent any care from being given to LGBTQ/transgendered patients at critical times during development.[8] This is supported by general exclusions of transgender medical care by insurance companies in 24 states and the District of Columbia. Only in Arkansas does the law explicitly permit insurers to directly refuse to cover transgender care.[9]

LGBT and transgender people are not going away, and they should not have to, so medical care for these marginalized populations requires prompt and meaningful action. What that looks like is not clear but easily implementable suggestions can be made across medical schools which often use nationally standardized programmatic content to prepare students for the US Medical Licensing Exam Steps I and II. First, block directors who are often highly accomplished basic scientists can easily add lecture content regarding the science of human sexuality and the extensions of that science into medical care.[10] Then, medical students would be receiving important training in the first and second years. During training, students can access videos via online learning platforms.[11] Then, students can incorporate into the professional patient cadre—paid and informed individuals used to train medical students in non-surgical medical procedures by providing immediate feedback to the students— LGBT/transgendered

"We have to remain visible. They have to see us, they have to know that we're not going [nowhere], that we've been here ever since God made man and woman, and they have to get over it."

 Miss Major Griffin-Gracy, Civil Rights Advocate

"standard" patients, too. This addition of a professional LGBT/transgendered patient was first done in 2017 and this individual was used to train residents in communication skills.[12] Adding real patients helps future clinicians understand that these skills are not theoretical; rather, being LGBTQ/transgendered individuals is their actual lived experience.

Data show that in the few medical schools in which this training is offered, clinicians emerge more confident and project less stigma onto these patients.[7] These early teachings also encouraged providers to seek more training via peer mentorship, independent learning/instruction through books, conferences, and online protocols such as the World Professional Association for Transgender Health and the Endocrine Society guidelines.[7] This may be instrumental in getting insurance coverage in alignment with the realities of LGBTQ/transgender patient needs. At this time, insurance companies can refuse all types of care, from drug therapy to reassignment surgeries.[13-17] Then, conscience clauses and profound ignorance is often responsible for pharmacists refusing to fill important prescriptions used in transgender care, even when a medical provider has been identified and insurance coverage of that care has been allowed.[18] We can do better for these patients, and it may begin with first-year medical students in our current training programs.

Writing Prompts

- When a parent denies a child's gender issue, is this abuse?
  - Can you distinguish gender NONCONFORMING from gender DYSPHORIA?
  - Can anyone?
  - Is it age-dependent?
  - Is all of this amenable to being outgrown?
- Does acknowledging this idea in childhood REINFORCE it for adulthood
  - Thus, should it be ignored?
- Should all transgender considerations be left until adulthood
  - Age of consent to sex differs among states
- Is this a type of sexual consent, literally the consent to CHANGE sex?
- Does this create another category of patient to discriminate against?
- Is seeking gender reassignment just another patient autonomy issue and not special?

- Is this just a run-of-the-mill medical issue, but simply new to us?
- Is the failure of healthcare professionals to use preferred pronouns bigoted or just lazy?
- When physicians blame all healthcare concerns on transition "issues", is this the same as blaming all health problems of the obese on their weight?
- Should politicians' opinions outweigh medical personnel's expertise?
- Should parents even consider consenting to therapy for their children?
- Should children get treatment without parental consent?
- Is childhood assent enough with parental consent?
  - Should this just be treated differently?
  - When would patient autonomy begin? Twelve? Sixteen? Eighteen?
    - Remember, puberty causes irreversible changes…which cannot be easily undone if you wait!
- Does depression cloud clarity for choice?
- Options to preserve fertility are real but overlooked by poorly trained MDs
  - What options should be made clear to transitioning patients about fertility and the potential to have a family?
- Insurance denies 25% of all trans requests to maintain "trans" status
  - Gender reassignment is expensive
- Trans populations have more suicide, substance abuse, anxiety, PTSD
  - But insurance denies them help…unless they revert to their original gender
- As trans, they cannot be covered like "nontrans" people with the same conditions
  - Insurers can call this a preexisting condition and raise premiums
  - But Affordable Care Act bars discrimination for this reason
- Should employer insurance pay for this or should these people acquire private insurance?
- Gender reassignment is not cancer treatment
  - Is it necessary or just desired?
  - Should this be a criterion for insurance coverage?

Works Cited

1. Moll J, Krieger P, Moreno-Walton L, et al. The prevalence of lesbian, gay, bisexual, and transgender health education and training in emergency medicine residency programs: what do we know? Acad Emerg Med. 2014;21(5):608-11.
2. Safer JD, Coleman E, Feldman J, et al. Barriers to healthcare for transgender individuals. Curr Opin Endocrinol Diabetes Obes. 2016;23(2):168-71.
3. Baldas T. Pediatrician Wouldn't Care for Baby with Two Moms. Detroit Free Press. February 18, 2015 ed. Detroit, MI: USA Today; 2015.
4. Jaffee KD, Shires DA, Stroumsa D. Discrimination and Delayed Health Care Among Transgender Women and Men: Implications for Improving Medical Education and Health Care Delivery. Med Care. 2016;54(11):1010-6.
5. Human Rights Watch. "All We Want is Equality" Religious Exemptions and Discrimination against LGBT People in the United States. 2018.
6. Stroumsa D. The state of transgender health care: policy, law, and medical frameworks. Am J Public Health. 2014;104(3):e31-8. Epub 20140116.
7. Soled KRS, Dimant OE, Tanguay J, et al. Interdisciplinary clinicians' attitudes, challenges, and success strategies in providing care to transgender people: a qualitative descriptive study. BMC Health Serv Res. 2022;22(1):1134. Epub 20220908.

8. Turban JL, Kraschel KL, Cohen IG. Legislation to Criminalize Gender-Affirming Medical Care for Transgender Youth. JAMA. 2021;325(22):2251-2.
9. Movement Advancement Project. Equality Maps: Healthcare Laws and Policies. 2022.
10. Kreines FM, Quinn GP, Cardamone S, et al. Training clinicians in culturally relevant care: a curriculum to improve knowledge and comfort with the transgender and gender diverse population. J Assist Reprod Genet. 2022. Epub 20221110.
11. Guss CE, Dahlberg S, Said JT, et al. Use of an Educational Video to Improve Transgender Health Care Knowledge. Clin Pediatr (Phila). 2022;61(5-6):412-7. Epub 20220331.
12. Greene RE, Hanley K, Cook TE, et al. Meeting the Primary Care Needs of Transgender Patients Through Simulation. J Grad Med Educ. 2017;9(3):380-1.
13. Gorton RN. Health care and insurance issues for transgender persons. Am Fam Physician. 2006;74(12):2022; author reply , 4.
14. Padula WV, Baker K. Coverage for Gender-Affirming Care: Making Health Insurance Work for Transgender Americans. LGBT Health. 2017;4(4):244-7. Epub 20170714.
15. Antommaria AHM. Accepting Things at Face Value: Insurance Coverage for Transgender Health Care. Am J Bioeth. 2018;18(12):21-3.
16. Dowshen NL, Christensen J, Gruschow SM. Health Insurance Coverage of Recommended Gender-Affirming Health Care Services for Transgender Youth: Shopping Online for Coverage Information. Transgend Health. 2019;4(1):131-5. Epub 20190411.
17. Carter SP, Cowan T, Snow A, et al. Health Insurance and Mental Health Care Utilization Among Adults Who Identify as Transgender and Gender Diverse. Psychiatr Serv. 2020;71(2):151-7. Epub 20191029.
18. Cicconi L. Pharmacist refusals and third-party interests: A proposed judicial approach to pharmacist conscience clauses. Ucla Law Rev. 2007;54(3):709-49.

Essay: Gender Dysphoria in Children

Is Gender-Affirming Medical Treatment the Best Option?

Faithe Elsberry

Gender Dysphoria and Transgenderism

Transgender hormone treatments and surgeries have become the most common solutions for treating gender dysphoria, which has significantly increased in prevalence in adults and children in recent decades. Gender dysphoria is defined as the distress one experiences when one feels his gender does not match his biological sex.[1] Those with gender dysphoria may experience severe discomfort in their bodies due to this gender incongruence. This discomfort is often accompanied by anxiety, depression, and a higher risk of suicide than that of the general population.[2] These psychological comorbidities are thought to be closely related to the severe distress as well as the societal, relational, and familial pressures on those with gender dysphoria. In 2017, it was found that approximately 0.5–1.3% of the population had gender dysphoria, including adults and children.[3] The percentage of the population diagnosed with gender dysphoria has increased significantly in the past two decades.[4] It is probable that this increase has been brought about by the normalization of the questioning of one's gender and making the medical solutions for gender dysphoria known, desirable, and even popular.

Now, instead of being viewed as a psychological disorder, gender dysphoria is widely viewed as an issue with the human body in relation to the mind, for which physical modifications to resemble and function as the opposite sex are the best solutions. Such modifications would qualify one to fall into the category of transgender, although transgender is a term used to describe anyone who identifies with a gender that does not align with his biological sex.[5] Being transgender ranges from solely changing one's pronouns to taking cross-sex hormones (testosterone for females and estrogen for males) and undergoing surgical procedures to resemble the opposite sex. Hormonal therapy and transgender surgery paired with psychotherapy are common treatments for gender dysphoria because they have been shown to improve mental health and reduce the risk of suicide in those with gender dysphoria in the short- to medium-term.[6,7]

Treatments for Gender Dysphoria

Psychotherapy, hormonal therapy, and gender-affirming surgeries are the general components of a gender transition, which is currently the main treatment for gender dysphoria.[8] In the beginning, patients may be required to go through psychotherapy for diagnosis and arrival at a decision regarding what treatment is best for them.[9] Psychotherapy may also consist of helping patients come out to their family and friends and providing support before and during hormonal therapy or surgical transition to improve their overall quality of life.[9]

After psychotherapy has begun and a diagnosis has been made, cross-sex hormone therapy is used to aid in the development of the desired secondary sex characteristics specific to the opposite sex.[10, 11] Biological males wishing to transition will be prescribed estrogen. This will initiate the development of female secondary sex characteristics such as the growth of breast tissue and desired fat deposition.[12] Exogenous estrogen also decreases secondary sex characteristics unique to males.[10] Over time, testicle size and sperm production will decrease, and with prolonged use, this will result in infertility.[13] Estrogen must be continued for life to maintain these feminine features.

Biological females wishing to transition will be prescribed testosterone. Similarly, masculine secondary sex characteristics such as body hair growth and deepening of the voice will occur while female secondary sex characteristics, such as ovary size and occurrence of the menstrual cycle, will decrease.[11] It has been shown that the menstrual cycle will return if testosterone use is discontinued after 1 year of use, but again, prolonged use is likely to result in permanent amenorrhea and infertility.[13] Testosterone also must be continued for life to maintain physical masculine features.

After cross-sex hormones have been used continuously for a minimum of 1 year, patients are eligible for surgical modifications.[14] Surgical procedures to remove sex organs and create new organs that match those of the desired gender usually go together. Biological males may undergo an orchiectomy, or the removal of the testes, to begin their surgical transition. Then, they may undergo vaginoplasty, the creation of a vagina from the existing phallus. For males, these two steps make up what is called bottom surgery.[14] The creation of the neovagina may come with complications, such as hair growth in the vagina or infection, although this can widely be avoided by permanent hair removal before vaginoplasty.[15] Other common surgical procedures for male-to-female transition include breast and gluteal augmentation and facial plastic surgery for further feminization.[8]

Bottom surgery for females begins with the removal of the female genitals and then phalloplasty, the creation of a phallus. The neophallus may either be created from vaginal tissue or a large patch of skin taken from the patient's non-dominant arm.[14] These procedures allow for urination from the neophallus, but not erection for penetrative intercourse. Penile implants to achieve erection may be surgically placed in the neophallus, but this procedure comes with many complications.[16] Complications with bottom surgery for females transitioning to males are common, especially regarding issues with urination.[17] Nearly half of the patients in one study who had penile implants had to undergo revision surgery, and the rate of infection was approximately 11%.[16] Some females may decide to undergo a hysterectomy or oophorectomy to remove the uterus and ovaries or just the ovaries, respectively, and some may desire to undergo a double mastectomy and facial plastic surgery for further masculinization.[8]

Gender Dysphoria in Children

The prevalence of gender dysphoria in children has drastically increased over the past decade.[18] There has been much debate regarding how to treat children with gender dysphoria. Just like adults with gender dysphoria, children with gender dysphoria are at a greater risk of committing suicide and are more likely to have depression and anxiety.[19] To begin treatment, children are usually first diagnosed with gender dysphoria, although this is not always seen as a necessary step.[20] Before undergoing cross-sex hormone therapy and surgery, pre- or early-pubescent children take puberty blockers to halt the progression of puberty.

Puberty blockers are GnRH analogs that halt the production of testosterone and estrogen in boys and girls, respectively, and halt the development of secondary sex characteristics and the process of sexual maturation.[20] It is recommended that children with gender dysphoria begin taking GnRH analogs at an early stage of puberty. This is thought to give the gender dysphoric child an opportunity to see what his body could look like if puberty continues while halting pubertal developments soon enough to mediate further distress associated with growing gender incongruence as the body matures.[20] The average recommended age to begin GnRH therapy, then, is 12 years-of-age. When the use of GnRH analogs is discontinued, puberty will resume, although the effects of long-term use on fertility are not fully known.[13] It is also possible that the use of GnRH analogs may result in incomplete skeletal development and adult height.[21]

Should Children Medically Transition?

Treating children with gender dysphoria in the same manner as adults does not account for the physical and psychological differences between children and adults or the role that puberty plays in the development of the adolescent body and brain. First, there is the issue of informed consent–can minors be fully informed of the consequences of gender-affirming medical care, and are they capable of making permanent, life-changing decisions? Then, there are questions regarding the efficacy of the current treatments for relieving the discomfort of gender dysphoria and the associated mental health issues and risks. Finally, and perhaps most compelling, there exists an extremely high rate of desistence of gender dysphoria as children move into adulthood.

The long-term effects of GnRH analogs, estrogen, and testosterone on pre-pubescent, pubescent, and post-pubescent adolescents are widely unknown.[19] These hormonal treatments have not been commonly used for physically healthy children during such a critical period of development as puberty until recently. Because of this, research has not been done to show the long-term outcomes, mental or physical, in children and adolescents. Children and their parents, therefore, cannot possibly be fully informed of the consequences of hormone treatment for gender dysphoria.

There has also been significant debate over whether children are capable of making decisions regarding the implementation of physical alterations that would undoubtedly drastically alter aspects of their adult life. Specifically, there is uncertainty over the average child's ability to make permanent or potentially permanent decisions regarding fertility.[19] The majority of children who wish to medically transition choose to give up their ability to sexually reproduce rather than choosing a route that would allow them to one day have biological children.[4] However, approximately 50% of transgender adults said that if they had known about the options for fertility preservation when they began their medical transitions, they would have chosen to do so.[13]

Children do not consider the significance of being able to have their own biological children as adults do.

Some studies show that gender-affirming medical treatments may not be significantly efficacious long-term treatments for gender dysphoria and the associated mental comorbidities. In a 2011 study in which the long-term mortality rate in patients (n=1,331) who had undergone medical transition beginning any time before July 1, 1997, was examined, it was found that the mortality rate of this population was 51% higher than that of the general population.[22]. The rate of suicide was six times higher in biological males who had transitioned and two times higher in biological females who had transitioned. Deaths from illicit drug use were also significantly higher in this population. In another follow-up study, it was found that those who had been using cross-sex hormones had a significantly higher mortality rate than that of the general population, partially attributable to suicide.[23] Therefore, treatment with testosterone or estrogen may not be the most efficacious long-term solution for gender dysphoria and the associated mental health issues. Hormone therapy may not significantly reduce the high risk of suicide seen in those with gender dysphoria before medical transition.

While informed consent, children's decision-making abilities, and treatment efficacy should be examined, it is vital to consider the extremely high desistance of childhood gender dysphoria. Approximately 73–98% of all children with gender dysphoria will not experience gender dysphoria in adulthood.[24] If children go through puberty and are still gender-dysphoric, it is more likely that this will persist into adulthood, although the use of puberty blockers in the first stages of puberty eliminates this assurance of persistence.

Conclusion
Children are not simply small adults and should not be considered as such when it comes to treating children who have gender dysphoria. It is naive to believe that children and their parents can make fully informed consent when the consequences of long-term use of cross-sex hormones and gender-affirming surgeries beginning in childhood are not yet known by anyone. It is also inappropriate to offer options to children that have been offered to adults and expect them to make decisions as adults do. Children lack the brain development, maturity, and experience that contribute to decisions made by adults, especially regarding fertility. The long-term studies on mortality rates in medically transitioned populations should raise concern for the long-term outcomes of these treatments when performed on children. The ultimate efficacy of current treatment methods should be closely examined and questioned. Finally, it is astounding that gender dysphoria in children, which is far more likely to be temporary than permanent, is mainly treated with permanent solutions, solutions that have significant implications that children are unable to fully understand. For children with gender dysphoria, alternatives to hormone therapy and gender-affirming surgeries should be considered and researched to identify a solution that is age-appropriate and efficacious in the long run.

Works Cited

1. Beek TF, Cohen-Kettenis PT, Kreukels BP. Gender incongruence/gender dysphoria and its classification history. Int Rev Psychiatry. 2016;28(1):5-12. Epub 20151119.
2. Dhejne C, Van Vlerken R, Heylens G, et al. Mental health and gender dysphoria: A review of the literature. Int Rev Psychiatry. 2016;28(1):44-57.

3. Zucker KJ. Epidemiology of gender dysphoria and transgender identity. Sex Health. 2017;14(5):404-11.
4. Bouman WP, de Vries AL, T'Sjoen G. Gender Dysphoria and Gender Incongruence: An evolving inter-disciplinary field. Int Rev Psychiatry. 2016;28(1):1-4. Epub 20160115.
5. Mueller SC, De Cuypere G, T'Sjoen G. Transgender Research in the 21st Century: A Selective Critical Review From a Neurocognitive Perspective. Am J Psychiatry. 2017;174(12):1155-62. Epub 20171020.
6. Baker KE, Wilson LM, Sharma R, et al. Hormone Therapy, Mental Health, and Quality of Life Among Transgender People: A Systematic Review. J Endocr Soc. 2021;5(4):bvab011. Epub 20210202.
7. Almazan AN, Keuroghlian AS. Association Between Gender-Affirming Surgeries and Mental Health Outcomes. JAMA Surg. 2021;156(7):611-8.
8. Anderson D, Wijetunge H, Moore P, et al. Gender Dysphoria and Its Non-Surgical and Surgical Treatments. Health Psychol Res. 2022;10(3):38358. Epub 20220923.
9. Hadj-Moussa M, Ohl DA, Kuzon WM, Jr. Evaluation and Treatment of Gender Dysphoria to Prepare for Gender Confirmation Surgery. Sex Med Rev. 2018;6(4):607-17. Epub 20180608.
10. Randolph JF, Jr. Gender-Affirming Hormone Therapy for Transgender Females. Clin Obstet Gynecol. 2018;61(4):705-21.
11. Moravek MB. Gender-Affirming Hormone Therapy for Transgender Men. Clin Obstet Gynecol. 2018;61(4):687-704.
12. Radix A. Hormone Therapy for Transgender Adults. Urol Clin North Am. 2019;46(4):467-73. Epub 20190819.
13. Cheng PJ, Pastuszak AW, Myers JB, et al. Fertility concerns of the transgender patient. Transl Androl Urol. 2019;8(3):209-18.
14. Pan S, Honig SC. Gender-Affirming Surgery: Current Concepts. Curr Urol Rep. 2018;19(8):62. Epub 20180607.
15. Horbach SE, Bouman MB, Smit JM, et al. Outcome of Vaginoplasty in Male-to-Female Transgenders: A Systematic Review of Surgical Techniques. J Sex Med. 2015;12(6):1499-512. Epub 20150326.
16. Hoebeke PB, Decaestecker K, Beysens M, et al. Erectile implants in female-to-male transsexuals: our experience in 129 patients. Eur Urol. 2010;57(2):334-40. Epub 20090310.
17. Nikolavsky D, Yamaguchi Y, Levine JP, et al. Urologic Sequelae Following Phalloplasty in Transgendered Patients. Urol Clin North Am. 2017;44(1):113-25.
18. Frisen L, Soder O, Rydelius PA. [Dramatic increase of gender dysphoria in youth]. Lakartidningen. 2017;114. Epub 20170222.
19. Vrouenraets LJ, Fredriks AM, Hannema SE, et al. Early Medical Treatment of Children and Adolescents With Gender Dysphoria: An Empirical Ethical Study. J Adolesc Health. 2015;57(4):367-73. Epub 20150625.
20. Rew L, Young CC, Monge M, et al. Review: Puberty blockers for transgender and gender diverse youth-a critical review of the literature. Child Adolesc Ment Health. 2021;26(1):3-14. Epub 20201215.
21. Vottero A, Pedori S, Verna M, et al. Final height in girls with central idiopathic precocious puberty treated with gonadotropin-releasing hormone analog and oxandrolone. J Clin Endocrinol Metab. 2006;91(4):1284-7. Epub 20060131.
22. Asscheman H, Giltay EJ, Megens JA, et al. A long-term follow-up study of mortality in transsexuals receiving treatment with cross-sex hormones. Eur J Endocrinol. 2011;164(4):635-42. Epub 20110125.

23. de Blok CJ, Wiepjes CM, van Velzen DM, et al. Mortality trends over five decades in adult transgender people receiving hormone treatment: a report from the Amsterdam cohort of gender dysphoria. Lancet Diabetes Endocrinol. 2021;9(10):663-70. Epub 20210902.
24. Wiepjes CM, Nota NM, de Blok CJM, et al. The Amsterdam Cohort of Gender Dysphoria Study (1972-2015): Trends in Prevalence, Treatment, and Regrets. J Sex Med. 2018;15(4):582-90. Epub 20180217.

About the Student Authors

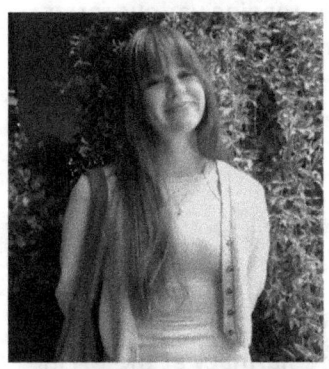

Inés Studer
Inés was born in Tucson and is following the family tradition started by her grandfather (UA alumnus). She loves hiking, indoor plants, traveling, and cooking. Inés is currently working towards a bachelor's degree in Pharmaceutical Sciences with a minor in biochemistry and at this time her academic goal is to earn a PhD in Pharmaceutical Sciences.

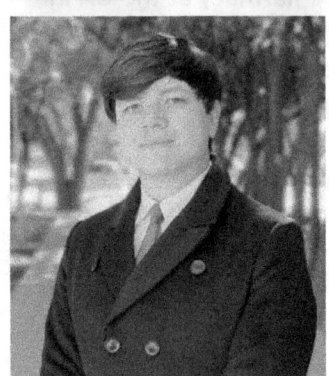

Jason Canizales
Although Jason was born in Phoenix, he grew up in the culturally diverse border town of Nogales, AZ. He enjoys spending time with family and friends, exercising, solving puzzles, and learning new languages. A first-generation college student, he is pursuing a BS in Pharmaceutical Sciences and Spanish literature with a minor in biochemistry. Having a keen interest in supporting the health of the community, his current academic goals are focused on receiving an MD and specializing in gastroenterology.

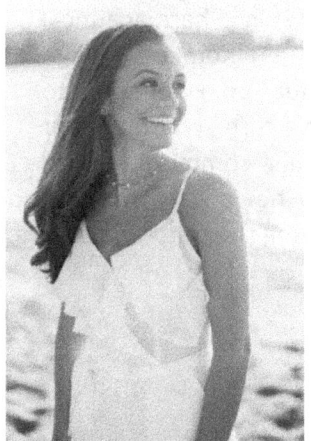

Lauren Thompson
Lauren was born in St. Louis, MO, and is a current junior studying Pharmaceutical Sciences at the University of Arizona. She will attend the R. Ken Coit College of Pharmacy in the fall of 2023, making her the fourth member of her family to attend pharmacy school. Outside of school, Lauren enjoys traveling, music, and spending time with her friends and family.

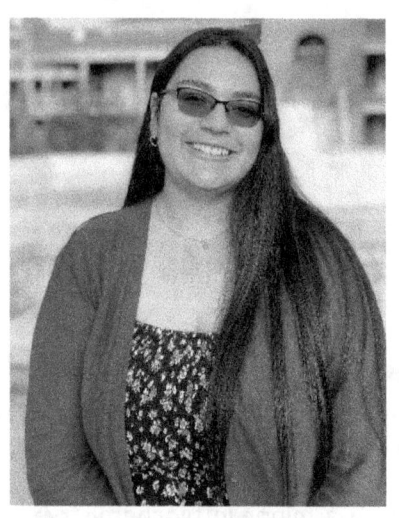

Teresa Noll
Teresa is currently a first-generation student at UA. She is pursuing a BS in Pharmaceutical Sciences. Once earned, she intends to pursue a PhD in Pharmacology and Toxicology. In addition, she aspires to become a Diplomat of the American Board of Toxicology. Outside the realm of academia, she enjoys exploring the great outdoors while discovering the diverse culture that makes up Tucson. She also enjoys reading various forms of literature, from scientific journals to fiction. Through all her interests and involvements, Teresa finds that every encounter allows her to learn something new and widen her perspective in life.

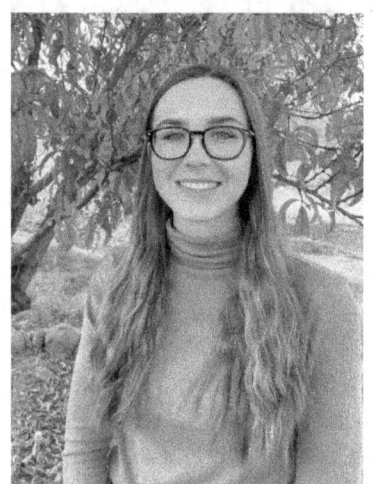

Alena LaBree
Alena is working towards a BS in Pharmaceutical Sciences and a minor in Biochemistry ('23). She hopes to attend the R. Ken Coit College of Pharmacy at the UA in fall of 2023 and achieve her goal of becoming a pharmacist. When she's not doing schoolwork, Alena loves to hike, travel, spend time with her dogs, and chat with her family and friends.

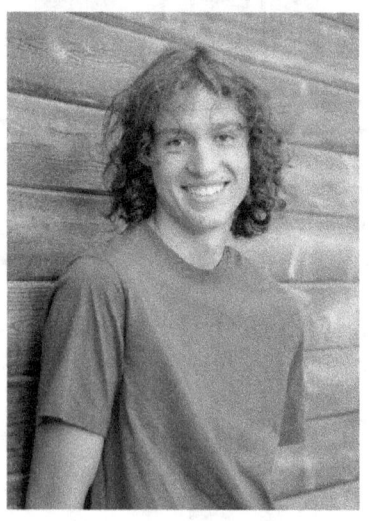

Baden Cruickshank
Baden is working towards a BS in Pharmaceutical Sciences and intends to apply to the R. Ken Coit College of Pharmacy at the UA after graduation. He intends to pursue a career in ambulatory care pharmacy or pediatric pharmacy and serve his community as a pharmacist. In his spare time, he enjoys reading, running, and spending time exploring the outdoors.

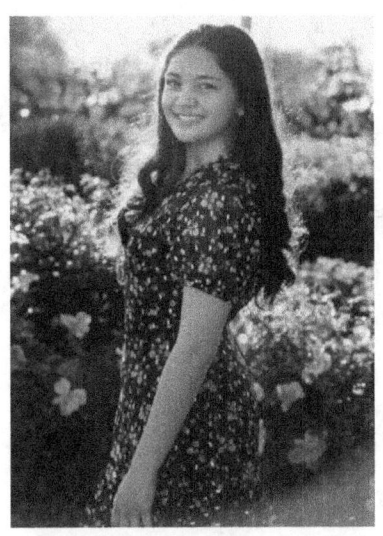

Hannah Ducasse
Hannah was born and raised in Mesa, AZ. She is an undergraduate at the UA currently pursuing a BS in Pharmaceutical Sciences. She hopes to attend the R. Ken Coit College of Pharmacy to earn a PharmD. In her spare time, she loves crocheting, drinking boba with her roommate, and singing in a collegiate a cappella group named Enharmonics. Her current career goal is to become a pharmacist specializing in oncology.

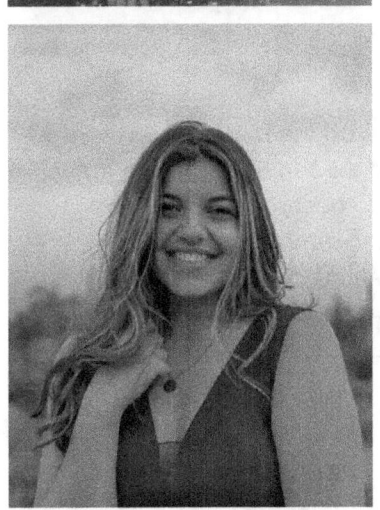

Sarah Wolff
Sarah grew up in El Mirage, AZ and is currently living in Tucson and is working towards her BS in Medicine—Basic Medical Sciences with a minor in Family Studies and Human Development at UA (Class of 2026). In her free time, she loves reading, spending time with her family and dogs, and trying new restaurants around Tucson. After graduation, she hopes to attend medical school.

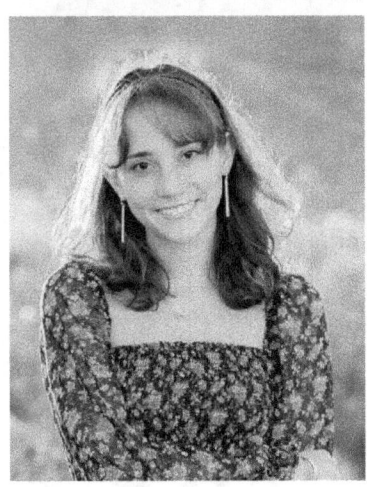

Brianna Hunt
Brianna was born in Tucson, AZ but grew up in Colorado Springs, CO. She is currently pursuing a BS in Pharmaceutical Sciences with a minor in French at UA. In her free time, she enjoys running, hiking, reading, and playing ultimate frisbee with her club team. With a passion for research, she intends to pursue a PhD in Pharmaceutical Sciences.

Erica Day

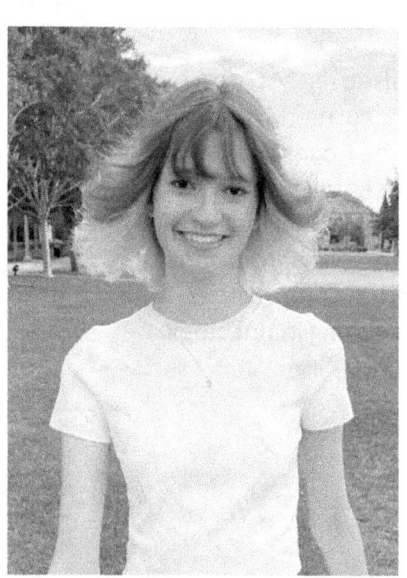

Erica Day was born in Denver, CO but grew up in Mesa, AZ. She is currently a student in the Early Assurance PharmD program at the UA and plans to attend the R. Ken Coit College of Pharmacy in the fall of 2024. Outside of university, Erica enjoys spending time with friends and reading fantasy novels. While her career goals are not figured out, Erica hopes to pursue a career in hospital pharmacy.

Faithe Elsberry

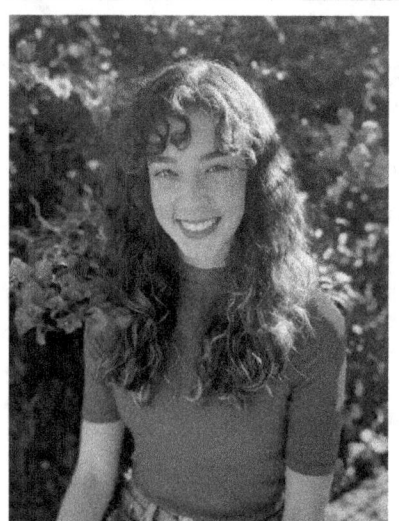

Faithe is a senior at the UA, working toward a BS in Pharmaceutical Sciences and a BA in Spanish. She grew up in Tucson, AZ and hopes to become a physical therapist, helping those in her community use movement to bring about healing. In her free time, she enjoys spending time with her family and friends, sketching, crocheting, and learning more about the human body.

Karlie Flader

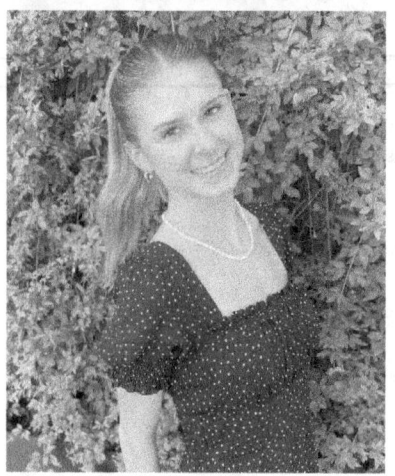

Karlie is a sophomore working towards a BS in Pharmaceutical Sciences. After graduation, she intends on pursuing a PhD in pharmacology. She enjoys reading, arts and crafts, and spending time outdoors.

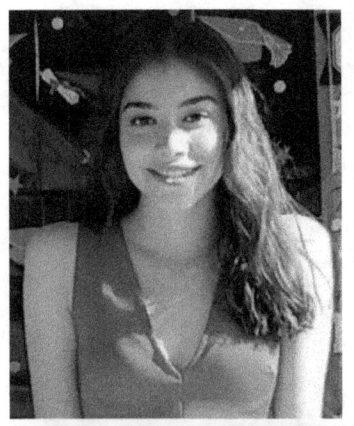

Aileen Muñoz

Aileen was born in Phoenix, AZ, and loves to travel to new places. She enjoys time with friends, music, and crafts in her free time. She is currently working on a BS in Pharmaceutical Sciences and minors in Spanish and psychology. Although her career goals are not ironed out, Aileen aspires to help those around her.

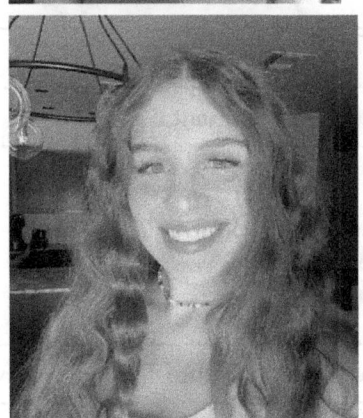

Gabbi Ciadella

Gabbi will earn her BS in Pharmaceutical Sciences in May of 2023 and attend the University of Arizona's R. Ken Coit College of Pharmacy in the fall. Now, Gabbi is uncertain which avenue of pharmacy she fits best, but she is eager to discover during pharmacy school. Outside of academics, Gabbi has a strong passion for dogs. Her ultimate goal is to own a dog rescue at some point later in her life.

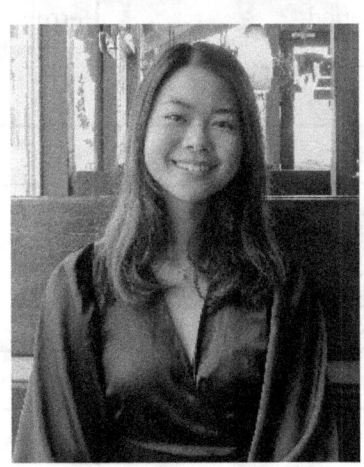

Nanase Toda

Nanase was born and raised in Tokyo, Japan, and has been living in AZ for the past several years. She is currently pursuing a BS in Pharmaceutical Sciences at the UA and will graduate in May 2023. In her spare time, she enjoys exploring local cafes and restaurants in Tucson.

Appendix

Below is the writing rubric used to evaluate essays.

WRITING RUBRIC

Score of 100 (BEST WRITING)—Clear understanding of task			
Position	**Complexity**	**Idea Development**	**Focus**
Takes position; offers critical context for discussion	Examines different perspectives; or evaluates implications and complications; or; responds to counter-arguments	Ample; specific; logical; elaborated	Clear
Organization	**Language**	**Sentence Structure**	**Conventions**
Clear; logically sequenced; integrated transitions; introduction and conclusion are well-developed	Good command; precise words	Varied	Few if any errors; does not distract reader
Score of 90 (ALMOST PERFECT)—Clear understanding of task			
Position	**Complexity**	**Idea Development**	**Focus**
Takes position; offers broad context for; offers a discussion	Partially evaluates implications and complications or responds to counterarguments	Specific; logical; most ideas are elaborated; general statements; specific reasons, examples, details	Maintained
Organization	**Language**	**Sentence Structure**	**Conventions**
Clear but predictable; logically sequenced; simple transitions; introduction and conclusion are generally well-developed	Competent word choice sometimes varied and precise	Somewhat varied	Few errors; rarely distracting
Score of 80 (PRETTY DARN GOOD...a budding essayist)—Understands task			
Position	**Complexity**	**Idea Development**	**Focus**

Takes position; Offers some; Context for Discussion	Some response to counterarguments	Adequate; Some specific reasons, examples, details	Maintained throughout most of the essay
Organization	**Language**	**Sentence Structure**	**Conventions**
Apparent but predictable; some evidence of logical sequencing; simple transitions; introduction and conclusion are somewhat developed	Adequate appropriate word choice	Some variety	Some distracting errors; but do not impede understanding

Score of 70 (Student is learning as he/she goes!)—Some understanding of task

Position	Complexity	Idea Development	Focus
Takes position; does not offer context for discussion	Acknowledges counterargument but brief or unclear	Limited; repetitious; limited specific reasons and examples	General topic maintained but the specific issue may not be maintained
Organization	**Language**	**Sentence Structure**	**Conventions**
Simple; little or no logical sequencing; transitions are simple and obvious; introduction and conclusion are under-developed	Basic control; word choice is appropriate	Little variety	Errors may be distracting; may occasionally impede understanding

Score of 60 (This needs work but it can be mastered!)—Weak understanding of task

Position	Complexity	Idea Development	Focus
May or may not take a position; states position but offers no reasons to support it (fails to support position)	Little or no recognition of a counterargument	Thinly developed; if examples—general and may not be relevant; repetition of ideas	General topic maintained but the specific issue may not be
Organization	**Language**	**Sentence Structure**	**Conventions**
Some indication of structure; grouping ideas in part of the essay; transitions simple and obvious; introduction and conclusion are minimal	Simple	Simple structure	Errors are frequently distracting; sometimes impede understanding

Score <60 (Someone had a terrible, very bad, no-good day! See me!)—Little/no understanding of task

Position	Complexity	Idea Development	Focus

	If there is a position, there is no support	May or may not take a position; states position but no reasons to support it; fails to support position	Minimally developed; excessive repetition of writer's ideas or of ideas in prompt	General topic maintained but the specific issue may not be
Organization		**Language**	**Sentence Structure**	**Conventions**
	General topic maintained but the specific issue may not be	No evidence of structure; no logical grouping of ideas; transitions are rare; introduction and conclusion not present or minimal	Simple	Simple

www.ingramcontent.com/pod-product-compliance
Lightning Source LLC
Chambersburg PA
CBHW080453220526
45465CB00006B/2260